THE
VITAMIN AND MINERAL FOOD COUNTER

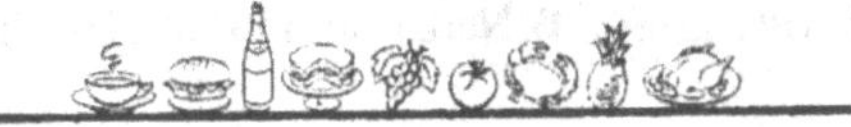

**Annette B. Natow, Ph.D., R.D.
and Jo-Ann Heslin, M.A., R.D.**

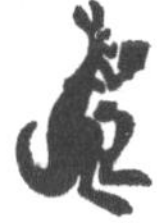

POCKET BOOKS
New York   London   Toronto   Sydney

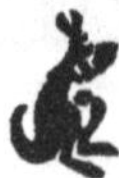 POCKET BOOKS, a division of Simon & Schuster, Inc.
1230 Avenue of the Americas, New York, NY 10020

Copyright © 2004 by Annette B. Natow and Jo-Ann Heslin

An *Original* Publication of POCKET BOOKS

All rights reserved, including the right to reproduce
this book or portions thereof in any form whatsoever.
For information address Pocket Books, 1230 Avenue
of the Americas, New York, NY 10020

ISBN 978-1-9821-6039-5

First Pocket Books printing April 2004

10 9 8 7 6 5 4 3 2 1

POCKET and colophon are registered trademarks of
Simon & Schuster, Inc.

Front cover photo © Photodisk

For information regarding special discounts for bulk purchases,
please contact Simon & Schuster Special Sales at 1-800-456-6798 or
business@simonandschuster.com.

THE VITAMIN AND MINERAL
FOOD COUNTER

VITAMIN A, THIAMIN, RIBOFLAVIN, NIACIN,
FOLIC ACID, VITAMIN C, CALCIUM, POTASSIUM,
SODIUM, IRON, AND ZINC—THEY ARE THE ELEVEN
FUNDAMENTAL OR "MARKER" VITAMINS AND MINERALS.
YET MOST DO NOT APPEAR ON FOOD LABELS.

Bearing that fact in mind, Annette B. Natow and Jo-Ann Heslin—the nutrition experts you can trust—have put together this all-new first edition of *THE VITAMIN AND MINERAL FOOD COUNTER*, so that health-conscious consumers can be fully informed about the vitamin and mineral value of the foods they buy and order out.

When we take in the recommended daily value of these eleven essential nutrients, we automatically get the recommended amounts of all the vitamins and minerals our bodies need for good health. Consult *THE VITAMIN AND MINERAL FOOD COUNTER*'s up-to-date, comprehensive listings for thousands of foods to enhance the level of valuable nutrients in the foods you eat each day.

THE VITAMIN AND MINERAL
FOOD COUNTER

An essential reference for healthy living!

Books by Annette B. Natow and Jo-Ann Heslin

The Antioxidant Vitamin Counter

Calcium Counts

The Calorie Counter (Third Edition)

The Carbohydrate, Sugar and Fiber Counter

The Cholesterol Counter (Sixth Edition)

The Complete Food Counter

Count on a Healthy Pregnancy

The Diabetes Carbohydrate and Calorie Counter
(Second Edition)

Eating Out Food Counter

The Fat Attack Plan

The Fat Counter (Fifth Edition)

The Food Shopping Counter (Second Edition)

Get Skinny the Smart Way

The Healthy Heart Food Counter

Megadoses

The Most Complete Food Counter

No-Nonsense Nutrition for Kids

The Pocket Encyclopedia of Nutrition

The Pocket Fat Counter (Second Edition)

The Pocket Protein Counter

The Pregnancy Nutrition Counter

The Protein Counter (Second Edition)

The Sodium Counter

The Vitamin and Mineral Food Counter

Published by POCKET BOOKS

To our families, who support us through every project: Harry, Allen, Irene, Sarah, Meryl, Laura, Marty, George, Emily, Steven, Joe, Kristen, Brian, Karen, and John.

ACKNOWLEDGMENTS

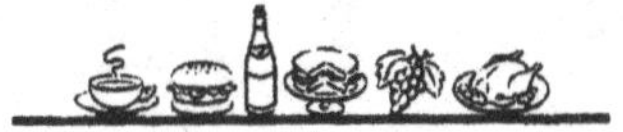

For graciously sharing their knowledge: Martin Lefkowitz, M.D. and Irene E. Rosenberg, M.D.

For all her support and help, our agent, Nancy Trichter.

For her suggestions and editing skills, Sara Clemence.

Without the tireless cooperation of Steven Natow, M.D., and Stephen Llano, *The Vitamin and Mineral Food Counter* would never have been completed.

A special thank you to our editor, Micki Nuding.

"... there are substances existing in minute quantities in food which exercise a profound influence upon nutrition."

Mary Swartz Rose, Ph.D.
Feeding the Family, Revised Edition
The Macmillan Company, 1925

CONTENTS

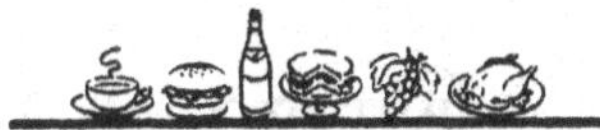

PART ONE
Vitamins in Food
49

PART TWO
Minerals in Food
249

INTRODUCTION

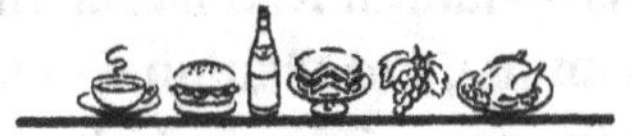

"Eat your vegetables."

Most of us heard it from our parents, and have said it to our own children.

Studies have shown that people who eat 5 to 9 servings of fruits and vegetables a day are healthier than those who eat fewer. Why? Because fruits and vegetables are rich in vitamins and minerals.

Vitamins and minerals are not only important to your health, they are big business. Enter any drugstore, supermarket, or health food store and you'll see aisles of bottles and boxes chock full of vitamins and minerals in varying combinations and doses. Billions are spent on these supplements each year.

Why are vitamins and minerals so important?

Unlike protein, fat and carbohydrate, vitamins and minerals have no calories and the body uses them in very small amounts. But that doesn't minimize their importance. They help you burn calories, build bones and tissues, and regulate the body's normal functions. Each one plays a vital role in health, the same way instruments in an orchestra all contribute to a song. Missing a vitamin or mineral can disrupt the body's normal functioning; sometimes, the consequences are serious.

In *The Vitamin and Mineral Food Counter* you will find out about 6 vitamins—vitamin A, thiamin, riboflavin, niacin, and folic acid (B vitamins), and vitamin C—and 5 minerals—calcium, iron, sodium, potassium, and zinc. Actually, over a dozen vitamins and 16 minerals are essential to health. Some are needed in very tiny amounts and most are found in combination in foods. It's hard to keep track of them all.

The 11 vitamins and minerals in *The Vitamin and Mineral Food Counter* are marker nutrients. If you meet your need for these marker nutrients, you can be pretty confident that you are getting enough of the others.

Studying vitamins and minerals can be complicated because they do a lot of their work inside cells, where they cannot be seen. Vitamins and minerals often work in groups, helping each other get a job done. You can think of them as a construction crew. Every member of the crew has a specialty—carpenter, electrician, plumber, mason—and their collective efforts build a house. The collective effort of vitamins and minerals keeps your body running smoothly.

Our goal is to help you understand how different vitamins and minerals work in your body; what are the best food sources of each; and how much you should be getting of each one every day.

Why can't I just take a supplement and not worry about vitamins and minerals in food?

That's one of the first questions we hear. We're not against supplements. We think of them like car insurance; wise to have, but no substitute for safe driving. Supplements are just that: a *supplement* to healthy eating, but not a *substitute* for healthy food.

Experts aren't in total agreement about who should take vitamin and mineral supplements, but they all agree we should be making smart food choices. So, we are going to turn the question back to you, and let you decide if you need a daily supplement. To help you decide, answer the following questions.

DO I NEED A DAILY VITAMIN AND MINERAL SUPPLEMENT?

Are you dieting to lose weight?	yes	no
Are you ill or recovering from an illness?	yes	no
Do you smoke?	yes	no
Do you regularly drink alcohol?	yes	no
Are you normally stressed or pressured?	yes	no
Are you a women of childbearing age?	yes	no
Are you pregnant or breastfeeding?	yes	no
Are you over 50?	yes	no
Do you rarely eat vitamin and mineral fortified foods such as cereal, juice, energy bars, soy beverages?	yes	no
Do you take prescription medicine daily?	yes	no
Do you regularly skip breakfast?	yes	no
Do you regularly skip meals?	yes	no
Is soda your usual beverage choice?	yes	no
Do you eat sweets (cookies, cake, candy, ice cream) daily	yes	no?
Do you eat less than 5 servings of fruits and vegetables a day?	yes	no
Do you eat less than 3 calcium-rich foods (milk, soy milk, yogurt, cheese) each day?	yes	no

The more times you answered "yes," the more likely you would benefit from a daily supplement. Next time you visit your doctor, discuss these answers with him and get his advice. In the meantime, a daily multivitamin-mineral supplement may be wise because there is some evidence that supplements may lower your risk for chronic diseases.

Almost everything recommended by health experts who advocate supplements can be found in a generic multivitamin-mineral, like a drugstore or supermarket brand. Women before menopause should pick one with iron; men and postmenopausal women should pick one without iron. We'll explain this more on page 34. The only nutrient that may not be covered adequately by a generic supplement is calcium. But we'll help you figure out what to do about that when we talk about calcium on page 24.

Whatever you decide about supplement use, always keep in mind that you should use multivitamin-mineral supplements in addition to eating well, rather than as an excuse not to bother eating well.

VITAMINS

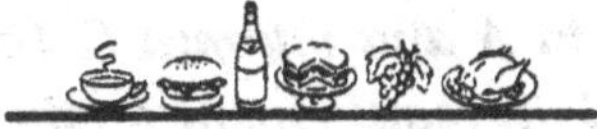

Just the word "vitamin" sounds healthy. Derived from the Latin *vita*, meaning "life," all vitamins are vital to life, even though they are needed by the body in very tiny amount. They help you absorb, digest, and use the fats, carbohydrates, and proteins found in food.

Vitamins can be destroyed or have their shape changed. This can be both good and bad. Cooking food at high temperatures, in a lot of water, for a long time, will reduce the amount of vitamins in food. But, your body can also change a vitamin's shape to make it more useful in certain situations.

Vitamins are divided into two groups—fat soluble and water soluble. Each is handled differently in the body. Fat soluble vitamins (like vitamin A) are carried into the body by foods containing fat and are stored in your fat tissues, waiting to be used. It isn't easy for your body to get rid of fat soluble vitamins, so they can build up if large doses are taken over a period of time. Water soluble vitamins (like thiamin, riboflavin, niacin, folic acid, and vitamin C) are absorbed directly into the blood and travel freely around the body through the bloodstream. If high amounts of a water soluble vitamin are detected as the blood passes through the kidneys, the vitamin will be filtered out and then leave your body through urine.

Labeling Law—Vitamins

Food labels in the U.S. are required to list % Daily Value (%DV) for vitamin A and vitamin C. The %DV is the amount of your daily requirement, for the vitamin, that you'll get from one serving of food.

Listing the %DV for thiamin, riboflavin, niacin, and folic acid is voluntary on food labels.

VITAMIN A

Will vitamin A help me see in the dark?

Vitamin A won't help you find your seat in a dim theater, but your eyes need it to adjust to changes between light and dark. Vitamin A maintains the health of the cornea, the clear outer window of the eye. *Night blindness*, an inability to adapt to dimming light, results from vitamin A deficiency. Vitamin A deficiency is rare in the U.S., because most healthy adults have up to a year's supply stored in their liver, but it is the leading cause of blindness in children worldwide.

Besides keeping my eyes healthy, what else does vitamin A do?

Vitamin A is crucial to maintaining healthy cells, particularly mucus, skin, and bone cells. It also boosts your immune function and helps your body fight infections. In men, vitamin A aids in the production of sperm, and in women it helps to maintain fertility. Provitamin A, *carotenoids*, may play a role in the prevention of cancer.

What's a provitamin?

Vitamin A is unique in that it comes from two sources, animal and plant foods, and in two forms, as retinoids and carotenoids. About half of the vitamin you need comes from animal foods—liver, cod liver oil, milk, butter, margarine, and eggs—in the form of retinoids. The body easily absorbs and uses this form of vitamin A.

The other half comes as carotenoids, or provitamin A, found in dark-green and deep-yellow fruits and vegetables like carrots, spinach, broccoli, sweet potato, cantaloupe, peaches, apricots, and mangos. Your body will convert carotenoids to vitamin A as needed. There are hundreds of different carotenoids in nature, but the one that your body changes most efficiently to active vitamin A is beta-carotene. The carotenoids that are not converted to active vitamin A help protect the body from harmful substances called *free radicals*. So, eating fruits and vegetables rich in carotenoids not only helps you meet your vitamin A requirement, but protects the body, as well. Scientists believe that is the main reason why people who eat a lot of fruits and vegetables seem to have a lower risk for cancer.

Which are richer in carotenoids, raw or cooked vegetables?

You might be surprised by this answer; it's cooked. A few minutes of cooking breaks down chemical bonds naturally found in food, releasing carotenoids and making them easier to absorb.

Should I take a carotenoid supplement?

That's hard to answer. Though people who eat more fruits and vegetables are healthier, experts have yet to connect carotenoid supplements with better health. This may be a case of nature at work: in other words, there may be other substances in plants that work with the carotenoids to protect your body. When the carotenoids are purified into a supplement, their helpful partners may be lost. Research has shown that a high intake of different carotenoids from fruits and vegetables appear to protect your body against certain illnesses. Isolated carotenoids don't show the same benefits. So the same advice holds: eat smart first, and take supplements as an insurance plan.

To help you understand—

The Dietary Reference Intakes *(DRIs) are nutrient reference values, based on the latest research, which are used to evaluate and plan diets for healthy people in the U.S. and Canada.*

How much vitamin A do I need each day?

The National Institute of Medicine sets daily recommendations for vitamins and minerals. In its latest edition of the Dietary Reference Intakes (DRIs), recommendations for vitamin A are:

900 REs	Men 14 and older
700 REs	Women 14 and older
770 REs	Pregnant women
1,300 REs	Breastfeeding women

Vitamin A Arithmetic

You may see vitamin A measured on your vitamin bottle as IUs (international units) or as REs (retinol equivalents).

1 RE = 1 microgram vitamin A
1 RE = 3.3 IUs of active vitamin A
~ or ~
1 RE = 10 IUs of beta carotene
~ or ~
1 RE = 5 IUs from varied sources

Using the equivalent of 1 RE = 5 IUs (because most of us get our vitamin A from varied sources), your daily need can be expressed as: 700 REs or 3,500 IUs for women, and 900 REs or 4,500 IUs daily for men.

Can you get too much vitamin A?

Unless you eat liver every day, it is hard to overdose on vitamin A from food. It is easier to get too much from a supplement. The experts have determined a tolerable upper limit (UL), a safe amount to take regularly. The UL for vitamin A is 3,000 REs. Taking more than this amount regularly can cause fatigue, vomiting, headache, bone and joint pain, hair loss, dry skin, loss of appetite, liver damage, and in extreme cases, death. Recent research has shown that a high intake of vitamin A weakens bones and increases the risk of broken hips. Excess vitamin A interferes with the cells that make new bone, stimulates cells that break down old bone, and disturbs the body's normal levels of calcium, a mineral essential for healthy bones. During pregnancy, high intake of vitamin A can cause birth defects.

You can't overdose on carotenoids because your body will not convert them to active vitamin A unless it is needed. Overdoing carotenoids can cause a yellowing of the skin, particularly the palms and soles of the feet. This condition is called *carotenodermia* and is harmless.

To help you understand—

The tolerable upper limit *(UL) is the highest average daily amount of a vitamin or mineral that you can take without causing harm. As intakes increase over the UL, the potential for harm increases.*

Can vitamin A be used to treat acne?

Two forms of vitamin A—*Retin-A* and *Accutane*—are used to effectively treat acne. Because these medications can accumulate in the body, women should not take them if they are pregnant or planning a pregnancy.

B VITAMINS

Scientists used to think that vitamin B was a single compound. But as they studied it, they realized that it was a family of compounds. To distinguish one B compound from another they gave each a number. Today we usually refer to each B vitamin by name, not number.

Bs BY THE NUMBERS

B_1 Thiamin
B_2 Riboflavin
B_3 Niacin
B_9 Folic Acid

The family of B vitamins is very important to the everyday work of your body. All of them help you change the calories in food to the fuel the body needs to operate. The B vitamins make sure that every step in this complex process goes smoothly so your body operates at peak performance.

Recognizing how important this group of vitamins was to good health, in the 1940's the U.S. government required that all milled grains be *enriched* with thiamin, riboflavin and niacin. This insured that the vitamins lost when the germ, bran, and husk are removed from the grain would be restored. In 1998, folic acid was added to the enrichment requirements.

Thiamin (B_1)

Why is thiamin important?

Like all other B vitamins, thiamin helps the body use energy, specifically the energy needed to fuel nerve tissues. It also helps to transmit messages throughout the nervous system. That's a pretty important responsibility.

In addition to enriched breads and cereals, what are the best sources of thiamin?

A small amount of thiamin is found in many foods, but pork, ham, and wheat germ are excellent sources, as are sunflower seeds, beans, watermelon, and nuts.

How much thiamin do I need each day?

This requirement is a good example of how a little goes a long way. The Dietary Reference Intakes (DRIs) for thiamin are:

      1.2 mg   Men 14 and older
      1.1 mg   Women 19 and older
      1.4 mg   Pregnant and breastfeeding women

To demonstrate just how small an amount this is, 1,000 mg (milligrams) = 1 g (gram), and 1 gram equals the weight of 1 small paper clip. Your daily thiamin requirement is approximately the weight of $\frac{1}{1000}$ of a paper clip.

Is taking too much thiamin dangerous?

There's no reason to take large amounts of thiamin, but even if you did, it would be harmless because your body gets rid of unneeded thiamin in your urine. The Food and Nutrition Board has not set a UL (tolerable upper level) for this vitamin because there has never been a report of a toxic intake in people.

Riboflavin (B_2)

Is it true that milk has no riboflavin?

The opposite is actually true: milk and yogurt contribute a good deal of your needed riboflavin, along with beef, pork, liver, and enriched and whole grain breads and cereals. The myth about milk having little riboflavin comes from the fact that it is destroyed by light. In the past, when the milkman delivered milk in glass bottles to a sunny doorstep, much of the riboflavin was destroyed. Today very little milk is home delivered, and most comes packaged in cardboard or opaque plastic bottles, protecting the riboflavin content.

Shopping Tip:

Buy pasta in boxes or opaque packages rather than clear plastic bags, to maximize the riboflavin content.

Does riboflavin do the same jobs as thiamin in the body?

It does similar jobs, because riboflavin is also very involved in the use of energy. Its main function is to pick up and drop off electrons. This transfer of microscopic particles is vital to the smooth operation of many systems in your body.

How much riboflavin do I need each day?

Like thiamin, your daily need for riboflavin is small. The Dietary Reference Intakes (DRIs) are:

1.3 mg	Men 14 and older
1.1 mg	Women 19 and older
1.4 mg	Pregnant women
1.6 mg	Breastfeeding women

If you take more riboflavin than necessary, your body excretes it through your urine, which becomes bright yellow. Because the body can easily get rid of excess riboflavin, the vitamin is not toxic and has no UL (tolerable upper limit).

Niacin (B₃)

Why is niacin important?

It's part of hundreds of chemical reactions in the body, especially in those tissues with very high energy demands like the heart, brain, liver, and muscles.

Can my body make niacin?

The strict definition of a vitamin is a substance that cannot not be made in the body in adequate amounts to meet our needs. Niacin can be made from a protein fragment, the amino acid *tryptophan*, but the conversion is very inefficient. It takes 60 mg (milligrams) of tryptophan to make 1 mg of niacin. This process supplies about half of your niacin need, the rest comes from food.

Which foods are rich in niacin?

Meat, poultry, fish, enriched and whole grain breads and cereals, mushrooms, peanuts, and liver are the best food sources. Very little niacin is lost when food is cooked.

How much niacin do I need each day?

The Dietary Reference Intakes (DRIs) for niacin are:

16 mg	Men 14 and older
14 mg	Women 14 and older
18 mg	Pregnant women
17 mg	Breastfeeding women

The UL (tolerable upper limit) is 35 mg (milligrams). Headache, itching, and flushing (increased blood flow to the skin) can occur with intakes as low as 100 mg.

Can niacin help lower my cholesterol?

Niacin can lower LDL (bad) cholesterol and raise HDL (good) cholesterol with doses of 1,000 to 5,000 mg (milligrams) daily. But at these levels, niacin is being used as a drug, not a vitamin, and should be taken only under a doctor's care. Large doses can cause flushing, headaches, cramps, nausea, itching, gastrointestinal upsets, high blood sugar, irregular heartbeat, and liver damage. Regular blood tests are needed to monitor this level of niacin.

Folic Acid (B$_9$)

Folate or folic acid, which is correct?

Folate is an all-encompassing term that includes both naturally occurring folates in food, and synthetic folic acid used in supplements and food fortification. Food sources include green leafy vegetables, orange juice, dried beans, liver, asparagus, broccoli, strawberries, wheat germ, and peanuts. Fortified sources are enriched bread, pasta, flour, breakfast cereal, and rice. The folic acid used to fortify foods is slightly more absorbable than what naturally occurs in foods like spinach. But that doesn't mean you should rely only on fortified foods for your folic acid needs. The natural food sources are rich in other important nutrients and protective compounds that are needed by your body. Most experts recommend getting folic acid from a variety of sources: food in which it is naturally found, fortified foods, and supplements, too.

> ## Fragile Folate
>
> *Cooking can destroy 50 to 90% of the folate in food. Experts recommend eating folate-rich foods uncooked, or else cooking them quickly by steaming, stir-frying, or microwaving in small amounts of water.*

Why is folic acid so important?

Folic acid is important to all cells that rapidly reproduce. It's involved in making the cells' genetic material and in the production of protein and red blood cells. When you don't have enough folic acid available, red blood cells develop abnormally and have a very short life span. The number of normal red blood cells then goes down and the body has trouble carrying enough oxygen. A type of anemia results, with weakness, fatigue, depression, irritability, forgetfulness, and disturbed sleep. Diarrhea and a depressed immune response can also result if folic acid deficiency continues. The good news is that the body normally stores 2 to 4 months of extra folate, and if you take a supplement a deficiency will correct itself within 24 hours.

Do most people get too little folic acid?

Scientists estimate that 10% of Americans are folate deficient. Others are not deficient but their normal intake is below the desirable level. Based on this evidence, fortification of bread, cereal, pasta, flour, and rice was begun in 1998. Since the fortification program started, it's estimated that the average American is getting 200 mcg (micrograms) more folic acid a day.

I'm thinking about getting pregnant and my doctor recommended a vitamin supplement with folic acid. Why?

Because folic acid helps to make the genetic material of every cell, it's essential to support the healthy growth of an unborn child. Pregnant women who take in too little folic acid have a higher risk for miscarriage and for birth defects involving the spinal cord and brain. These organs begin to develop very soon after conception, even before you are aware that you are pregnant. That's why most experts recommend all women of childbearing age get adequate folic acid. Unfortunately, many still fall short.

How much folic acid do I need each day?

The Dietary Reference Intakes (DRIs) for folic acid are:

400 mcg	Men 14 and older
400 mcg	Women 14 and older
600 mcg	Pregnant women
500 mcg	Breastfeeding women

In the U.S., women get about 325 mcg of folic acid a day; men average 420 mcg a day. The UL (tolerable upper limit) for folic acid is 1,000 mcg (micrograms) from fortified foods and supplements. It's hard to take in too much folate from natural food sources.

Is folic acid important for men, too?

Absolutely. Everyone needs this vitamin to insure that new cells reproduce and develop correctly. Research has shown that men with low sperm counts and more fragile sperm have low intakes of folic acid. So when it comes to a healthy pregnancy, adequate folic acid levels are important for both parents.

Why did my cardiologist recommend more folic acid after my last checkup?

If your doctor took blood tests, perhaps your results showed elevated levels of homocysteine (a byproduct of using protein), which is a risk factor for heart attacks and strokes. Folic acid and other B vitamins help to lower homocysteine levels by converting it to a harmless compound. As folic acid intake increases, homocysteine levels decrease, lowering your risk for heart disease.

Evolving research also shows that keeping homocysteine levels in check may slow the onset of Alzheimer's and other memory problems associated with aging. Those with high homocysteine levels were twice as likely to be diagnosed with Alzheimer's or other forms of dementia.

VITAMIN C

Does vitamin C cure colds?

Though the evidence is inconclusive, some studies do report a slightly lower incidence of colds in those people who regularly get enough vitamin C. The vitamin helps the immune system function properly, which in turn keeps you healthy. But vitamin C actually can shorten a cold's duration and make the symptoms more tolerable. This is due to the antihistamine properties of the vitamin.

Isn't vitamin C an antioxidant?

Vitamin C is one of many substances in the body that act as antioxidants. Like a police force, they help protect the body against harmful substances, called *free radicals*, that damage healthy cells. Free radicals result from smoking, air pollution, and sun exposure. They are also by-products of normal body functions. Antioxidants scoop up free radicals and prevent them from causing damage that may lead to heart disease and cancer.

What else does vitamin C do?

Lack of vitamin C was the major downfall of early ocean explorers. At sea for months at a time, with no source of fresh fruits and vegetables, many sailors developed and died from scurvy. The sailors suffered from bleeding gums and aching joints because they were unable to make collagen. Vitamin C plays a critical role in the formation of collagen, the connective tissue that holds together the structures of the body. It's found in most of the tissues throughout your body, especially in the heart, brain, pancreas, adrenal glands, thymus, lungs, pituitary gland, and lens of the eyes.

Vitamin C also protects many other nutrients—vitamin E, folic acid, and iron—so they can work effectively in the body.

Do smokers need more vitamin C?

Yes, they do, because smoking depletes the body's stores of vitamin C by promoting free radicals. Smokers are encouraged to get an extra 35 mg (milligrams) of vitamin C each day.

> ## Unlikely but possible—
>
> *A young college student who went to the doctor with swelling, bruising, bleeding gums, and a rapid heartbeat was diagnosed with scurvy, even though he was eating plenty of calories. He admitted to doctors that he ate no fruits or vegetables. In fact, he ate very few foods, mostly cheese, crackers, soda, cookies, chocolate, and water. Only 4 days after starting a multivitamin with vitamin C, his symptoms began to disappear, and he recovered completely.*

How much vitamin C do I need each day?

The Dietary Reference Intakes (DRIs) for vitamin C are:

90 mg	Men 19 and older
125 mg	Men who smoke
75 mg	Women 19 and older
110 mg	Women who smoke
85 mg	Pregnant women
120 mg	Breastfeeding women

Excellent food sources are: citrus fruits, potatoes, broccoli, strawberries, kiwi, cabbage, spinach and other leafy greens, cantaloupe, green peppers, and vitamin-fortified juices.

My friend recommended I take 1,000 mg of vitamin C every day. Is that a good idea?

Many people firmly believe that large amounts of vitamin C are beneficial, but research has never proven this. Here are a

> ## Hot & C
>
> *An estimated one-quarter of the world's adults eat chili peppers every day. By weight, they are one of the richest sources of both vitamin C and vitamin A.*

few reasons why you may want to rethink your friends recommendation. When you take in 100 mg (milligrams) of vitamin C, your body absorbs 80 to 90% of the vitamin. When you take in very large amounts at one time, the absorption rate falls as low as 20%. As vitamin C intake increases, absorption decreases, with most of the excess being excreted through the urine. Some experts also believe that large amounts of vitamin C can reverse its normal antioxidant effect, and stimulate free radical damage, instead. Very large amounts, over 2,000 mg daily, may cause nose bleeds, abdominal cramps, and diarrhea. High levels of vitamin C can also cause a false-positive result when testing for diabetes. In people prone to kidney stones, high intakes may contribute to the problem. And for people with *hemochromotosis*, a condition that causes excess accumulation of iron, too much vitamin C, which enhances iron absorption, is problematic. The UL (tolerable upper limit) for vitamin C has been set at 2,000 mg.

Which type of orange juice is the best source of vitamin C?

Orange juice is the most important source of vitamin C for Americans. Most types—fresh squeezed, frozen, or refrigerated—all start out with about the same amount of the vitamin. Heat and light destroy vitamin C, so the way juice is packaged and handled affects its vitamin content. Opaque cardboard cartons are better than clear plastic or glass bottles. Pouring a glassful and promptly returning the juice container to the cool, dark refrigerator is better than leaving the juice on the sunny breakfast table. Estimates suggest that 2% of the vitamin C is lost each day from reconstituted frozen or refrigerated juice. For the best vitamin retention, don't buy juice that is close to its expiration date, and drink all the orange juice you buy within a week.

MINERALS

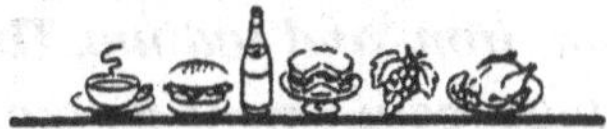

Minerals never change. Unlike vitamins, minerals cannot be destroyed or have their shape changed. The calcium that is in seashells, milk, and your bones is the same. Iron is iron, whether it's in a cast-iron frying pan or your red blood cells. And, your body absorbs most minerals in proportion to its need. Growing children absorb calcium more efficiently than adults. If you are anemic (low iron stores), your body will absorb iron from food more efficiently than when your iron stores are adequate.

Minerals, like vitamins, are divided into two groups—major minerals and trace minerals. If your body needs more than 100 mg (milligrams) a day (like calcium, potassium, and sodium), the mineral is classified *major. Trace* minerals, like iron and zinc, are needed in amounts less than 100 mg a day. Classification as a *major* or *trace* mineral has nothing to do with the mineral's importance in your body.

Labeling Law—Minerals

Food labels in the U.S. are required to list % Daily Value (%DV) for calcium, iron, and sodium. The %DV is the amount of your daily requirement, for the mineral, that you'll get from one serving of food.

Listing the %DV for potassium and zinc is voluntary on food labels.

CALCIUM

Why is calcium so important?

We've all heard that calcium builds strong teeth and bones, and protects us against *osteoporosis* (adult bone thinning), but it does much more than that.

Calcium:
- helps blood clot
- helps nerves work normally
- helps muscles work and the heart beat
- helps lower high blood pressure
- aids in weight loss
- helps prevent mid-life weight gain in women
- relieves PMS (premenstrual syndrome)
- protects against complications in pregnancy
- lowers the risk for some cancers
- may help increase HDL (good) cholesterol in post-menopausal women

- lowers the risk for periodontal disease, a leading cause of tooth loss

- protects against infertility

- reduces the risk for kidney stones

Calcium may even influence behavior. A study with rats showed that they became frantic on a low-calcium diet but calmed down when they were fed adequate amounts.

And the winner is?

Calcium—depending on your size and weight, your body contains up to 3 pounds of it, more than any other mineral.

Why do bones thin as we age?

Most of us think our bones are solid, unchanging structures. Bone, in fact, is a living tissue that changes in response to stress. Your bones and teeth contain 99% of your body's calcium. The remaining 1% is in your blood and tissues. Your body protects that 1% at all costs because calcium has so many important functions in the body, not the least of which is to keep your heart beating!

The calcium in your bones serves as a reservoir for the calcium needed in your body. To keep blood levels constant, your body will sacrifice bone strength. Over time, if more calcium is taken from the bones than is replaced, they become fragile and likely to break. But because bones are living tissue, they can take up calcium to replace the loss, and they will thicken and rebuild if you do weight-bearing exercises like walking and lifting weights. Bone thinning does not have to be a natural consequence of getting older.

> ## Not for Women Only—
>
> *Most women know they need to get enough calcium every day, but according to recent statistics the average guy over 40 doesn't get enough.*
>
> *A Harvard University study found that men over 40 with a calcium-rich diet had the lowest risk of colon and rectal cancer.*

What are the best food sources of calcium?

More than half of the calcium in the American diet comes from dairy products—milk, cheese, yogurt, ice cream. A glass of nonfat milk provides more than one-third of your calcium for the day. Calcium-fortified soy milk is the best nondairy source. Other good sources are canned sardines and salmon with bones, oysters, clams, tofu, molasses, almonds, calcium-fortified foods, beans, and dark green leafy vegetables like Chinese cabbage, kale, mustard and turnip greens. And as much as 25% of your daily calcium comes from mineral-rich bottled water!

> ## Shopping Tips:
>
> *Choose nonfat and lowfat milk—fewer calories and more calcium than whole milk.*
>
> *Lowfat or nonfat ricotta cheese has twice the calcium of cottage cheese.*
>
> *Lowfat chocolate milk has the same amount of calcium as regular chocolate milk.*

Should I be drinking calcium-fortified orange juice?

Orange juice, soymilk, cereal, yogurt, cottage cheese, bread, cereal, breakfast bars, and energy bars are just some of the ever-expanding selection of calcium-fortified foods you can buy. Should you eat them? Maybe yes, maybe no.

If you don't regularly drink milk, calcium-fortified orange juice and soymilk are good substitutes. If you normally eat calcium-rich foods and take a supplement, you might not need these fortified foods. For teenagers, who can drink a quart of orange juice at a time, or children, who may eat 3 bowls of cereal at a sitting, highly fortified choices may be overdoing it. As with any food, calcium-fortified products are fine in moderation. Experts recommend getting calcium first from traditional rich food sources, second from fortified foods, and last from supplements.

How much calcium do I need each day?

The Dietary Reference Intakes (DRIs) for calcium are:

1,000 mg	Men 19 to 50
1,200 mg	Men 51 and older
1,000 mg	Women 19 to 50
1,200 mg	Women 51 and older

There is no additional need for calcium, over and above the normal requirement, during pregnancy and breastfeeding. Growing children, between the ages of 9 and 18 should be getting slightly more—1,300 mg (milligrams)—to help them form strong bones.

In the U.S., men average 830 mg of calcium a day; women 735 mg. Both fall short of the recommended DRI.

> ## Out With Milk—In With Soda
>
> *Surveys show we drink more soda than milk in the U.S. At age 12, 78% of kids drink milk daily; by age 19, only 36% do.*

Can you take too much calcium?

The UL (tolerable upper limit) has been set at 2,500 mg (milligrams) a day. There is no evidence that higher levels have any benefit. High intakes of calcium will reduce the absorption of iron and zinc, cause constipation, and force the kidneys to work harder in getting rid of the excess.

Someone told me a high protein diet will strip my body of calcium.

It's a complicated process for your body to turn protein into fuel, which is exactly what happens on a high protein diet. When protein is burned as fuel, an unused part of the protein is removed from your body by the kidneys. Minerals, including calcium, potassium, and sodium, escort this unneeded material out of the body. In the process, they are eliminated, too.

A very recent study challenged this idea, showing that high protein intakes do not deplete the body of calcium unless calcium intakes are low. So if you are considering a high protein diet, be sure to get adequate calcium.

Why does my antibiotic say, "Do Not Take with Milk"?

Many antibiotics, like *Cipro, Tequin,* and *Levaquin,* interact with the minerals calcium, iron, and zinc, causing the body to absorb less of the medication. Getting less of the drug could be the difference between staying sick and getting well. Drug labels often warn users not to take these medications with milk, mineral supplements, or antacids, but don't say anything about calcium fortified foods like orange juice and cereal.

POTASSIUM

Why do athletes refer to bananas as "potassium sticks"?

Bananas, along with tomato juice, orange juice, lima beans, spinach, cantaloupe, potatoes, and apricots, are rich sources of potassium. All fruits and vegetables contain some. Milk, meats, whole grains, coffee, and tea are other good sources.

Endurance athletes, who lose potassium in sweat, especially in hot weather, often rely on bananas, orange juice, or fortified sports drinks to replenish this important mineral.

Why is potassium so important?

As the third most abundant mineral in your body, potassium is found inside the fluid of every cell. It's important to the firing of nerves and working of muscles. Potassium allows the heart muscle to relax—the opposite of calcium, which makes it contract. Potassium also helps to regulate high blood pressure. People with high blood pressure usually see their pressure come down when they increase their intake of potassium-rich fruits and vegetables.

More Fruits and Vegetables = Strong Bones

If you want stronger bones, eat potassium-rich fruits and vegetables. Researches found that as fruit and vegetable intake went up, bones got stronger. They believe that high potassium levels encourage the body to hang on to calcium instead of excreting it—the net result, stronger bones.

Why did my doctor tell me to take my diuretic with orange juice?

Diuretics are used to control high blood pressure by removing water from your body. Along with the water, you body loses potassium. Orange juice is an excellent source to replace the lost potassium. You could also drink a glass of tomato juice, eat a wedge of cantaloupe, or top your morning cereal with a banana for the same effect.

How much potassium do I need each day?

Potassium is so abundant in food, that no Dietary Reference Intake (DRI) has been set. Experts have set an adult daily minimum requirement at 1,600 to 2,000 mg (milligrams) a day. A healthy diet supplies 2,000 to 4,000 mg daily. Most people get enough.

Is it possible to get too little potassium?

Unlikely, but it could happen. People with eating disorders, those who abuse laxatives, people taking diuretics, endurance athletes, physical laborers, and those sick with vomiting and diarrhea, could have their potassium drop too low. *Hypokalemia,* low potassium, results in muscle weakness, cramping, and fatigue, which can progress to an irregular heart beat and paralysis. Most cases are mild and can be easily handled by eating potassium-rich foods or taking a supplement.

Can I take too much potassium?

The risk of eating too much potassium is slim, because the kidneys monitor and excrete any excess. *Hyperkalemia,* a high concentration of potassium in the blood, can't happen as long as your kidneys are healthy.

SODIUM

Isn't sodium bad for you?

There isn't a "yes" or "no" answer to this question. Most of us associate too much sodium with high blood pressure. With all the bad press sodium gets, it's hard to think about it as an important essential mineral. Too much sodium is actually a recent problem. For centuries, salt was highly valued and hard to come by. In fact, our word *salary* comes from the Latin word for salt.

Sodium regulates your body's fluid level both outside and inside cells. This monitors your blood volume, blood pressure, and the acidity of your body. The movement of sodium into and out of cells allows other important substances to make this journey, too, helping to transmit nerve impulses and electrical messages vital to your body's minute-by-minute functioning.

What's the difference between salt and sodium?

It's easy to confuse the two. Sometimes the terms are used interchangeably, but they truly are two different things. Table salt is actually a mixture of two minerals—sodium and chloride. In a teaspoon of salt (which equals 5,000 milligrams), 2,000 are sodium and 3,000 are chloride. Sodium is also found in MSG (mono*sodium* glutamate), food additives (*sodium* benzoate, *sodium* propionate), artificial sweeteners (*sodium* saccharin), medications (*sodium* citrate), and water (*sodium*).

Salt by any name—

Sea salt, kosher salt, and rock salt differ from regular table salt in taste and texture, but they all have the same amount of sodium.

Don't we all eat too much sodium?

Most of us eat 3,000 to 6,000 mg (milligrams) of sodium daily. There is no Dietary Reference Intake (DRI) for sodium, but experts estimate that healthy adults could do nicely on as little as 500 mg a day. Authorities recommend 2,400 mg or less daily (approximately 1 teaspoon of salt).

When people are told to eat less sodium, most stop salting their food. That's not the best approach, because your total daily sodium intake comes from:

Salt and **sodium** containing additives used in food processing	75%
Sodium naturally occurring in food	10%
Salt added in cooking and at the table	15%

Which foods should I limit if I need to cut down on sodium?

Restaurant and processed foods have the most sodium— luncheon meats, hot dogs, cheeses, soups, gravies, snack chips, french fries, and prepared meals. You don't have to totally eliminate high sodium foods, but you should eat them less frequently and in smaller amounts. Many food manufacturers and some restaurants are now offering low salt or no salt options. You can even request your french fries without salt from your local burger chain. In 2002, the American Public Health Association asked restaurants and food processors to join them in a 10-year initiative to reduce the sodium content of foods by 50%. They estimate this could prevent 150,000 premature deaths a year from high blood pressure.

And the label says—

Label language	Sodium per serving
Sodium Free	Contains 5 mg or less
Very Low Sodium	Contains 35 mg or less
Low Sodium	Contains 140 mg or less
Reduced Sodium	At least 25% less sodium than original
Unsalted ~or~ No Added Salt	No salt added to recipe

Does too much sodium cause high blood pressure?

Worldwide, studies have shown that in places where little salt is used, blood pressure does not go up with age the way it does in the U.S. Reducing sodium can lower high blood pressure in people who have it, and even, to a lesser extent, in people who have normal blood pressure. About 10 to 15% of people with high blood pressure are particularly sensitive to salt. If they decrease their salt intake, their blood pressure improves remarkably. People who are not salt-sensitive do not get the same dramatic results, but their blood pressure does go down.

Is it possible to get too little sodium?

Because sodium is found is so many foods—even water—it's very unlikely. On rare occasions, as when someone sweats profusely or has chronic diarrhea, sodium levels can dip, but even then a deficiency would be rare. Simply eating foods and drinking fluids, especially soups or sports drinks, would replace the lost sodium.

Is it true that too much sodium can act like a poison in the body?

Too much of anything can be harmful. Your kidneys maintain the exact amount of sodium your body needs, and excretes the rest in urine. But getting rid of excess sodium wastes water. If you eat a lot of salt, which normally makes you thirsty, you should also drink enough water to help your kidneys do their job. Still, only in people with congestive heart failure or kidney disease, would getting rid of excess sodium cause a problem. Over time, high intakes of sodium can contribute to high blood pressure and weaken bones by causing calcium loss in the urine.

IRON

Does spinach really have a lot of iron?

Popeye was right, spinach does have iron. But the story is a little more complicated than simply gulping down a canful, like the cartoon character regularly did. Iron in food comes in two forms—heme iron and nonheme iron.

Heme iron is found only in animal tissue. You eat it in meat, fish and poultry, and your body absorbs it efficiently. Nonheme iron is found in plants and iron-fortified foods. You eat it as green leafy vegetables (like spinach), beans, soy, and fortified breads and cereals. Your body absorbs this type less efficiently. Plus, what you eat with nonheme iron foods affects how easily your body makes use of this type of iron. Combine beans with tomatoes (high in vitamin C), and the iron in the beans is more easily absorbed. Have spinach with chicken, and the iron from the spinach is more easily absorbed.

Easy Does It—On Antacids

Regular use of antacids can reduce the amount of iron your body absorbs. Absorption of iron depends on adequate stomach acids, which antacids neutralize.

Does too little iron cause anemia?

Yes. Iron deficiency is the most common nutritional deficiency in the world, affecting 500 to 600 million people. In the U.S., infants, toddlers, teenage girls, young women, and pregnant women are at risk. If left untreated, iron deficiency can lead to a more serious condition, iron-deficiency anemia, which interferes with the production of normal red blood cells.

Why is it important to get enough iron?

Iron carries oxygen in the blood, in *hemoglobin*, and moves oxygen into muscles as *myoglobin*. Without enough iron, hemoglobin and myoglobin cannot be made and the body is deprived of needed oxygen. Besides transporting oxygen, iron is part of hundreds of enzymes needed to make the body function, and it plays a role in brain development and immune function.

If iron is so important, does my body contain a lot of it?

The opposite is true. Iron is a *trace* mineral and most people have less than a teaspoon of iron in their body. About 80% of the iron in your body is found in your bloodstream, and the rest is in your muscles and enzymes. The cells in your intestines act as the body's gatekeepers of iron, carefully maintaining the right amount. If your iron gets low, more is absorbed. When you have enough, less is absorbed and any excess is excreted.

Your body is also very good at recycling iron. When old red blood cells are broken down, your body produces new cells using 95% recycled iron. Food sources and iron stores make up the rest.

How much iron do I need each day?

The Dietary Reference Intakes (DRIs) for iron are:

11 mg	Men 14 to 18
8 mg	Men 19 and older
15 mg	Women 14 to 18
18 mg	Women 19 to 50
8 mg	Women 50 and older
27 mg	Pregnant women
9 mg	Breastfeeding women

Iron requirements are based on growth and need. Younger people and pregnant women are growing. Women between the ages of 19 and 50 need more iron because they lose it monthly through menstruation. After menopause, the iron requirement for men and women is the same. Men in the U.S. more than meet their daily need, averaging 17.5 mg a day. Women fall short, averaging only 13.5 mg a day.

Can too much iron be dangerous?

It's hard to overdose on iron in food because your body simply turns away the iron it does not need. Iron supplements, however, can be hard on your digestive tract. The UL (tolerable upper limit) of 45 mg (milligrams) is the level that causes digestive discomfort in most people. Too much iron can also cause constipation.

A hereditary condition, *hemochromatosis,* causes excessive iron absorption. Without treatment, it can lead to organ damage and even death. Though it was once thought of as rare, doctors now realize that as many as 12 of every 1,000 people of European descent may have this genetic condition.

> ## Poison Alert
>
> *Accidental iron overdose from supplements is the leading cause of poisoning deaths in children under 6. Just a few pills can poison a small child.*

ZINC

Can zinc prevent colds?

Prevent—no. But 50% of the studies on zinc and the common cold say the mineral can make the symptoms less severe and can help cold suffers recover faster. The other 50% say it doesn't work. It could be that not everyone responds to zinc lozenges, the typical "cold remedy." Using zinc lozenges, as directed, when you feel a cold coming on surely will not hurt you, and you may feel better. Colds are a viral infection and some scientists believe that zinc can slow down viral growth, which, in theory, should make you feel better faster. A note of caution, though: zinc can't keep you from catching colds, so don't use supplements preventively, and don't take extra zinc for longer than 5 to 7 days.

What does zinc do in the body?

Even though you have less than half a teaspoon of zinc in your entire body, it's in every one of your cells and is involved in more than 200 chemical reactions that normally occur. It helps protect cells from free radical damage, and when levels of zinc are too low, cells fail to duplicate correctly. That's why zinc is so important in normal growth and sexual maturation. Without zinc, your body can't fight off viruses, bacteria, and fungi. Even a mild deficiency puts you at risk for infection. Zinc helps vitamin A keep your eyes healthy. And a number of studies show that zinc is important in taste and appetite regulation.

Which foods contain zinc?

Your muscles are rich in zinc, as are the muscles of animals, which is why meat, liver, eggs, and seafood, especially oysters, are excellent sources. Dark meat in poultry is higher in zinc than white meat. And the zinc in animal foods is very well absorbed. Whole grain breads and cereals, fortified cereals, wheat germ, bran, and beans all have a fair amounts of zinc, but your body does not absorb it as well from plant foods.

The absorption of zinc is very similar to that of iron. You absorb more when you need more or when you're growing. You absorb less when you need less. As with iron, cells in the intestine act as gatekeepers, carefully monitoring zinc absorption to maintain correct body levels. The body gets rid of unneeded zinc in your stools and you lose small amounts in urine, sweat, skin, hair, semen, and menstrual fluids.

Hair Analysis

This test is wrongly recommended as a way to tell if you are zinc deficient. The amount of zinc in your hair has little to do with the level in your body. Hair zinc is influenced by hair dyes; perming agents; shampoos; the color, diameter, and rate of growth of your hair; the season of the year; where you live; and your age and sex.

How much zinc do I need each day?

Surveys in the U.S. show that most people get enough zinc. The Dietary Reference Intakes (DRIs) for zinc are:

11 mg	Men 14 and older
9 mg	Women 14 to 18
8 mg	Women 19 and older
11 mg	Pregnant women
12 mg	Breastfeeding women

Both men and women in the U.S. meet their daily zinc requirement. Men take in almost 14 mg a day; women average close to 10 mg a day.

Can too much zinc be dangerous?

Because your body absorbs only the amount of zinc it needs, getting too much from food is pretty hard. Overdoing supplements is another issue. Intakes of 100 to 150 mg (milligrams) of zinc a day, for just a few days, will depress your immune system. Excess zinc also depresses HDL (good) cholesterol and elevates LDL (bad) cholesterol. Levels of 200 mg or more a day will make you nauseous and cause vomiting. The UL (tolerable upper limit) for zinc is 40 mg a day.

Can extra zinc increase my sexuality?

Though it's been reported that Casanova ate 50 raw oysters a day—one of the richest food sources of zinc—we can't guarantee you the same results. Most of the research done on zinc and fertility used infertile men as subjects. Supplementing their zinc resulted in increased sperm counts and fertility.

USING YOUR VITAMIN AND MINERAL FOOD COUNTER

The Vitamin and Mineral Food Counter lists the calories, portion size, vitamin A, thiamin, riboflavin, niacin, folic acid, vitamin C, calcium, potassium, sodium, iron, and zinc content of over 7,000 foods. These are key nutrients for you to consider when you're choosing foods. Recommended intakes for all vitamins and minerals counted are given in the introduction. There are still other vitamins and minerals needed for good health, but when you eat a variety of foods containing the nutrients listed in this counter, you will automatically get the other necessary nutrients.

Now you will be able to compare your usual food selections with others that are available, so you can make the best choices. With this information at your fingertips, you'll find it easy to eat healthy. A dash (—) appears in some entries. This means that no analysis was done for that vitamin or mineral. It is not the same as "0," which means the vitamin or mineral is not in that food.

The Vitamin and Mineral Food Counter lists foods alphabetically. For each category, you will find nonbranded (generic) foods listed first in alphabetical order, followed by an alphabetical listing of brand name foods. The nonbranded listing will help you find values for foods when you do not see your favorite brand.

The Vitamin and Mineral Food Counter is divided into two sections, Part 1, Vitamins in Foods, and Part 2, Minerals in Foods.

Most foods are listed alphabetically, but in some cases, foods are grouped by category. For example, a tuna salad sandwich is found in the sandwich category. Other group categories include:

ASIAN FOOD   **Page 52**
    includes all types of Asian foods except
    egg rolls and sushi, which are found in
    separate categories

DELI MEATS/COLD CUTS   **Page 118**
    includes all sandwich meats except
    beef, chicken, ham, and turkey, which
    are found in separate categories

DINNER   **Page 119**
    includes all by brand name, except
    pasta dinners, which are found in a
    separate category

LIQUOR/LIQUEUR   **Page 163**
    includes all alcoholic beverages except
    beer, champagne, and wine, which are
    found in separate categories

NUTRITION SUPPLEMENTS   **Page 176**
    includes all meal replacers and drinks,
    except energy bars and energy drinks,
    which are found in separate categories

SANDWICHES   **Page 223**
   includes popular sandwich choices

SPANISH FOOD   **Page 233**
   includes all types of Spanish and
   Mexican foods except salsa and
   tortillas, which are found in separate
   categories

DEFINITIONS

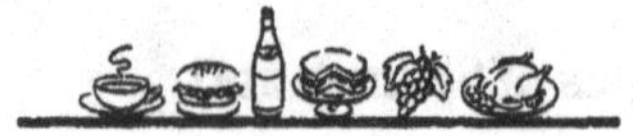

as prep (as prepared): refers to food that has been prepared according to   package   directions

lean and fat: describes meat with some fat on its edges that is not cut away before cooking, or poultry prepared with skin and fat as purchased

lean only: refers to lean meat that is trimmed of all visible fat or poultry without skin

shelf stable: refers to prepared products found on the supermarket shelf that are ready-to-eat or are ready to be heated and do not require refrigeration

take-out: describes prepared dishes that you purchase ready-to-eat; those included serve as a guide to the calories, vitamin A, thiamin, riboflavin, niacin, folic acid, vitamin C, calcium, potassium, sodium, iron, and zinc in products you may purchase.

ABBREVIATIONS

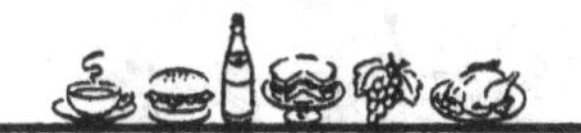

avg	=	average
diam	=	diameter
fl	=	fluid
frzn	=	frozen
g	=	gram
in	=	inch
lb	=	pound
lg	=	large
med	=	medium
mg	=	milligram
oz	=	ounce
pkg	=	package
pt	=	pint
prep	=	prepared
qt	=	quart
reg	=	regular
sec	=	second
serv	=	serving
sm	=	small
sq	=	square
tbsp	=	tablespoon
tr	=	trace
tsp	=	teaspoon
w/	=	with
w/o	=	without
<	=	less than

NOTES

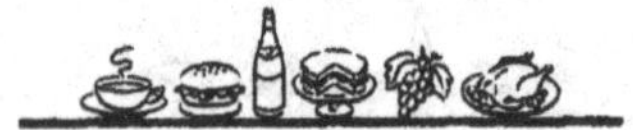

Cals = Calories

vit A = vitamin A
   All vitamin A values are given in International Units (IUs)

thia = thiamin
   All thiamin values are given in milligrams (mg)

ribo = riboflavin
   All riboflavin values are given in milligrams (mg)

niacin = niacin
   All niacin values are given in milligrams (mg)

folic = folic acid
   All folic acid values are given in micrograms (mcg)

vit C = vitamin C
   All vitamin C values are given in milligrams (mg)

calci = calcium
   All calcium values are given in milligrams (mg)

potas = potassium
   All potassium values are given in milligrams (mg)

sod = sodium
   All sodium values are given in milligrams (mg)

iron = iron
   All iron values are given in milligrams (mg)

zinc = zinc

All zinc values are given in milligrams (mg)

tr (trace) = less than 1 IU of vitamin A; less than 1 mg of thiamin, riboflavin, niacin, vitamin C, calcium, potassium, sodium, iron, or zinc; and less than 1 microgram of folic acid

- (dash) indicates data was not available.

0 (zero) indicates that there is none of the vitamin or mineral in that food.

Discrepancies in figures are due to rounding, product reformulation, and reevaluation. Labeling law allows rounding of values. Because much of the data is analysis data, obtained directly from manufacturers and not from labels, in some cases our values may not be exactly the same as label information because they have not been rounded.

PART ONE

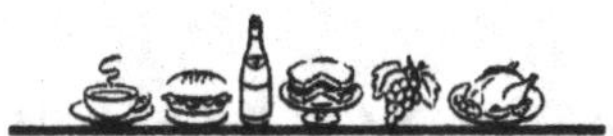

Vitamins in Food

FOOD	PORTION	CALS	VIT A	THIA	RIBO	NIACIN	FOLIC	VIT C
ACEROLA								
fresh	1	2	37	tr	tr	tr	—	81
ACEROLA JUICE								
juice	1 cup	51	1232	tr	0.1	1	—	3872
ADZUKI BEANS								
dried cooked	1 cup	294	13	0.3	0.1	1.6	—	0
AKEE								
fresh	3.5 oz	223	1	0.1	0.2	1.4	—	26
ALFALFA								
sprouts	1 tbsp	1	5	tr	tr	tr	1	tr
ALLSPICE								
ground	1 tsp	5	10	tr	tr	0.1	—	1
ALMONDS								
almond butter	1 tbsp	101	0	tr	0.1	0.5	10	tr
almond paste	1 oz	127	0	0.1	0.2	0.8	16	tr
dry roasted salted	1 oz	167	0	tr	0.2	0.8	18	tr
oil roasted salted	1 oz	174	0	tr	0.1	1.1	18	tr
toasted	1 oz	167	0	tr	0.2	0.8	18	tr
AMARANTH								
uncooked	1 cup (6.8 oz)	729	0	0.2	0.4	2.5	96	8
ANCHOVY								
fresh fillets	3 (0.4 oz)	21	0	0	0	0	—	0
APPLE								
apple	1	81	74	tr	tr	0.1	4	8
baked	1 (5.3 oz)	126	37	tr	tr	0.1	4	8
rings	10	155	0	0	0.1	0.6	—	3
APPLE JUICE								
juice	1 cup	116	2	0.1	tr	0.2	tr	2
Eden								
Organic Juice	8 oz	80	0	—	—	—	—	0
Hansen's								
Junior Juice 100%	1 box (4.23 oz)	60	0	—	—	—	—	60

FOOD	PORTION	CALS	VIT A	THIA	RIBO	NIACIN	FOLIC	VIT C
Mott's								
100% Juice	8 fl oz	120	0	–	–	–	–	2
APPLESAUCE								
sweetened	½ cup	97	14	tr	tr	0.2	1	2
unsweetened	½ cup	53	35	tr	tr	0.2	1	2
Eden								
Organic	½ cup	50	0	0	0	0	0	0
Organic Sweet Cinnamon	½ cup	50	0	0	0	0	0	2
APRICOT JUICE								
nectar	1 cup	141	3304	tr	tr	0.7	3	1
APRICOTS								
apricots	3	51	2769	tr	tr	0.6	9	11
halves, dried	10	83	2534	tr	0.1	1	4	1
halves heavy syrup pack w/ skin	1 cup (9.1 oz)	214	3174	0.1	0.1	1.0	4	8
halves water pack w/ skin	1 cup (8.5 oz)	65	3142	0.1	0.1	1.0	4	8
halves water pack w/o skin	1 cup (8 oz)	51	4109	tr	0.1	1.0	4	4
halves cooked w/o sugar	½ cup	106	2954	tr	tr	1.2	0	2
heavy syrup w/ skin	3 halves	70	1046	tr	tr	0.3	1	3
juice pack w/ skin	3 halves	40	1421	tr	tr	0.3	–	4
light syrup w/ skin	3 halves	54	1124	tr	tr	0.3	1	2
puree from heavy syrup pack w/ skin	¾ cup (9.1 oz)	214	3174	0.1	0.1	1.0	4	8
puree from light pack w/ skin	¾ cup (8.9 oz)	160	3344	tr	0.1	0.8	4	7
puree from water pack w/ skin	¾ cup (8.5 oz)	65	3142	0.1	0.1	1.0	4	8
puree juice pack w/ skin	1 cup (8.7 oz)	119	4195	tr	0.1	0.9	–	12
sweetened	½ cup	119	2033	tr	tr	1	–	11
water pack w/ skin	3 halves	22	1086	tr	tr	0.3	2	3
water pack w/o skin	4 halves	20	1629	tr	tr	0.4	2	2

FOOD	PORTION	CALS	VIT A	THIA	RIBO	NIACIN	FOLIC	VIT C
Chiquita								
Apricots	3 med (4 oz)	60	2250	–	–	–	–	12
Del Monte								
Halves Unpeeled Lite	½ cup (4.3 oz)	60	1500	–	–	–	–	5
Orchard Select Halves Unpeeled	½ cup (4.4 oz)	80	1500	–	–	–	–	48
ARROWROOT								
flour	1 cup (4.5 oz)	457	0	tr	0	0	9	0
ARTICHOKE								
boiled	1 med (4 oz)	60	212	0.1	0.1	1.2	61	12
cooked	1 pkg (9 oz)	108	394	0.1	0.4	2.2	285	12
hearts cooked	½ cup	42	149	0.1	0.1	0.8	42	8
Birds Eye								
Hearts	½ cup	40	100	–	–	–	–	6
S&W								
Marinated Hearts	2 pieces (1 oz)	20	0	–	–	–	–	6
ASIAN FOOD								
buddha's delight w/ cellophane noodles fat choi jai	1 serv (7.6 oz)	211	1920	0.3	0.4	2.7	36	59
cha siu bao steamed buns w/ chicken filling	1 (2.3 oz)	160	0	–	–	–	–	0
chicken teriyaki	¾ cup	399	443	0.1	0.2	8	14	tr
chicken teriyaki w/ rice	1 serv (11 oz)	430	2000	–	–	–	–	12
chop suey w/ beef & pork	1 cup	300	600	0.3	0.4	5	–	33
chop suey w/ pork	1 cup	375	215	0.4	0.4	9.1	24	58
chow mein chicken	1 cup	255	280	0.1	0.2	4.3	–	10

FOOD	PORTION	CALS	VIT A	THIA	RIBO	NIACIN	FOLIC	VIT C
chow mein chicken, canned	1 cup	95	150	0.1	0.1	1	—	tr
chow mein pork	1 cup	425	214	0.7	0.5	10	27	15
chow mein shrimp	1 cup	221	236	0.1	0.3	5.4	28	15
chow mein vegetable	1 serv (8 oz)	90	1250	—	—	—	—	9
filipino chicken adobo	1 serv (15 oz)	555	1080	0.5	0.2	12.9	15	3
fried rice	6.6 oz	249	0	0.1	tr	1.5	—	2
fried rice w/ egg	6.7 oz	395	335	0.1	0.2	2.7	—	tr
phad thai	1 serv (9.2 oz)	232	505	0.1	0.1	1	27	21
sesame seed paste bun	1 (2.5 oz)	220	0	—	—	—	—	0
shrimp chips	1¼ cups (1 oz)	140	0	—	—	—	—	0
shu mai chicken & vegetable dumplings	6 (3.6 oz)	160	1000	—	—	—	—	5
sweet & sour pork	1 serv (8 oz)	250	200	—	—	—	—	9
sweet red bean bun	1 (2.5 oz)	130	0	—	—	—	—	0
szechuan chicken w/ lo mein	1 cup (5.3 oz)	190	200	—	—	—	—	1
wonton fried	½ cup (1 oz)	111	356	0.1	0.1	0.4	5	1
wonton soup	1 cup	205	807	0.2	0.2	4.8	15	5
wonton wrappers	1	23	1	tr	tr	0.4	1	0
Annie Chun's								
Chow Mein Noodles w/ Garlic Scallion Sauce	1 serv	240	0	—	—	—	—	9
Azumaya								
Round Wraps	10	160	0	—	—	—	—	0
Square Wraps	6	160	0	—	—	—	—	0
Wrappers Large Square	3	170	0	—	—	—	—	0
Banquet								
Fried Rice w/ Chicken & Egg Rolls	1 meal (8.5 oz)	330	1000	—	—	—	—	0

FOOD	PORTION	CALS	VIT A	THIA	RIBO	NIACIN	FOLIC	VIT C
Birds Eye								
Easy Recipe Creations Oriental Lo Mein	2¼ cups	230	750	–	–	–	–	9
Easy Recipe Creations Sesame Ginger Teriyaki	2¼ cups	140	3000	–	–	–	–	42
Easy Recipe Creations Spicy Szechuan Cashews	2¼ cups	180	2500	–	–	–	–	27
Lean Cuisine								
Everyday Favorites Oriental Style Dumplings	1 pkg (9 oz)	300	1500	–	–	–	–	15
Everyday Favorites Teriyaki Stir Fry	1 pkg (10 oz)	290	3000	–	–	–	–	0
Nasoya								
Egg Roll Wrapper	3	170	0	–	–	–	–	0
Won Ton Wrappers	8	160	0	–	–	–	–	0

ASPARAGUS

FOOD	PORTION	CALS	VIT A	THIA	RIBO	NIACIN	FOLIC	VIT C
cooked	½ cup	22	485	0.1	0.1	1	132	18
cooked	4 spears	14	323	0.1	0.1	0.6	88	7
cooked	1 pkg (10 oz)	82	2397	0.2	0.3	3	395	72
raw	½ cup	16	390	0.1	0.1	0.8	86	9
raw	4 spears	14	338	0.1	0.1	0.7	74	8
Birds Eye								
Cuts	½ cup	25	750	–	–	–	–	24
Jumbo Spears	3 oz	20	500	–	–	–	–	21
Del Monte								
Cuts & Tips	½ cup (4.4 oz)	20	400	–	–	–	–	15
Spears Extra Long	½ cup (4.4 oz)	20	400	–	–	–	–	15
Spears Tender Young	½ cup (4.4 oz)	20	400	–	–	–	–	15
Tips Hand Selected	½ cup (4.4 oz)	20	400	–	–	–	–	15

FOOD	PORTION	CALS	VIT A	THIA	RIBO	NIACIN	FOLIC	VIT C
S&W								
Green	6 pieces (4.5 oz)	15	500	–	–	–	–	21
ATEMOYA								
fresh	½ cup	94	10	–	–	–	–	9
AVOCADO								
fresh	1	324	1230	0.2	0.2	3.9	124	16
fresh mashed	1 cup	370	1407	0.2	0.3	4.4	142	18
guacamole	1 serv (2.2 oz)	105	215	0.1	0.1	1.1	38	7
Chiquita								
Fresh	⅓ med (1 oz)	55	0	–	–	–	–	2
BACON								
breakfast strips cooked	3 strips	156	0	0.3	0.1	2.6	1	0
gammon lean & fat grilled	4.2 oz	274	0	1.1	0.3	14.2	–	0
pan fried	3 strips	109	0	0.1	0.1	1.4	1	0
BACON SUBSTITUTES								
bacon substitute	1 strip	25	7	0.4	tr	0.6	3	0
BAGEL								
cinnamon raisin	1 (3½ in)	194	52	0.3	0.2	2.2	–	1
cinnamon raisin toasted	1 (3½ in)	194	47	0.2	0.2	2	–	tr
egg	1 (3½ in)	197	77	0.4	0.2	2.4	16	tr
egg toasted	1 (3½ in)	197	70	0.3	0.2	2.2	11	tr
mini onion	1 (1.4 oz)	100	0	–	–	–	–	0
oat bran	1 (3½ in)	181	3	0.2	0.2	2.1	–	tr
oat bran toasted	1 (3½ in)	181	3	0.2	0.2	1.9	–	tr
onion	1 (3½ in)	195	0	0.4	0.2	3.2	16	0
plain	1 (3½ in)	195	0	0.4	0.2	3.2	16	0
plain toasted	1 (3½ in)	195	0	0.3	0.2	2.9	11	0
poppy seed	1 (3½ in)	195	0	0.4	0.2	3.2	16	0
Pepperidge Farm								
Mini	1 (1.4 oz)	120	0	–	–	–	–	0
Plain	1 (3.5 oz)	290	0	–	–	–	–	0

FOOD	PORTION	CALS	VIT A	THIA	RIBO	NIACIN	FOLIC	VIT C
Sara Lee								
Egg	1 (2.8 oz)	210	200	–	–	–	–	0
Thomas'								
Everything	1 (3.6 oz)	300	0	–	–	–	–	0
Multi-Grain	1 (3.6 oz)	280	0	–	–	–	–	0
Plain	1 (3.6 oz)	280	0	–	–	–	–	0
BAKING POWDER								
baking powder	1 tsp	2	0	0	0	0	0	0
low sodium	1 tsp	5	0	0	0	0	0	0
BAKING SODA								
baking soda	1 tsp	0	0	0	0	0	0	0
BALSAM PEAR								
leafy tips cooked	½ cup	10	503	tr	0.1	0.3	25	16
leafy tips raw	½ cup	7	416	tr	0.1	0.3	–	21
pods cooked	½ cup	12	70	tr	tr	0.2	–	21
BAMBOO SHOOTS								
canned sliced	1 cup	25	11	tr	tr	0.2	–	1
fresh	½ cup	21	15	0.1	0.1	0.5	–	3
fresh cooked	½ cup	15	0	tr	0.1	0.4	–	0
BANANA								
fresh	1	105	92	0.1	0.1	0.6	22	10
fresh mashed	1 cup	207	182	0.1	0.2	1.2	43	20
powder	1 tbsp	21	19	tr	tr	0.2	–	tr
BARBECUE SAUCE								
barbecue	1 cup	188	2170	0.1	0.1	2.3	–	18
Muir Glen								
Garlic Mesquite	2 tbsp (1.3 oz)	40	300	–	–	–	–	5
Hot & Smoky	2 tbsp (1.2 oz)	40	300	–	–	–	–	5
Original	2 tbsp (1.2 oz)	40	300	–	–	–	–	5
BARLEY								
flour	1 cup (5.2 oz)	511	0	0.5	0.2	9.3	12	0

FOOD	PORTION	CALS	VIT A	THIA	RIBO	NIACIN	FOLIC	VIT C
malt flour	1 cup (5.7 oz)	585	31	0.5	0.5	9.1	62	1
pearled cooked	1 cup (5.5 oz)	193	11	0.1	0.1	3.2	25	0
Quaker								
Medium Pearled	¼ cup	172	11	0.1	0.1	2.2	32	0
Quick Pearled	¼ cup	172	11	0.1	0.1	1.2	32	0
Scotch								
Medium Pearled	¼ cup	172	11	0.1	0.1	2.2	32	0
Quick Pearled	¼ cup	172	11	0.1	0.1	1.2	32	0
BARRACUDA								
fresh	3 oz	122	135	0.1	0.1	2.6	–	0
BASIL								
ground	1 tsp	4	131	tr	tr	0.1	–	1
BAY LEAF								
crumbled	1 tsp	2	37	tr	tr	tr	–	tr
BEANS								
baked beans	½ cup	190	0	0.2	0.1	0.5	61	1
baked beans w/ beef	½ cup	161	283	0.1	0.1	1.3	–	2
baked beans w/ franks	½ cup	182	197	0.1	0.1	1.2	38	3
baked beans w/ pork	½ cup	133	225	0.1	tr	0.6	46	3
baked beans w/ pork & sweet sauce	½ cup	140	144	0.1	0.1	0.4	47	4
baked beans w/ pork & tomato sauce	½ cup	123	156	0.1	0.1	0.6	28	4
barbecue beans	3.5 oz	120	200	0.1	0.1	2	–	2
four bean salad	3.5 oz	100	500	0.1	tr	1.6	–	5
refried beans	½ cup	43	231	tr	tr	0.2	9	0
three bean salad	¾ cup	230	220	0.1	0.1	0.7	5	3
Bush's								
Barbecue	½ cup (4.6 oz)	160	1500	–	–	–	–	0

FOOD	PORTION	CALS	VIT A	THIA	RIBO	NIACIN	FOLIC	VIT C
Maple Cured Bacon	½ cup (4.6 oz)	150	0	–	–	–	–	1
Vegetarian	½ cup (4.6 oz)	130	500	–	–	–	–	2
Eden								
Organic Baked w/ Sorghum & Mustard	½ cup (4.6 oz)	150	0	0.1	0.1	0.8	0	0
Pringles								
Vegetarian	1 cup (7.9 oz)	250	200	–	–	–	–	0
BEEF								
bottom round lean & fat trim ¼ in Choice braised	3 oz	241	0	0.1	0.2	3.2	8	0
bottom round lean & fat trim ¼ in Choice roasted	3 oz	221	0	0.1	0.2	3.2	10	0
brisket flat half lean & fat trim ¼ in braised	3 oz	309	0	0.1	0.2	2.7	5	0
brisket point half lean & fat trim ¼ in braised	3 oz	343	0	0.1	0.2	2.5	5	0
brisket whole lean & fat trim ¼ in braised	3 oz	327	0	0.1	0.2	2.6	5	0
chuck arm pot roast lean & fat trim ¼ in braised	3 oz	282	0	0.1	0.2	2.7	8	0
chuck blade roast lean & fat trim ¼ in braised	3 oz	293	0	0.1	0.2	2.1	5	0
eye of round lean & fat trim ¼ in Choice roasted	3 oz	205	0	0.1	0.1	3	6	0
eye of round lean & fat trim ¼ in Select roasted	3 oz	184	0	0.1	0.1	3	6	0

FOOD	PORTION	CALS	VIT A	THIA	RIBO	NIACIN	FOLIC	VIT C
porterhouse steak lean & fat trim ¼ in Choice broiled	3 oz	260	0	0.1	0.2	3.4	6	0
rib large end lean & fat trim ¼ in broiled	3 oz	295	0	0.1	0.1	2.3	5	0
rib large end lean & fat trim ¼ in roasted	3 oz	310	0	0.1	0.2	3.1	6	0
rib small end lean & fat trim 0 in broiled	3 oz	252	0	0.1	0.2	3.6	6	0
rib small end lean & fat trim ¼ in broiled	3 oz	285	0	0.1	0.2	3.4	6	0
rib small end lean & fat trim ¼ in roasted	3 oz	295	0	0.1	0.1	2.7	5	0
rib whole lean & fat trim ¼ in Choice broiled	3 oz	306	0	0.1	0.1	2.7	5	0
rib whole lean & fat trim ¼ in Choice roasted	3 oz	320	0	0.1	0.2	2.9	6	0
rib whole lean & fat trim ¼ in Prime roasted	3 oz	348	0	0.1	0.2	2.8	6	0
shank crosscut lean & fat trim ¼ in Choice simmered	3 oz	224	0	0.1	0.2	4.5	8	0
short loin top loin lean & fat trim ¼ in Choice braised	3 oz	253	0	0.1	0.2	4	6	0
short loin top loin lean & fat trim ¼ in Choice broiled	1 steak (6.3 oz)	536	0	0.1	0.3	8.4	13	0
short loin top loin lean & fat trim ¼ in Prime broiled	1 steak (6.3 oz)	582	0	0.1	0.3	8.4	13	0

FOOD	PORTION	CALS	VIT A	THIA	RIBO	NIACIN	FOLIC	VIT C
short loin top loin lean only trim ¼ in Choice broiled	1 steak (5.2 oz)	314	0	0.1	0.3	7.9	12	0
t-bone steak lean & fat trim ¼ in Choice broiled	3 oz	253	0	0.1	0.2	3.5	6	0
tenderloin lean & fat trim ¼ in Choice broiled	3 oz	259	0	0.1	0.2	3	5	0
tenderloin lean & fat trim ¼ in Choice roasted	3 oz	288	0	0.1	0.2	3.3	7	0
tenderloin lean & fat trim ¼ in Choice broiled	3 oz	208	0	0.1	0.2	3.2	6	0
tenderloin lean & fat trim ¼ in Prime broiled	3 oz	270	0	0.1	0.2	3	5	0
tenderloin lean & fat trim ¼ in Select roasted	3 oz	275	0	0.1	0.2	2.5	6	0
tenderloin lean only trim ¼ in Choice broiled	3 oz	188	0	0.1	0.3	3.3	6	0
tip round lean & fat trim ¼ in Choice roasted	3 oz	210	0	0.1	0.2	3	6	0
tip round lean & fat trim ¼ in Prime roasted	3 oz	233	0	0.1	0.2	2.9	6	0
tip round lean & fat trim ¼ in Select roasted	3 oz	191	0	0.1	0.2	3	6	0
top round lean & fat trim 0 in Choice braised	3 oz	184	0	0.1	0.2	3.2	8	0
top round lean & fat trim 0 in Select braised	3 oz	170	0	0.1	0.2	3.2	8	0

FOOD	PORTION	CALS	VIT A	THIA	RIBO	NIACIN	FOLIC	VIT C
top round lean & fat trim ¼ in Choice braised	3 oz	221	0	0.1	0.2	3.1	7	0
top round lean & fat trim ¼ in Choice broiled	3 oz	190	0	0.1	0.2	4.9	10	0
top round lean & fat trim ¼ in Choice fried	3 oz	235	0	0.1	0.2	4.3	10	0
top round lean & fat trim ¼ in Prime broiled	3 oz	195	0	0.1	0.2	5	10	0
top sirloin lean & fat trim ¼ in Choice broiled	3 oz	228	0	0.1	0.2	3.3	8	0
top sirloin lean & fat trim ¼ in Choice fried	3 oz	277	0	0.1	0.2	3.2	7	0
top sirloin lean & fat trim ¼ in Select broiled	3 oz	208	0	0.1	0.2	3.4	8	0
tripe raw	4 oz	111	0	tr	0.2	0.1	2	4
Alpine Lace								
Roast Beef 97% Fat Free	2 oz	70	0	—	—	—	—	0
Boar's Head								
Corned Beef Brisket	2 oz	80	0	—	—	—	—	0
Eye Round Pepper Seasoned	2 oz	90	0	—	—	—	—	0
Italian Style Oven Roasted Top Round	2 oz	80	100	—	—	—	—	0
Roast Beef Cajun	2 oz	80	0	—	—	—	—	0
Top Round Deluxe	2 oz	90	0	—	—	—	—	0
Top Round Oven Roasted No Salt Added	2 oz	90	0	—	—	—	—	0

FOOD	PORTION	CALS	VIT A	THIA	RIBO	NIACIN	FOLIC	VIT C
BEEF DISHES								
beef bourguignon	1 serv (7 oz)	254	100	0.2	0.2	4.6	—	2
bubble & squeak	5 oz	186	180	0.1	tr	1.2	—	10
bulgoghi korean grilled beef	1 serv (5.2 oz)	256	125	0.1	0.2	3.9	10	3
cornish pasty	1 (8 oz)	847	0	0.3	0.2	8.4	—	0
greek moussaka	1 serv (8.5 oz)	450	960	0.1	0.5	3.5	25	4
irish stew	1 cup (7 oz)	280	10	0.2	0.3	5.4	—	11
kebab indian	1 (5.4 oz)	553	495	0.3	0.6	20.2	—	3
kheena	6.7 oz	781	780	tr	0.3	9.5	—	2
koftas	5	280	250	tr	0.1	5.6	—	2
samosa	2 (4 oz)	652	155	0.1	0.1	2.3	—	1
shepherds pie	1 serv (7 oz)	282	110	tr	0.1	2	20	4
steak & kidney pie w/ top crust	1 slice (5 oz)	400	700	0.2	0.7	9.5	—	3
stew	6 oz	208	2335	0.1	0.2	6.7	—	0
stew w/ vegetables	1 cup	220	5690	0.2	0.2	4.7	—	17
stroganoff	¾ cup	260	692	0.1	0.2	5	12	3
swiss steak	4.6 oz	214	684	0.1	0.2	4.8	9	14
toad in the hole	1 (4.7 oz)	383	155	0.1	0.2	3.8	—	0
Banquet								
Sandwich Toppers Creamed Chipped Beef	1 pkg (4 oz)	120	0	—	—	—	—	0
Sandwich Toppers Gravy & Salisbury Steak	1 pkg (5 oz)	210	0	—	—	—	—	1
Sandwich Toppers Gravy & Sliced Beef	1 pkg (4 oz)	70	0	—	—	—	—	0
Hamburger Helper								
BBQ Beef as prep	1 cup	320	500	0.3	0.3	5	60	0
Beef Pasta as prep	1 cup	270	0	0.2	0.3	5	60	0
Beef Romanoff as prep	1 cup	280	0	0.3	0.3	5	60	0
Beef Stew as prep	1 cup	260	500	0.1	0.1	4	8	0
Beef Taco as prep	1 cup	280	500	0.3	0.3	5	80	0
Beef Teriyaki as prep	1 cup	290	500	0.2	0.1	5	40	0

FOOD	PORTION	CALS	VIT A	THIA	RIBO	NIACIN	FOLIC	VIT C
Cheddar & Broccoli as prep	1 cup	350	0	0.3	0.3	4	60	0
Cheddar Melt as prep	1 cup	310	0	0.3	0.3	4	60	0
Cheddar'n Bacon as prep	1 cup	330	100	0.2	0.4	5	60	0
Cheeseburger Macaroni as prep	1 cup	360	0	0.3	0.4	5	80	0
Cheesy Italian as prep	1 cup	320	200	0.3	0.3	5	60	0
Cheesy Shells as prep	1 cup	330	0	0.3	0.4	5	100	0
Chili Macaroni as prep	1 cup	290	1000	0.2	0.3	5	40	0
Fettuccine Alfredo as prep	1 cup	300	0	0.3	0.3	5	120	0
Four Cheese Lasagne as prep	1 cup	330	200	0.3	0.3	4	60	0
Italian Parmesan w/ Rigatoni as prep	1 cup	300	300	0.3	0.3	5	60	0
Lasagne as prep	1 cup	270	0	0.2	0.3	5	60	0
Meat Loaf as prep	⅛ loaf	270	0	0.1	0.3	4	16	0
Meaty Spaghetti & Cheese as prep	1 cup	290	300	0.3	0.3	5	60	0
Mushroom & Wild Rice as prep	1 cup	310	100	0.2	0.3	5	40	0
Nacho Cheese as prep	1 cup	320	0	0.3	0.3	5	60	0
Pizza Pasta w/ Cheese Topping as prep	1 cup	280	200	0.3	0.3	4	40	0
Pizzabake as prep	⅛ pie	270	200	0.2	0.2	4	40	0
Potatoes Au Gratin as prep	1 cup	280	100	0.1	0.3	4	0	0
Potatoes Stroganoff as prep	1 cup	250	0	0.1	0.2	5	0	0
Reduced Sodium Cheddar Spirals as prep	1 cup	300	300	0.3	0.3	4	60	0

FOOD	PORTION	CALS	VIT A	THIA	RIBO	NIACIN	FOLIC	VIT C
Reduced Sodium Italian Herby as prep	1 cup	270	200	0.3	0.3	5	60	0
Reduced Sodium Southwestern Beef as prep	1 cup	300	200	0.3	0.3	5	60	0
Rice Oriental as prep	1 cup	280	0	0.2	0.1	3	40	0
Salisbury as prep	1 cup	270	300	0.2	0.3	4	60	0
Spaghetti as prep	1 cup	270	500	0.3	0.3	5	60	0
Stroganoff as prep	1 cup	320	100	0.2	0.3	5	60	0
Swedish Meatballs as prep	1 cup	290	400	0.3	0.3	5	80	0
Three Cheeses as prep	1 cup	340	100	0.3	0.3	5	60	0
Zesty Italian as prep	1 cup	300	300	0.3	0.3	5	60	0
Zesty Mexican as prep	1 cup	280	200	0.2	0.3	5	80	0
TastyBite								
Beef Roganjosh	1 pkg (9.5 oz)	270	700	–	–	–	–	15
Meatballs Vindaloo	1 pkg (9.5 oz)	270	1000	–	–	–	–	12
Tyson								
Roast Beef In Brown Gravy	1 serv + gravy (3.5 oz)	160	0	–	–	–	–	0

BEER AND ALE

FOOD	PORTION	CALS	VIT A	THIA	RIBO	NIACIN	FOLIC	VIT C
ale brown	10 oz	77	0	0	tr	1.1	–	0
ale pale	10 oz	88	0	0	0.1	1.4	–	0
beer light	12 oz can	100	0	0	0.1	1.4	15	0
beer regular	12 oz can	146	0	tr	0.1	1.6	21	0
lager	10 oz	80	0	0	0.1	1.5	–	0
stout	10 oz	102	0	0	0.1	1.4	–	0

BEETS

FOOD	PORTION	CALS	VIT A	THIA	RIBO	NIACIN	FOLIC	VIT C
greens cooked	½ cup	20	3672	0.1	0.2	0.4	–	18
pickled	½ cup	75	7	tr	0.1	0.3	–	3
raw sliced	½ cup (2.4 oz)	29	26	tr	tr	0.2	74	3
sliced cooked	½ cup (3 oz)	38	30	tr	tr	0.3	68	3

FOOD	PORTION	CALS	VIT A	THIA	RIBO	NIACIN	FOLIC	VIT C
whole cooked	2 (3.5 oz)	44	35	tr	tr	0.3	80	4
whole raw	2 (5.7 oz)	70	61	0.1	0.1	0.5	178	8
Del Monte								
Pickled Crinkle Style Sliced	½ cup (4.5 oz)	80	0	–	–	–	–	4
Sliced	½ cup (4.3 oz)	35	0	–	–	–	–	2
Whole	½ cup (4.3 oz)	35	0	–	–	–	–	2
S&W								
Julienne	½ cup (4.3 oz)	30	0	–	–	–	–	0
Pickled Sliced	1 oz	15	0	–	–	–	–	0
Pickled Whole	1 oz	15	0	–	–	–	–	0
Sliced	½ cup (4.3 oz)	30	0	–	–	–	–	0
Whole Small	½ cup (4.3 oz)	30	0	–	–	–	–	0
Veg-All								
Small Sliced	½ cup	40	0	–	–	–	–	0

BISCUIT

FOOD	PORTION	CALS	VIT A	THIA	RIBO	NIACIN	FOLIC	VIT C
buttermilk	1 (2 oz)	212	49	0.2	0.2	1.8	7	tr
oatcakes	2 (4 oz)	115	0	0.1	tr	0.8	–	0
tea biscuit	1 (3 oz)	210	200	–	–	–	–	0
w/ egg	1 (4.8 oz)	316	649	0.3	0.3	0.7	61	0
w/ egg & bacon	1 (5.2 oz)	458	191	0.1	0.2	2.4	60	3
w/ egg & ham	1 (6.7 oz)	442	874	0.7	0.6	2	65	0
w/ egg & sausage	1 (6.3 oz)	581	635	0.5	0.5	3.6	65	0
w/ egg & steak	1 (5.2 oz)	410	704	0.4	0.5	3.1	56	tr
w/ egg cheese & bacon	1 (5.1 oz)	477	648	0.3	0.4	2.3	53	2
w/ ham	1 (4 oz)	386	133	0.5	0.3	3.5	38	tr
w/ sausage	1 (4.4 oz)	485	56	0.4	0.3	3.3	46	tr
w/ steak	1 (4.9 oz)	455	65	0.4	0.4	4.2	63	tr

BLACK BEANS

FOOD	PORTION	CALS	VIT A	THIA	RIBO	NIACIN	FOLIC	VIT C
dried cooked	1 cup	227	10	0.4	0.1	0.9	256	0
Bean Cuisine								
Pasta & Beans Mediterranean Black Beans & Fusilli	1 serv	210	750	–	–	–	–	6
Eden								
Organic	½ cup (4.6 oz)	100	0	0.1	0.1	0.4	0	0

FOOD	PORTION	CALS	VIT A	THIA	RIBO	NIACIN	FOLIC	VIT C
BLACKBERRIES								
canned in heavy syrup	½ cup	118	280	tr	0.1	0.4	34	4
fresh	½ cup	37	119	tr	tr	0.3	–	15
unsweetened frzn	1 cup	97	172	tr	0.1	1.8	51	5
BLACKEYE PEAS								
cooked	1 cup	198	26	0.3	0.1	0.8	356	1
w/pork	½ cup	199	0	0.2	0.1	1	–	1
Birds Eye								
Blackeye Peas	½ cup	110	0	–	–	–	–	1
Eden								
Organic	½ cup (4.6 oz)	90	0	0.5	0.1	0.1	24	0
BLINTZE								
cheese	1 (2.7 oz)	160	4500	–	–	–	–	0
Golden								
Cheese	1 (2.1 oz)	80	0	–	–	–	–	0
BLUEBERRIES								
canned in heavy syrup	1 cup	225	164	0.1	0.1	0.3	4	3
fresh	1 cup	82	145	0.1	0.1	0.5	9	19
unsweetened frzn	1 cup	78	126	0.1	0.1	0.8	10	4
Tree Of Life								
Organic	1 cup (5 oz)	80	100	–	–	–	–	6
BLUEFIN								
fillet baked	4.1 oz	186	537	0.1	0.1	8.5	2	tr
BLUEFISH								
fresh baked	3 oz	135	390	0.1	0.1	6.2	2	tr
BORAGE								
fresh chopped	½ cup	9	1848	tr	0.1	0.4	–	15
fresh chopped cooked	3½ oz	25	4385	0.1	0.2	0.9	–	33
BOYSENBERRIES								
in heavy syrup	1 cup	226	102	0.1	0.1	0.6	88	16
unsweetened frzn	1 cup	66	89	0.1	tr	1	84	4
BRAINS								
beef pan-fried	3 oz	167	0	0.1	0.2	3.2	5	3

FOOD	PORTION	CALS	VIT A	THIA	RIBO	NIACIN	FOLIC	VIT C
beef simmered	3 oz	136	0	0.1	0.1	1.9	6	1
lamb braised	3 oz	124	0	0.1	0.2	2.1	4	10
lamb fried	3 oz	232	0	0.1	0.3	3.9	6	20
pork braised	3 oz	117	0	0.1	0.2	2.8	3	12
veal braised	3 oz	115	0	0.1	0.2	2.1	3	11
veal fried	3 oz	181	0	0.1	0.3	4.9	5	12

BRAN

FOOD	PORTION	CALS	VIT A	THIA	RIBO	NIACIN	FOLIC	VIT C
corn	1 cup (2.7 oz)	170	18	tr	0.1	2.1	3	0
oat	½ cup (1.6 oz)	116	0	0.5	0.1	0.4	25	0
oat cooked	½ cup (3.8 oz)	44	0	0.2	tr	0.2	7	0
rice	½ cup (2.1 oz)	187	0	1.6	0.1	20.1	37	0
wheat	½ cup (2 oz)	63	0	0.2	0.2	3.9	23	0
Hodgson Mill								
Oat	¼ cup (1.4 oz)	120	0	–	–	–	–	0
Kretschmer								
Toasted Wheat Bran	⅓ cup	57	0	0.3	0.1	5.1	49	0
Quaker								
Unprocessed	2 tbsp	8	0	tr	tr	1.5	9	0

BRAZIL NUTS

FOOD	PORTION	CALS	VIT A	THIA	RIBO	NIACIN	FOLIC	VIT C
dried	1 oz	186	0	0.3	tr	0.5	1	tr

BREAD

FOOD	PORTION	CALS	VIT A	THIA	RIBO	NIACIN	FOLIC	VIT C
boston brown	1 slice (1.6 oz)	88	39	tr	0.1	0.5	3	0
challah	1 slice (2 oz)	160	200	–	–	–	–	0
chapatis as prep w/ fat	1 bread (1.6 oz)	95	221	0.1	0.1	1.6	11	0
chapatis as prep w/o fat	1 (2½ oz)	141	0	0.2	tr	2.1	–	0
cornbread	1 piece (2 oz)	189	123	0.1	0.2	1.2	7	tr
cornstick	1 (1.3 oz)	101	52	0.1	0.1	0.3	4	tr
egg	1 slice (1.4 oz)	115	30	0.2	0.2	1.9	28	0
focaccia	1 piece (2 oz)	130	0	–	–	–	–	0
focaccia onion	1 piece (4.6 oz)	282	5	0.4	0.3	3.3	43	2
focaccia rosemary	1 piece (3.5 oz)	251	2	0.4	0.3	3.3	38	tr

FOOD	PORTION	CALS	VIT A	THIA	RIBO	NIACIN	FOLIC	VIT C
focaccia tomato olive	1 piece (4.7 oz)	270	85	0.4	0.3	3.5	39	3
french	1 slice (1 oz)	78	0	0.1	0.1	1.3	9	0
french	1 loaf (1 lb)	1270	tr	2.1	1.6	18.2	–	tr
garlic bread	2 slices (2 oz)	190	0	–	–	–	–	0
irish soda bread	1 slice (2 oz)	174	116	0.2	0.2	1.4	6	1
italian	1 loaf (1 lb)	1255	0	1.8	1.1	15	–	0
italian	1 slice (1 oz)	81	0	0.1	0.1	1.3	9	0
naan	1 bread (3.5 oz)	286	1400	0.5	0.4	3.5	53	tr
navajo fry	1 (10.5 in diam)	527	0	0.7	0.5	5.8	20	0
navajo fry	1 (5 in diam)	296	0	0.4	0.3	3.4	11	0
paratha	1 bread (2.1 oz)	201	1995	0.2	0.1	1.9	11	0
pita	1 reg (2 oz)	165	0	0.4	0.2	2.8	14	0
pita	1 sm (1 oz)	78	0	0.2	0.1	1.3	7	0
pita whole wheat	1 sm (1 oz)	76	0	0.1	tr	0.8	–	0
pita whole wheat	1 reg (2 oz)	170	0	0.2	0.1	1.8	–	0
pumpernickel	1 slice	80	0	0.1	0.1	1	11	0
seven grain	1 slice	65	0	0.1	0.1	1.1	12	tr
sourdough	1 slice (1 oz)	78	0	0.1	0.1	1.3	9	0
vienna	1 slice (1 oz)	78	0	0.1	0.1	1.3	9	0
wheat berry	1 slice	65	0	0.1	0.1	1	–	0
white	1 slice	67	0	0.1	0.1	1	8	0
white toasted	1 slice	67	0	0.1	0.1	0.9	6	0
white cubed	1 cup	80	tr.	0.1	0.1	1.1	–	tr
Arnold								
Bran'nola Country Oat	1 slice (1.3 oz)	110	0	–	–	–	–	0
Country Buttermilk	1 slice (1.3 oz)	110	0	–	–	–	–	0
Country Wheat	1 slice (1.3 oz)	100	0	–	–	–	–	0
Country White	1 slice (1.3 oz)	110	0	0.2	0.1	1.6	60	0
Natural 100% Whole Wheat	1 slice (1.3 oz)	90	0	–	–	–	–	0

FOOD	PORTION	CALS	VIT A	THIA	RIBO	NIACIN	FOLIC	VIT C
Raisin Cinnamon	1 slice (1 oz)	80	0	–	–	–	–	0
Bread Du Jour								
French	3 in slice (2 oz)	140	0	0.3	0.2	2	40	0
Damascus								
Wraps Honey Wheat	½ wrap (2 oz)	130	0	0.2	0.1	2	60	0
Wraps Plain	½ wrap (2 oz)	130	0	0.3	0.2	2	60	0
Wraps Spinach	1 (2 oz)	280	400	0.5	0.3	4	160	0
Wraps Tomato	1 12-inch (4 oz)	240	0	0.5	0.3	4	120	0
Gold Medal								
100% Whole Wheat	1 slice	70	0	0.1	tr	0.8	–	0
Hodgson Mill								
European Cheese & Herb	¼ cup (1.2 oz)	130	0	–	–	–	–	0
Home Pride								
Wheat	1 slice (1 oz)	80	0	0.1	0.1	0.8	16	0
Marie Callender's								
Cornbread & Honey Butter	1 piece + butter	210	100	–	–	–	–	0
Original Garlic	1 piece	190	200	–	–	–	–	0
Parmesan & Romano Garlic	1 piece	200	300	–	–	–	–	0
Pepperidge Farm								
Farmhouse Country Wheat	1 slice	110	0	0.2	0.1	1.6	40	0
Farmhouse Hearty White	1 slice (1.5 oz)	110	0	0.1	0.1	1.2	24	0
Farmhouse Sesame Wheat	1 slice	110	0	0.2	0.1	1.2	32	0
Farmhouse Sourdough	1 slice (1.5 oz)	110	0	0.2	0.2	2	60	0
Natural Whole Grain Whole Wheat	1 slice (1.2 oz)	90	0	0.1	0	0.8	8	0
Natural Whole Grain Honey Oat	1 slice (1.2 oz)	90	0	0.1	tr	1.2	16	0

FOOD	PORTION	CALS	VIT A	THIA	RIBO	NIACIN	FOLIC	VIT C
Stroehmann								
100% Whole Wheat	1 slice (1.3 oz)	90	0	0.1	tr	1.2	8	0
D'Italiano Italian No Seeds	1 slice (1 oz)	80	0	0.2	0.1	1.2	32	0
D'Italiano Italian Seeded	1 slice (1 oz)	80	0	0.2	0.1	1.2	32	0
Family White	1 slice (0.8 oz)	65	0	0.1	0.1	0.8	24	0
Homestyle Split Top Wheat	1 slices (0.8 oz)	60	0	0.1	0.1	0.8	24	0
Homestyle Split Top White	1 slice (0.8 oz)	65	0	0.1	0.1	0.8	24	0
Honey Cracked Wheat	1 slice (1.2 oz)	80	0	0.1	0.1	1.2	32	0
King White	1 slice (0.8 oz)	65	0	0.1	0.1	0.8	24	0
Potato	1 slice (1.2 oz)	100	0	0.2	0.1	1.2	32	0
Ranch White	1 slice (0.8 oz)	65	0	0.1	0.1	0.8	24	0
Rye	1 slice (1.1 oz)	80	0	0.1	0.1	0.8	24	0
Rye w/ Caraway	1 slice (1.1 oz)	80	0	0.1	0.1	0.8	24	0
Twelve Grain	1 slice (1.2 oz)	90	0	0.2	0.1	1.2	32	0
TastyBite								
Nan Kontos Massala	½ loaf (1.4 oz)	120	0	–	–	–	–	0
Nan Kontos Onion	½ loaf (1.4 oz)	120	0	–	–	–	–	0
Nan Kontos Roghani	½ loaf (1.4 oz)	125	0	–	–	–	–	0
Nan Kontos Tandoori	½ loaf (1.4 oz)	120	0	–	–	–	–	0
Roti Kontos Missy	½ loaf (1.4 oz)	125	0	–	tr	–	–	0

FOOD	PORTION	CALS	VIT A	THIA	RIBO	NIACIN	FOLIC	VIT C
BREAD COATING								
Don's Chuck Wagon								
Chicken Baking Mix	¼ cup (1 oz)	95	0	0.1	0.1	0.8	–	0
Fish & Chips Mix	¼ cup (1 oz)	100	0	0.2	0.1	1.2	–	0
Fish Mix	¼ cup (1 oz)	95	0	0.1	0.1	0.8	–	0
Mushroom Batter Mix	¼ cup (1 oz)	95	0	0.2	0.1	1.2	–	0
Onion Ring Mix	¼ cup (1 oz)	100	0	0.2	0.1	1.2	–	0
Seafood Bake & Fry Mix	¼ cup (1 oz)	95	0	0.1	0.1	0.8	–	0
Luzianne								
Cajun Chicken Coating Mix	2 tbsp (1 oz)	100	75	–	–	–	–	0
BREADCRUMBS								
fresh	⅔ cup	76	0	0.1	0.1	1.1	10	0
BREADFRUIT								
fresh	¼ small	99	38	0.1	tr	0.9	–	28
seeds raw	1 oz	54	73	0.1	0.1	0.1	–	2
BREADSTICKS								
plain	1 sm	25	0	0.1	0.1	0.5	–	0
Bread Du Jour								
Original	1 (1.9 oz)	130	0	0.3	0.2	2	40	0
Sourdough	1 (1.9 oz)	130	0	0.2	0.1	2	40	0
Stella D'Oro								
Original	1 (0.4 oz)	45	0	–	–	–	–	0
Roasted Garlic	1 (0.4 oz)	45	0	–	–	–	–	0
Snack Stix Cracked Pepper	4 (0.5 oz)	70	0	–	–	–	–	0
BREAKFAST DRINKS								
orange drink powder	3 rounded tsp	93	1490	tr	tr	0	116	98
orange drink powder as prep w/water	6 oz	86	1376	tr	tr	0	107	91
Carnation								
Instant Breakfast French Vanilla as prep w/ 2% milk	1 serv	250	2250	–	–	–	100	30

FOOD	PORTION	CALS	VIT A	THIA	RIBO	NIACIN	FOLIC	VIT C
Instant Breakfast French Vanilla as prep w/ fat free milk	1 serv	220	2250	–	–	–	100	30
Instant Breakfast French Vanilla as prep w/ whole milk	1 serv	280	2250	–	–	–	100	30
BROAD BEANS								
canned	1 cup	183	26	0.1	0.1	2.5	84	5
dried cooked	1 cup	186	26	0.2	0.2	1.2	177	1
fresh cooked	3½ oz	56	270	0.1	0.1	1.2	–	20
BROCCOFLOWER								
fresh raw	½ cup (1.8 oz)	16	76	tr	0.1	0.4	29	44
BROCCOLI								
chinese broccoli (gai lan) cooked	1 cup (3.1 oz)	19	1441	0.1	0.1	0.4	87	0
chopped cooked	½ cup	25	1741	0.1	0.1	0.4	52	37
raw chopped	½ cup	12	678	tr	0.1	0.3	31	41
spears cooked	½ cup	25	1741	0.1	0.1	0.4	28	37
spears cooked	10 oz pkg	69	4730	0.1	0.2	1.1	76	100
Birds Eye								
Chopped	⅓ cup	25	1250	–	–	–	–	42
Cuts	½ cup	25	500	–	–	–	–	60
Florets	1 cup	25	750	–	–	–	–	54
Fresh Like								
Spear	3.5 oz	26	2084	0.1	0.1	0.5	–	57
Health Is Wealth								
Broccoli Munchees	2 (1 oz)	60	200	–	–	–	–	2
Tree Of Life								
Cuts	1 cup (3.1 oz)	25	500	–	–	–	–	36
BROWNIE								
plain	1 2 in sq (2.1 oz)	243	11	0.1	0.1	0.6	17	3
plain low calorie	1 (0.8 oz)	84	0	tr	tr	0.2	1	0
w/ nuts	1 (1 oz)	100	70	0.1	0.1	0.3	–	tr

FOOD	PORTION	CALS	VIT A	THIA	RIBO	NIACIN	FOLIC	VIT C
No Pudge!								
Original Fudge	1	100	0	–	–	–	–	0
BRUSSELS SPROUTS								
cooked	½ cup	30	561	0.1	0.1	0.5	47	48
cooked	1 sprout	8	151	tr	tr	0.1	13	13
raw	½ cup	19	389	0.1	tr	0.3	27	37
raw	1 sprout	8	168	tr	tr	0.1	12	16
Birds Eye								
Brussels Sprouts	11 sprouts	35	500	–	–	–	–	54
BUCKWHEAT								
groats roasted cooked	1 cup (5.9 oz)	647	0	0.1	0.1	1.6	24	0
groats roasted uncooked	1 cup (5.7 oz)	567	0	0.4	0.4	8.4	69	0
BULGUR								
cooked	1 cup (6.3 oz)	151	0	0.1	0.1	1.8	33	0
uncooked	1 cup (4.9 oz)	479	0	0.3	0.2	7.2	38	0
Hodgson Mill								
Bulgur w/ Soygrits	¼ cup (1.4 oz)	120	0	0.1	0.1	1.6	–	0
BURDOCK ROOT								
fresh	1 cup	85	0	tr	tr	0.4	–	4
BUTTER								
clarified butter	3½ oz	876	3750	–	–	–	–	0
ghee cow's milk	1 tbsp	126	475	0	–	–	0	0
stick	1 stick (4 oz)	813	3468	tr	tr	tr	3	0
stick	1 pat (5 g)	36	153	tr	tr	tr	tr	0
whipped	4 oz	542	2312	tr	tr	tr	2	0
Cormau								
Light	1 tbsp	55	400	–	–	–	–	0
Crystal								
Salted Stick	1 tbsp (0.5 oz)	102	422	0	0	0	0	tr
Unsalted Stick	1 tbsp (0.5 oz)	102	422	0	0	0	0	tr
BUTTER BEANS								
Birds Eye								
Speckled	½ cup	100	0	–	–	–	–	2

FOOD	PORTION	CALS	VIT A	THIA	RIBO	NIACIN	FOLIC	VIT C
BUTTER BLENDS								
stick	1 stick	811	3624	tr	tr	tr	2	tr
BUTTER SUBSTITUTE								
Olivio								
Spread	1 tbsp	80	500	–	–	–	–	0
BUTTERBUR								
canned fuki chopped	1 cup	3	0	tr	tr	0.2	–	15
fresh fuki	1 cup	13	47	tr	tr	0.2	–	30
CABBAGE								
chinese bok choy shredded cooked	½ cup	10	2183	tr	0.1	0.4	–	22
chinese pak-choi raw shredded	½ cup	5	1050	tr	tr	0.2	–	16
chinese pe-tsai raw shredded	1 cup	12	912	tr	tr	0.3	60	21
chinese pe-tsai shredded cooked	1 cup	16	1151	0.1	0.1	0.6	64	19
danish raw	1 head (2 lbs)	228	1210	0.5	0.4	2.7	392	292
danish raw shredded	½ cup (1.2 oz)	9	47	tr	tr	0.1	15	11
danish shredded cooked	½ cup (2.6 oz)	17	99	tr	tr	0.2	15	15
green raw	1 head (2 lbs)	228	1210	0.5	0.4	2.7	392	292
green raw shredded	½ cup (1.2 oz)	9	47	tr	tr	0.1	15	11
green shredded cooked	½ cup (2.6 oz)	17	99	tr	tr	0.2	15	15
korean kimchee	½ cup	22	60	tr	0.1	0.4	–	16
napa cooked	1 cup (3.8 oz)	13	96	tr	tr	0.5	47	0
red raw shredded	½ cup	10	14	tr	tr	0.1	7	20
red shredded cooked	½ cup	16	20	tr	tr	0.2	9	26
savoy raw shredded	½ cup	10	350	tr	tr	0.1	–	11

FOOD	PORTION	CALS	VIT A	THIA	RIBO	NIACIN	FOLIC	VIT C
savoy shredded cooked	½ cup	18	649	tr	tr	tr	–	12
stuffed cabbage	1 (6 oz)	373	776	0.4	0.4	2.9	22	7
sweet & sour red cabbage	4 oz	61	170	tr	tr	tr	–	14

CACTUS

FOOD	PORTION	CALS	VIT A	THIA	RIBO	NIACIN	FOLIC	VIT C
napoles fresh sliced	½ cup (1.5 oz)	7	178	tr	tr	0.2	1	6
pricklypear fresh	1 cup (5.3 oz)	56	75	0.1	0.1	0.3	–	29

CAKE

FOOD	PORTION	CALS	VIT A	THIA	RIBO	NIACIN	FOLIC	VIT C
angelfood	1/12 cake (1.9 oz)	142	0	0.1	0.2	0.4	2	0
apple crisp	½ cup (5 oz)	230	193	0.1	0.2	1.1	7	3
baklava	1 oz	126	219	tr	0.1	0.4	8	1
battenburg cake	1 slice (2 oz)	204	125	tr	0.1	1	–	0
boston cream pie	⅙ cake (3.3 oz)	293	180	0.1	0.2	1.0	8	tr
cannoli w/ cannoli cream	1	369	0	0	0	0	–	0
carrot w/ cream cheese icing	1/12 cake (3.9 oz)	484	3827	0.2	0.2	1.1	14	1
cheesecake	1/12 cake (4.5 oz)	456	1354	tr	0.3	0.5	16	1
cheesecake w/ cherry topping	1/12 cake (5 oz)	359	1122	tr	0.2	0.4	12	1
cherry fudge w/ chocolate frosting	⅛ cake (2.5 oz)	187	158	tr	0.1	0.4	–	10
chocolate w/o frosting	1/12 cake (3.3 oz)	340	133	0.1	0.2	1.1	9	tr
coffeecake crumb topped cinnamon	1/12 cake (2.1 oz)	240	383	0.1	0.1	0.7	9	tr
coffeecake fruit	⅛ cake (1.8 oz)	156	70	tr	0.1	1.3	9	tr
cream puff shell	1 (2.3 oz)	239	763	0.1	0.2	1.0	14	0

FOOD	PORTION	CALS	VIT A	THIA	RIBO	NIACIN	FOLIC	VIT C
cream puff w/ custard filling	1 (4.6 oz)	336	968	0.2	0.4	1.1	20	tr
devil's food cupcake w/ chocolate frosting	1	120	50	tr	tr	0.3	–	tr
devil's food w/ creme filling	1 (1 oz)	105	20	0.1	0.1	0.7	–	0
eccles cake	1 slice (2 oz)	285	185	0.1	tr	1	–	0
eclair	1 (3 oz)	262	718	0.1	0.3	0.8	14	tr
french apple tart	1 (3.5 oz)	302	345	tr	tr	0.2	2	3
fruitcake	1/36 cake (2.9 oz)	302	60	0.1	0.1	0.9	8	4
gingerbread	1/9 cake (2.6 oz)	264	36	0.1	0.1	1.3	6	tr
jelly roll lemon filled	1 slice (3 oz)	210	100	0	tr	0	0	1
pineapple upside down	1/9 cake (4 oz)	367	291	0.2	0.2	1.4	8	1
pound fat free	1 oz	80	27	tr	0.1	0.2	1	0
pound cake	1 slice (1 oz)	120	200	0.1	0.1	0.5	–	tr
sheet cake w/ white frosting	1/9 cake	445	240	0.1	0.2	1.1	–	tr
sponge	1/12 cake (1.3 oz)	110	59	0.1	0.1	0.7	5	0
strudel apple	1 piece (2½ oz)	195	21	tr	tr	0.2	–	1
tiramisu	1 piece (5.1 oz)	409	1580	0.2	0.4	0.6	16	1
treacle tart	1 slice (2.5 oz)	258	210	0.1	tr	0.9	–	0
trifle w/ cream	6 oz	291	665	0.1	0.2	1.1	–	7
white w/ coconut frosting	1/12 cake (3.9 oz)	399	43	0.1	0.2	1.2	6	tr
white w/o frosting	1/12 cake (2.6 oz)	264	42	0.1	0.2	1.1	5	tr
white w/ white frosting	1/16 cake	260	40	0.2	0.1	1.7	–	0
yellow w/o frosting	1/12 cake (2.4 oz)	245	94	0.1	0.2	1.0	7	tr

FOOD	PORTION	CALS	VIT A	THIA	RIBO	NIACIN	FOLIC	VIT C
Kellogg's								
Pop-Tarts Apple Cinnamon	1 (1.8 oz)	210	500	0.2	0.2	2	40	0
Pop-Tarts Blueberry	1 (1.8 oz)	210	500	0.2	0.2	2	40	0
Pop-Tarts Brown Sugar Cinnamon	1 (1.8 oz)	210	500	0.2	0.2	2	40	0
Pop-Tarts Cherry	1 (1.8 oz)	200	500	0.2	0.2	2	40	0
Pop-Tarts Chocolate Graham	1 (1.8 oz)	210	500	0.2	0.2	2	40	0
Pop-Tarts Frosted Apple Cinnamon	1 (1.8 oz)	190	500	0.2	0.2	2	40	0
Pop-Tarts Frosted Blueberry	1 (1.8 oz)	200	500	0.2	0.2	2	40	0
Pop-Tarts Frosted Brown Sugar Cinnamon	1 (1.8 oz)	210	500	0.2	0.2	2	40	0
Pop-Tarts Frosted Cherry	1 (1.8 oz)	200	500	0.2	0.2	2	40	0
Pop-Tarts Frosted Chocolate Vanilla Creme	1 (1.8 oz)	200	500	0.2	0.2	2	40	0
Pop-Tarts Frosted Chocolate Fudge	1 (1.8 oz)	200	500	0.2	0.2	2	40	0
Pop-Tarts Frosted Grape	1 (1.8 oz)	200	500	0.2	0.2	2	40	0
Pop-Tarts Frosted Raspberry	1 (1.8 oz)	210	500	0.2	0.2	2	40	0
Pop-Tarts Frosted S'mores	1 (1.8 oz)	200	500	0.2	0.2	2	40	0
Pop-Tarts Frosted Strawberry	1 (1.8 oz)	200	500	0.2	0.2	2	40	0
Pop-Tarts Frosted Wild Berry	1 (2 oz)	210	500	0.2	0.2	2	40	0
Pop-Tarts Frosted Wild Watermelon	1 (2 oz)	210	500	0.2	0.2	2	40	0
Pop-Tarts Low Fat Blueberry	1 (1.8 oz)	190	500	0.2	0.2	2	40	0
Pop-Tarts Low Fat Cherry	1 (1.8 oz)	190	500	0.2	0.2	2	40	0

FOOD	PORTION	CALS	VIT A	THIA	RIBO	NIACIN	FOLIC	VIT C
Pop-Tarts Low Fat Frosted Brown Sugar Cinnamon	1 (1.8 oz)	190	500	0.2	0.2	2	40	0
Pop-Tarts Low Fat Frosted Chocolate Fudge	1 (1.8 oz)	190	500	0.2	0.2	2	40	0
Pop-Tarts Low Fat Frosted Strawberry	1 (1.8 oz)	190	500	0.2	0.2	2	40	0
Pop-Tarts Low Fat Strawberry	1 (1.8 oz)	190	500	0.2	0.2	2	40	0
Pop-Tarts Strawberry	1 (1.8 oz)	200	500	0.2	0.2	2	40	0

CANADIAN BACON

FOOD	PORTION	CALS	VIT A	THIA	RIBO	NIACIN	FOLIC	VIT C
grilled	1 pkg (6 oz)	257	0	1.2	0.3	9.6	6	0

CANDY

FOOD	PORTION	CALS	VIT A	THIA	RIBO	NIACIN	FOLIC	VIT C
butterscotch	1 piece (6 g)	24	8	0	tr	tr	0	0
candied cherries	1 (4 g)	12	7	tr	tr	tr	–	0
candied pineapple slice	1 slice (2 oz)	179	59	0.1	tr	0.2	–	13
candy corn	1 oz	105	0	tr	tr	tr	–	0
dark chocolate	1 oz	150	10	tr	tr	0.1	–	tr
fruit pastilles	1 tube (1.4 oz)	101	0	0	0	0	–	0
fudge brown sugar w/ nuts	1 piece (0.5 oz)	56	11	tr	tr	tr	1	tr
fudge chocolate marshmallow	1 piece (0.7 oz)	84	66	tr	tr	tr	0	0
fudge chocolate marshmallow w/ nuts	1 piece (0.8 oz)	96	67	tr	tr	tr	1	tr
fudge chocolate w/ nuts	1 piece (0.7 oz)	81	38	tr	tr	tr	2	tr
fudge peanut butter	1 piece (0.6 oz)	59	6	tr	tr	0.2	2	0
fudge vanilla w/ nuts	1 piece (0.5 oz)	62	30	tr	tr	tr	2	tr
jelly beans	10 sm (0.4 oz)	40	0	0	0	0	–	0

FOOD	PORTION	CALS	VIT A	THIA	RIBO	NIACIN	FOLIC	VIT C
marzipan	1 oz	128	0	tr	0.1	0.5	16	tr
milk chocolate	1 bar (1.55 oz)	226	82	tr	0.1	0.1	4	tr
milk chocolate crisp	1 bar (1.45 oz)	203	23	tr	0.1	0.2	3	tr
milk chocolate w/ almonds	1 bar (1.45 oz)	215	30	tr	0.2	0.3	–	tr
peanut brittle	1 oz	128	54	0.1	tr	1	20	0
peanuts chocolate covered	10 (1.4 oz)	208	0	tr	0.1	1.7	3	0
praline	1 piece (1.4 oz)	177	18	0.1	tr	0.1	6	tr
taffy	1 piece (0.5 oz)	56	20	tr	tr	tr	0	0
toffee	1 piece (0.4 oz)	65	152	tr	tr	tr	0	0
truffles	1 piece (0.4 oz)	59	62	tr	tr	tr	0	tr
Body Smarts								
Chocolate Peanut Crunch	2 bars (1.8 oz)	210	500	0.4	0.5	6	–	6

CANTALOUPE

FOOD	PORTION	CALS	VIT A	THIA	RIBO	NIACIN	FOLIC	VIT C
fresh cubed	1 cup	57	5158	0.1	tr	0.9	27	68
fresh half	½	94	8608	0.1	0.1	1.5	46	113

CARDOON

FOOD	PORTION	CALS	VIT A	THIA	RIBO	NIACIN	FOLIC	VIT C
fresh shredded	½ cup	36	107	tr	tr	0.3	–	2

CARISSA

FOOD	PORTION	CALS	VIT A	THIA	RIBO	NIACIN	FOLIC	VIT C
fresh	1	12	8	tr	tr	tr	–	8

CAROB

FOOD	PORTION	CALS	VIT A	THIA	RIBO	NIACIN	FOLIC	VIT C
flour	1 cup	185	15	0.1	0.5	2	30	tr

CARROT JUICE

FOOD	PORTION	CALS	VIT A	THIA	RIBO	NIACIN	FOLIC	VIT C
canned	6 oz	73	47381	0.2	0.1	0.7	7	16

CARROTS

FOOD	PORTION	CALS	VIT A	THIA	RIBO	NIACIN	FOLIC	VIT C
baby raw	1 (½ oz)	6	296	tr	–	0.1	5	1
raw	1 (2.5 oz)	31	20253	0.1	tr	0.7	10	7
raw shredded	½ cup	24	15471	0.1	tr	0.5	8	5
slices	½ cup	17	10055	tr	tr	0.4	7	2

FOOD	PORTION	CALS	VIT A	THIA	RIBO	NIACIN	FOLIC	VIT C
CASABA								
cubed	1 cup	45	51	0.1	tr	0.7	—	27
fresh	1/10	43	49	0.1	tr	0.7	—	26
CASHEWS								
cashew butter w/o salt	1 tbsp	94	0	0.1	tr	0.3	11	0
dry roasted salted	1 oz	163	0	0.1	0.1	0.4	20	0
oil roasted salted	1 oz	163	0	0.1	0.1	0.5	19	0
CASSAVA								
fresh	3½ oz	120	10	0.2	0.1	1.4	—	48
CAULIFLOWER								
cooked	½ cup (2.2 oz)	14	19	tr	tr	0.3	27	28
flowerets raw	3 (2 oz)	14	11	tr	tr	0.3	32	26
green cooked	1½ cup (3.2 oz)	29	127	0.1	0.1	0.6	40	0
green raw	1 cup (2.2 oz)	20	97	0.1	0.1	0.5	36	22
raw	½ cup (1.8 oz)	13	10	tr	tr	0.3	28	23
Fresh Like								
Florets	3.5 oz	26	23	0.1	0.1	0.4	—	52
CELERIAC								
fresh cooked	3½ oz	25	0	tr	tr	0.4	—	4
raw	½ cup	31	0	tr	tr	0.5	—	6
CELERY								
diced cooked	½ cup	13	99	tr	tr	0.2	16	5
fresh	1 stalk (1.3 oz)	6	54	tr	tr	0.1	11	3
raw diced	½ cup	10	80	tr	tr	0.2	17	4
CELTUCE								
raw	3½ oz	22	3500	0.1	0.1	0.6	—	20
CEREAL								
bran flakes	¾ cup (1 oz)	90	1250	0.4	0.4	5	—	0
corn flakes	1¼ cup (1 oz)	110	1250	0.4	0.4	5	—	15

FOOD	PORTION	CALS	VIT A	THIA	RIBO	NIACIN	FOLIC	VIT C
farina as prep w/ water	¾ cup (6.1 oz)	88	0	0.1	0.1	1	40	0
farina not prep	1 tbsp (0.4 oz)	40	0	0.1	tr	0.4	19	0
granola	½ cup (2.1 oz)	285	23	0.5	0.2	1.3	53	1
puffed rice	1 cup (0.5 oz)	56	0	0.4	0.3	4.9	3	0
puffed wheat	1 cup (0.4 oz)	44	0	0.3	0.2	4.2	4	0
shredded mini wheats	1 cup (1.1 oz)	107	0	0.1	0.1	1.6	14	0
shredded wheat rectangular	1 biscuit (0.8 oz)	85	0	0.1	0.1	1.1	12	0
Alpen								
Corn Flakes	1 serv (1 oz)	110	0	tr	0.1	0.1	–	0
Regular	1 serv (2 oz)	200	0	0.1	0.3	1.2	–	3
General Mills								
Basic 4	1 cup (1.9 oz)	200	500	0.4	0.4	5	100	0
Boo Berry	1 cup (1 oz)	120	0	0.4	0.4	5	100	6
Cheerios	1 cup (1 oz)	110	500	0.4	0.4	5	200	6
Cheerios Apple Cinnamon	¾ cup (1 oz)	120	500	0.4	0.4	5	100	6
Cheerios Frosted	1 cup (1 oz)	120	500	0.4	0.4	5	200	6
Cheerios Honey Nut	1 cup (1 oz)	120	500	0.4	0.4	5	200	6
Cheerios Multi Grain	1 cup (1 oz)	110	500	1.5	1.7	20	400	15
Cheerios Team	1 cup (1 oz)	120	500	0.4	0.4	5	200	6
Chex Corn	1 cup (1 oz)	110	500	0.4	0.4	5	200	6
Chex Honey Nut	¾ cup	120	0	0.4	–	5	100	6
Chex Morning Mix Cinnamon	1 pkg (1.1 oz)	130	400	0.2	0.3	3	180	0
Chex Morning Mix Fruit & Nut	1 pkg (1.1 oz)	180	0	0.2	0.3	3	180	0
Chex Morning Mix Honey Nut	1 pkg (1.1 oz)	130	0	0.2	0.3	3	180	0
Chex Multi-Bran	1 cup (2 oz)	200	500	0.4	tr	5	400	6
Chex Rice	1¼ cup (1.1 oz)	120	500	0.4	0.4	5	200	6
Cinnamon Grahams	¾ cup (1 oz)	120	500	0.4	0.4	5	100	6

FOOD	PORTION	CALS	VIT A	THIA	RIBO	NIACIN	FOLIC	VIT C
Cinnamon Toast Crunch	¾ cup (1 oz)	130	500	0.4	0.4	5	100	6
Cocoa Puffs	1 cup (1 oz)	120	0	0.4	0.4	5	100	6
Cookie Crisp	1 cup (1 oz)	120	500	0.4	0.4	5	100	6
Count Chocula	1 cup (1 oz)	120	0	0.4	0.4	5	100	6
Country Corn Flakes	1 cup (1 oz)	120	500	0.4	0.4	5	200	6
Fiber One	½ cup (1 oz)	60	0	0.4	0.4	5	100	6
Franken Berry	1 cup (1 oz)	120	0	0.4	0.4	5	100	6
French Toast Crunch	¾ cup (1 oz)	120	500	0.4	0.4	5	100	6
Gold Medal Raisin Bran	1⅓ cups (1.9 oz)	170	500	0.4	0.9	10	400	0
Golden Grahams	¾ cup (1 oz)	120	500	0.4	0.4	5	100	6
Harmony	1¼ cups (1.9 oz)	200	500	1.5	0.9	10	400	30
Honey Nut Clusters	1 cup (1.9 oz)	210	0	0.4	0.4	5	100	6
Kaboom	1¼ cup (1 oz)	120	500	0.4	0.4	5	200	6
Kix	1⅓ cup (1 oz)	120	500	0.4	0.4	5	200	6
Kix Berry Berry	¾ cup (1 oz)	120	500	0.4	0.4	5	100	6
Lucky Charms	1 cup (1 oz)	120	500	0.4	0.4	5	200	6
Nature Valley Low Fat Fruit Granola	⅔ cup (1.9 oz)	210	0	0.1	tr	—	—	0
Newquick	¾ cup (1 oz)	120	500	0.4	0.4	5	100	6
Oatmeal Crisp Almond	1 cup (1.9 oz)	220	0	0.4	0.4	5	100	6
Oatmeal Crisp Apple Cinnamon	1 cup (1.9 oz)	210	0	0.4	0.4	5	100	6
Oatmeal Crisp Raisin	1 cup (1.9 oz)	210	0	0.4	0.4	5	100	0
Para Su Familia Cinnamon Stars	1 cup (1 oz)	120	500	0.4	0.4	5	200	6
Para Su Familia Fruitis	1 cup (1 oz)	120	500	0.4	0.4	5	200	6
Para Su Familia Raisin Bran	1¼ cups (2 oz)	170	500	0.4	0.9	10	400	0
Raisin Nut Bran	¾ cup (1.9 oz)	200	0	0.4	0.4	5	100	0
Reese's Puffs	¾ cup	130	500	0.4	0.4	5	100	6

FOOD	PORTION	CALS	VIT A	THIA	RIBO	NIACIN	FOLIC	VIT C
Snack 'N Dash Cinnamon Toast Crunch	1 pkg (1.2 oz)	140	500	0.4	0.7	5	100	6
Snack 'N Dash Honey Nut Cheerios	1 pkg (1 oz)	110	400	0.3	0.4	4	180	4
Snack 'N Dash Lucky Charms	1 pkg (1 oz)	110	400	0.3	0.3	4	180	4
Sunrise Organic	¾ cup (1 oz)	110	0	tr	0.4	5	100	6
Total Brown Sugar & Oat	¾ cup (1 oz)	110	500	1.5	1.7	20	400	60
Total Corn Flakes	1⅓ cup (1 oz)	110	500	1.5	1.7	20	400	60
Total Raisin Bran	1 cup (1.9 oz)	170	500	1.5	1.7	20	400	0
Total Whole Grain	¾ cup (1 oz)	110	500	1.5	1.7	20	400	60
Trix	1 cup (1 oz)	120	500	0.4	0.4	5	100	6
Wheaties	1 cup (1 oz)	110	500	0.8	0.9	10	200	6
Wheaties Energy Crunch	1 cup (1.9 oz)	210	1000	1.5	1.7	20	400	12
Wheaties Frosted	¾ cup (1 oz)	110	500	0.8	0.9	10	400	6
Wheaties Raisin Bran	1 cup (1.9 oz)	180	500	0.8	0.9	10	200	0
Grainfield's								
Brown Rice	1 serv (1 oz)	110	0	tr	0.1	1.8	–	0
Crisp Rice	1 serv (1 oz)	112	0	tr	0.1	0.6	–	0
Raisin Bran	1 serv (1 oz)	90	0	tr	tr	1.3	–	3
Wheat Flakes	1 serv (1 oz)	100	0	tr	0.1	1.7	–	1
Hansen's								
Orange & Chocolate	½ cup	230	2250	1.8	1.6	9	340	36
Straberry & Yogurt	½ cup	230	2250	1.8	1.6	9	340	36
Toasted Nut Crunch	½ cup	230	2250	1.8	1.6	9	340	60
Tropical Cluster	½ cup	210	2250	1.8	1.4	9	340	36
Healthy Choice								
Almond Crunch With Raisins	1 cup (2 oz)	210	500	0.5	0.6	7	100	0
Golden Multi-Grain Flakes	¾ cup (1.1 oz)	110	500	0.5	0.6	7	100	0
Toasted Brown Sugar Squares	1 cup (2 oz)	190	500	0.5	0.6	7	100	0

FOOD	PORTION	CALS	VIT A	THIA	RIBO	NIACIN	FOLIC	VIT C
Hodgson Mill								
Cracked Wheat	¼ cup (1.4 oz)	110	0	0.2	tr	1.6	—	0
Kashi								
Go Apple Spice	½ cup (4.9 oz)	270	0	0.1	0.1	2	8	0
Go Banana Almond	½ cup (4.9 oz)	280	0	0.1	0.1	2	8	1
Go Berry Tart	½ cup (4.9 oz)	260	0	0.1	0.1	1.6	8	1
Go Blueberry Bliss	½ cup (4.9 oz)	260	0	0.1	0.1	1.6	8	1
Go Cherry Vanilla	½ cup (4.9 oz)	260	0	0.1	0.1	1.6	8	1
Go Just Peachy	½ cup (4.9 oz)	260	100	0.1	0.1	2	8	1
Good Friends	¼ cup (1 oz)	90	0	0.1	tr	0.8	8	0
Honey Puffed	1 cup (1 oz)	120	0	0.1	tr	0.8	8	0
Medley	½ cup (1 oz)	100	0	0.1	0.1	1.2	8	0
Pillows Chocolate	¾ cup (1.9 oz)	200	0	tr	0.1	1.2	8	0
Kellogg's								
All-Bran	½ cup (1.1 oz)	80	750	0.4	0.4	5.0	100	15
All-Bran Bran Buds	⅓ cup (1 oz)	80	750	0.4	0.4	5	100	15
All-Bran Extra Fiber	½ cup (0.9 oz)	50	750	0.4	0.4	5	100	15
Apple Jacks	1 cup (1.2 oz)	120	750	0.4	0.4	5	100	15
Cocoa Frosted Flakes	¾ cup (1.1 oz)	120	750	0.4	0.4	5	100	15
Cocoa Krispies	¾ cup (1.1 oz)	120	750	0.4	0.4	5	100	15
Complete Oat Bran Flakes	¾ cup (1 oz)	110	750	0.4	0.4	5	100	0
Complete Wheat Bran Flakes	¾ cup (1 oz)	90	1250	0.4	0.4	5	100	15
Corn Flakes	1 cup (1 oz)	100	750	0.4	0.4	5	100	15
Cracklin' Oat Bran	¾ cup (1.7 oz)	190	750	0.4	0.4	5	100	15
Crispix	1 cup (1 oz)	110	750	0.4	0.4	5	100	15

FOOD	PORTION	CALS	VIT A	THIA	RIBO	NIACIN	FOLIC	VIT C
Frosted Flakes	¾ cup (1.1 oz)	120	750	0.4	0.4	5	100	15
Granola Low Fat	½ cup (1.7 oz)	190	750	0.4	0.4	5	100	2
Honey Crunch Corn Flakes	¾ cup (1.1 oz)	120	750	0.4	0.4	5	100	15
Just Right Crunchy Nuggets	1 cup (2 oz)	210	500	0.4	0.4	5	100	0
Just Right Fruit & Nut	1 cup (2.1 oz)	220	500	0.4	0.4	5	100	0
Low Fat With Raisins	⅔ cup (2.1 oz)	220	750	0.4	0.4	5	100	4
Mini-Wheat Frosted	1 cup (1.8 oz)	180	0	0.4	0.4	5	100	0
Mini-Wheat Strawberry Squares	¾ cup (1.8 oz)	170	0	0.4	0.4	5	100	0
Mini-Wheats Apple Cinnamon Squares	¾ cup (1.9 oz)	180	0	0.4	0.4	5	100	0
Mini-Wheats Blueberry Squares	¾ cup (1.9 oz)	180	0	0.4	0.4	5	100	0
Mini-Wheats Frosted Bite Size	24 pieces (2.1 oz)	200	0	0.4	0.4	5	100	0
Mini-Wheats Raisin Squares	¾ cup (1.9 oz)	180	0	0.4	0.4	5	100	0
Mueslix Apple & Almond Crunch	¾ cups (1.9 oz)	200	750	0.4	0.4	5	100	0
Mueslix Raisin & Almond	⅔ cup (1.9 oz)	200	200	0.4	0.4	5	100	0
Nutri-Grain Almond Raisin	1¼ cup (1.7 oz)	180	0	0.4	0.4	5	100	0
Nutri-Grain Golden Wheat	¾ cup (1 oz)	100	0	0.4	0.4	5	100	0
Product 19	1 cup (1 oz)	100	750	1.5	1.7	20	400	60
Raisin Bran	1 cup (2.1 oz)	200	750	0.4	0.4	5	100	0

FOOD	PORTION	CALS	VIT A	THIA	RIBO	NIACIN	FOLIC	VIT C
Rice Krispies	1¼ cup (1.2 oz)	120	750	0.4	0.4	5	100	15
Rice Krispies Razzle Dazzle	¾ cup (1 oz)	110	500	0.4	0.4	5	100	15
Rice Krispies Treats	¾ cup (1 oz)	120	750	0.4	0.4	5	100	15
Smacks	¾ cup (1 oz)	100	750	0.4	0.4	5	100	15
Smart Start	1 cup (1.8 oz)	180	750	1.5	1.7	20	400	15
Special K	1 cup (1.1 oz)	110	750	0.5	0.6	7	140	15
McCann's								
Irish Oatmeal Instant Apples & Cinnamon	1 pkg (1 oz)	130	1250	0.5	0.2	3	100	0
Irish Oatmeal Instant Maple & Brown Sugar	1 pkg (1 oz)	160	1250	0.5	0.2	3	100	0
Irish Oatmeal Instant Regular	1 pkg (1 oz)	100	1250	0.5	0.2	3	100	0
Morning Traditions								
Banana Nut Crunch	1 cup (2 oz)	250	750	0.4	0.4	5	100	0
Blueberry Morning	1¼ cup (1.9 oz)	220	750	0.4	0.4	5	100	0
Cranberry Almond Crunch	1 cup (1.9 oz)	220	750	0.4	0.4	5	100	0
Great Grains Crunchy Pecan	⅔ cup (1.9 oz)	220	750	0.4	0.4	5	100	0
Great Grains Raisins Dates & Pecans	⅔ cup (1.9 oz)	210	750	0.5	0.5	6	120	0
Mueslix								
Crispy Blend	⅔ cup (1.9 oz)	200	200	0.4	0.4	5	100	0
Nabisco								
100% Bran	⅓ cup (1 oz)	80	750	0.4	0.4	5	100	0
Frosted Shredded Wheat Bite Size	1 cup (1.8 oz)	190	0	0.4	0.4	5	100	0
Honey Nut Shredded Wheat Bite Size	1 cup (1.8 oz)	200	0	0.4	0.4	5	100	0
Original Shredded Wheat	2 biscuits (1.6 oz)	160	0	0.1	0	2	16	0

FOOD	PORTION	CALS	VIT A	THIA	RIBO	NIACIN	FOLIC	VIT C
Original Shredded Wheat 'N Bran	1¼ cup (2.1 oz)	200	0	0.2	tr	4	24	0
Original Shredded Wheat Spoon Size	1 cup (1.7 oz)	170	0	0.1	tr	3	16	0
Post								
Alpha-Bits	1 cup (1 oz)	130	750	0.4	0.4	5	100	0
Alpha-Bits Marshmallow	1 cup (1 oz)	120	750	0.4	0.4	5	100	0
Bran Flakes	¾ cup (1 oz)	100	750	0.4	0.4	5	100	0
Cocoa Pebbles	¾ cup (1 oz)	120	750	0.4	0.4	5	100	0
Fruit & Fibre Dates Raisins & Walnuts	1 cup (1.9 oz)	210	750	0.5	0.5	6	120	0
Fruit & Fibre Peaches Raisins & Almonds	1 cup (1.9 oz)	210	750	0.5	0.5	6	120	0
Fruity Pebbles	¾ cup (1 oz)	110	750	0.4	0.4	5	100	0
Golden Crisp	¾ cup (1 oz)	110	750	0.4	0.4	5	100	0
Grape-Nuts	¾ cup (1 oz)	100	750	0.4	0.4	5	100	0
Grape-Nuts Flakes	¾ cup (1 oz)	100	750	0.4	0.4	5	100	0
Honey Bunches Of Oats	¾ cup (1 oz)	120	750	0.4	0.4	5	100	0
Honey Bunches Of Oats With Almonds	¾ cup (1.1 oz)	130	750	0.4	0.4	5	100	0
Honeycomb	1⅓ cups (1 oz)	110	750	0.4	0.4	5	100	0
Post Toasties	1 cup (1 oz)	100	750	0.4	0.4	5	100	0
Raisin Bran	1 cup (2 oz)	190	750	0.5	0.6	7	140	0
Waffle Crisp	1 cup (1 oz)	130	750	0.4	0.4	5	100	0
Quaker								
Oatmeal Instant Cinnamon & Spice	1 pkg (1.6 oz)	170	1000	0.3	0.3	4	80	0
Oatmeal Instant Maple & Brown Sugar	1 pkg (1.5 oz)	160	1000	0.3	0.3	4	80	0
Oatmeal Nutrition for Women Golden Brown Sugar	1 pkg (1.6 oz)	170	1000	0.4	0.4	4	140	0

FOOD	PORTION	CALS	VIT A	THIA	RIBO	NIACIN	FOLIC	VIT C
Uncle Sam								
Cereal	1 cup (1.9 oz)	190	0	0.8	0.9	10	—	1
Weetabix								
Cereal	2 biscuits (1.2 oz)	100	0	0.1	0.6	2.9	—	1

CEREAL BARS

FOOD	PORTION	CALS	VIT A	THIA	RIBO	NIACIN	FOLIC	VIT C
Dolly Madison								
Apple	1 (1.3 oz)	120	1250	0.4	0.4	5	120	0
Blueberry	1 (1.3 oz)	120	1250	0.4	0.4	5	120	0
Raspberry	1 (1.3 oz)	120	1250	0.4	0.4	5	120	0
Strawberry	1 (1.3 oz)	120	1250	0.4	0.4	5	120	0
Entenmann's								
Apple Cinnamon	1 (1.3 oz)	140	750	0.4	0.2	5	120	0
Blueberry	1 (1.3 oz)	140	750	0.4	0.2	5	120	0
Oatmeal Apple Cinnamon	1 (1.3 oz)	140	750	0.4	0.2	5	120	0
Oatmeal Apple Raisin	1 (1.3 oz)	140	750	0.4	0.2	5	120	0
Raspberry	1 (1.3 oz)	140	750	0.4	0.2	5	120	0
Strawberry	1 (1.3 oz)	140	750	0.4	0.2	5	120	0
General Mills								
Milk 'N Cereal Bars Chex	1 bar (1.6 oz)	160	750	0.5	0.6	6	200	9
Milk 'N Cereal Bars Cinnamon Toast Crunch	1 bar (1.6 oz)	180	750	0.5	0.6	6	200	9
Hershey's								
Crisy Rice Snacks Peanut Butter	1 bar (0.5 oz)	60	100	—	—	—	—	1
Hostess								
Apple	1 (1.3 oz)	120	1250	0.4	0.4	5	120	0
Banana Nut	1 (1.3 oz)	120	1250	0.5	0.5	5	120	0
Blueberry	1 (1.3 oz)	120	1250	0.4	0.4	5	120	0
Raspberry	1 (1.3 oz)	120	1250	0.4	0.4	5	120	0
Strawberry	1 (1.3 oz)	120	1250	0.4	0.4	5	120	0
Kellogg's								
Nutri-Grain Apple Cinnamon	1 (1.3 oz)	140	750	0.4	0.4	5	40	0

FOOD	PORTION	CALS	VIT A	THIA	RIBO	NIACIN	FOLIC	VIT C
Nutri-Grain Peach	1 (1.3 oz)	140	750	0.4	0.4	5	40	0
Nutri-Grain Raspberry	1 (1.3 oz)	140	750	0.4	0.4	5	40	0
Nutri-Grain Strawberry	1 (1.3 oz)	140	750	0.4	0.4	5	40	0
Nutri-Grain								
Blueberry	1 (1.3 oz)	140	750	0.4	0.4	5	40	0
Cherry	1 (1.3 oz)	140	750	0.4	0.4	5	40	0
Fruit-full Squares Apple	1 (1.7 oz)	180	500	0.2	0.2	2	40	0
Fruit-full Squares Banana	1 (1.7 oz)	190	500	0.2	0.2	2	40	0
Fruit-full Squares Cinnamon Raisin	1 (1.7 oz)	180	500	0.2	0.2	2	40	0
Minis Strawberry	1 pkg (1.5 oz)	160	750	0.4	0.4	5	40	0
Mixed Berry	1 (1.3 oz)	140	750	0.4	0.4	5	40	0
Quaker								
Fruit & Oatmeal Bites Apple Crisp	1 pkg	140	1000	0.2	0.4	5	100	0
Fruit & Oatmeal Bites Strawberry	1 pkg	140	1000	0.2	0.4	5	100	0
Fruit & Oatmeal Bites Very Berry	1 pkg	140	1000	0.2	0.2	5	100	0
Rice Krispies								
Treats	1 (0.8 oz)	90	200	0.2	0.2	2	20	0
Treats Peanut Butter Chocolate	1 (0.8 oz)	110	200	0.2	0.2	2	32	0

CHAYOTE

FOOD	PORTION	CALS	VIT A	THIA	RIBO	NIACIN	FOLIC	VIT C
fresh cooked	1 cup	38	75	tr	0.1	0.7	—	13

CHEESE

FOOD	PORTION	CALS	VIT A	THIA	RIBO	NIACIN	FOLIC	VIT C
american	1 oz	93	259	tr	0.1	tr	—	0
beaufort	1 oz	115	314	tr	tr	tr	1	0
blue	1 oz	100	204	tr	0.1	0.3	10	0
blue crumbled	1 cup (4.7 oz)	477	973	tr	0.5	1.4	49	0
brick	1 oz	105	307	tr	0.1	tr	6	0
brie	1 oz	95	189	tr	0.1	0.1	18	0
caerphilly	1.4 oz	150	700	tr	0.2	2.2	—	tr

FOOD	PORTION	CALS	VIT A	THIA	RIBO	NIACIN	FOLIC	VIT C
camembert	1 oz	85	262	tr	0.1	0.2	18	0
cantal	1 oz	105	256	tr	0.1	tr	6	0
caraway	1 oz	107	299	tr	0.1	0.1	–	0
chabichou	1 oz	95	443	tr	0.2	0.4	36	0
chaource	1 oz	83	486	tr	0.2	0.3	27	0
cheddar	1 oz	114	300	tr	0.1	tr	5	0
cheddar reduced fat	1.4 oz	104	365	tr	0.2	3	–	tr
cheddar shredded	1 cup	455	1197	tr	0.4	0.1	21	0
cheshire	1 oz	110	279	tr	0.1	–	–	0
colby	1 oz	112	293	tr	0.1	tr	–	0
comte	1 oz	114	319	tr	tr	tr	1	0
coulommiers	1 oz	88	280	tr	tr	0.3	19	0
derby	1.4 oz	161	755	tr	0.2	2.3	–	tr
edam	1 oz	101	260	tr	tr	tr	5	0
fontina	1 oz	110	333	tr	0.1	tr	–	0
frais	1.6 oz	51	225	tr	0.2	0.8	–	tr
gloucester double	1.4 oz	162	755	tr	0.2	2.4	–	tr
gouda	1 oz	101	183	tr	0.1	tr	6	0
gruyere	1 oz	117	346	tr	0.1	tr	3	0
lancashire	1.4 oz	149	720	tr	0.2	2.2	–	tr
leicester	1.4 oz	160	730	tr	0.2	2.3	–	tr
limburger	1 oz	93	363	tr	0.1	tr	16	0
lymeswold	1.4 oz	170	990	tr	0.2	1.7	–	tr
maroilles	1 oz	97	226	tr	tr	tr	3	0
morbier	1 oz	99	1000	tr	0.1	tr	6	0
mozzarella	1 oz	80	225	tr	0.1	tr	1	0
muenster	1 oz	104	318	tr	0.1	tr	3	0
parmesan grated	1 tbsp (5 g)	23	35	tr	tr	tr	tr	0
parmesan hard	1 oz	111	171	tr	0.1	0.1	2	0
pont l'eveque	1 oz	86	795	tr	0.1	tr	3	0
port du salut	1 oz	100	378	–	0.1	tr	5	0
provolone	1 oz	100	231	tr	0.1	tr	3	0
pyrenees	1 oz	101	915	tr	tr	tr	7	0
queso anego	1 oz	106	63	tr	0.1	tr	0	0
queso asadero	1 oz	101	63	tr	0.1	0.1	2	0
queso chichuahua	1 oz	106	64	tr	0.1	tr	1	0
queso fresco	1 oz	41	100	tr	0.1	tr	–	0
queso panela	1 oz	74	70	tr	0.1	0.1	–	0
raclette	1 oz	102	1000	tr	tr	tr	15	0

FOOD	PORTION	CALS	VIT A	THIA	RIBO	NIACIN	FOLIC	VIT C
reblochon	1 oz	88	1130	tr	tr	tr	7	0
ricotta part skim	½ cup (4.4 oz)	171	536	tr	0.2	0.1	—	0
ricotta whole milk	½ cup (4.4 oz)	216	608	tr	0.2	0.1	—	0
romano	1 oz	110	162	—	0.1	tr	2	0
roquefort	1 oz	105	297	tr	0.2	0.2	14	0
rouy	1 oz	95	790	tr	tr	tr	—	0
saint nectaire	1 oz	97	780	tr	tr	tr	6	0
saint paulin	1 oz	85	900	tr	tr	tr	6	0
stilton blue	1.4 oz	164	770	tr	0.2	2.3	—	tr
stilton white	1.4 oz	145	685	tr	0.2	1.9	—	tr
swiss	1 oz	107	240	tr	0.1	tr	2	0
tilsit	1 oz	96	296	tr	0.1	0.1	—	0
tome	1 oz	92	1000	tr	tr	tr	6	0
triple creme	1 oz	113	1925	tr	tr	tr	3	tr
vacherin	1 oz	92	90	tr	tr	tr	3	0
wensleydale	1.4 oz	151	635	tr	0.2	2.2	—	tr
whey cheese	1 oz	126	356	tr	0.8	2.2	—	1
Di Giorno								
Parmesan Grated	2 tsp (5 g)	25	0	0	0	0	0	0
Parmesan Shredded	2 tsp (5 g)	20	0	0	0	0	0	0
Romano Grated	2 tsp (5 g)	25	0	0	0	0	0	0
Romano Shredded	2 tsp (5 g)	20	0	0	0	0	0	0
Lactaid								
American	3.5 oz	328	913	tr	0.4	0.1	0	0
Land O Lakes								
Cheese Spread Golden Velvet	1 oz	80	80	—	—	—	—	0
Colby	1 oz	110	110	—	—	—	—	0

CHEESE DISHES

FOOD	PORTION	CALS	VIT A	THIA	RIBO	NIACIN	FOLIC	VIT C
cheese omelette as prep w/ 2 eggs	1 (6.8 oz)	519	2750	0.1	0.6	8.4	—	tr
fondue	½ cup (3.8 oz)	247	447	tr	0.2	0.2	5	0
souffle	1 serv (7 oz)	504	1000	0.1	0.5	0.4	38	tr
welsh rarebit	1 slice	228	825	0.1	0.1	2.5	—	tr

CHEESE SUBSTITUTES

FOOD	PORTION	CALS	VIT A	THIA	RIBO	NIACIN	FOLIC	VIT C
Sargento								
Mozzarella Shredded	¼ cup (1 oz)	80	400	0	0.3	0	40	0

FOOD	PORTION	CALS	VIT A	THIA	RIBO	NIACIN	FOLIC	VIT C
Yves								
Good Slice American	1 slice (0.7 oz)	35	300	–	0.1	–	–	0
Good Slice Cheddar	1 slice (0.7 oz)	35	300	–	0.1	–	–	0
Good Slice Jalapeno Jack	1 slice (0.7 oz)	35	300	–	0.1	–	–	0
Good Slice Mozzarella	1 slice (0.7 oz)	30	300	–	0.1	–	–	0
Good Slice Swiss	1 slice (0.7 oz)	35	300	–	0.1	–	–	0

CHERIMOYA

FOOD	PORTION	CALS	VIT A	THIA	RIBO	NIACIN	FOLIC	VIT C
fresh	1	515	55	0.5	0.6	7.1	–	49

CHERRIES

FOOD	PORTION	CALS	VIT A	THIA	RIBO	NIACIN	FOLIC	VIT C
sour	1 cup	51	1321	tr	tr	0.4	8	10
sour in heavy syrup	½ cup	232	1827	tr	0.1	0.4	19	5
sour unsweetened	1 cup	72	1349	0.1	0.1	0.2	7	3
sour water packed	1 cup	87	1840	tr	0.1	0.4	20	5
sweet	10	49	146	tr	tr	0.3	3	5
sweet in heavy syrup	½ cup	107	199	tr	0.1	0.5	–	5
sweet in light syrup	½ cup	85	197	tr	0.1	0.5	–	5
sweet juice pack	½ cup	68	156	tr	tr	0.5	–	3

CHESTNUTS

FOOD	PORTION	CALS	VIT A	THIA	RIBO	NIACIN	FOLIC	VIT C
creme de marrons	1 oz	73	0	tr	tr	0.1	9	0
japanese dried	1 oz	102	24	0.2	0.1	1	–	17
japanese roasted	1 oz	57	21	0.1	0.1	0.2	–	8
roasted	2 to 3 (1 oz)	70	7	0.1	0.1	0.4	10	7

CHEWING GUM

FOOD	PORTION	CALS	VIT A	THIA	RIBO	NIACIN	FOLIC	VIT C
bubble gum	1 block (8 g)	27	0	0	0	0	–	0
stick	1 (3 g)	10	0	0	0	0	–	0

CHICKEN

FOOD	PORTION	CALS	VIT A	THIA	RIBO	NIACIN	FOLIC	VIT C
broiler/fryer back w/ skin batter dipped & fried	½ back (2.5 oz)	238	85	0.1	0.2	4.2	6	0

FOOD	PORTION	CALS	VIT A	THIA	RIBO	NIACIN	FOLIC	VIT C
broiler/fryer back w/ skin floured & fried	1.5 oz	146	54	tr	0.1	3.2	3	0
broiler/fryer back w/ skin roasted	1 oz	96	111	tr	0.1	2.2	2	0
broiler/fryer back w/ skin stewed	½ back (2.1 oz)	158	188	tr	0.1	2.6	3	0
broiler/fryer back w/o skin fried	½ back (2 oz)	167	57	0.1	0.1	4.5	5	0
broiler/fryer breast w/ skin batter dipped & fried	2.9 oz	218	56	0.1	0.1	8.8	5	0
broiler/fryer breast w/ skin batter dipped & fried	½ breast (4.9 oz)	364	94	0.2	0.2	14.7	8	0
broiler/fryer breast w/ skin roasted	½ breast (3.4 oz)	193	91	0.1	0.1	12.5	3	0
broiler/fryer breast w/ skin roasted	2 oz	115	54	tr	0.1	7.4	2	0
broiler/fryer breast w/ skin stewed	½ breast (3.9 oz)	202	90	tr	0.1	8.6	3	0
broiler/fryer breast w/o skin fried	½ breast (3 oz)	161	20	0.1	0.1	12.7	4	0
broiler/fryer breast w/o skin roasted	½ breast (3 oz)	142	18	0.1	0.1	11.8	3	0
broiler/fryer breast w/o skin stewed	2 oz	86	11	tr	0.1	4.8	2	0
broiler/fryer drumstick w/ skin batter dipped & fried	1 (2.6 oz)	193	62	0.1	0.2	3.7	6	0
broiler/fryer drumstick w/ skin floured & fried	1 (1.7 oz)	120	41	tr	0.1	3	4	0
broiler/fryer drumstick w/ skin roasted	1 (1.8 oz)	112	52	tr	0.1	3.1	4	0
broiler/fryer drumstick w/ skin stewed	1 (2 oz)	116	52	tr	0.1	2.4	4	0

FOOD	PORTION	CALS	VIT A	THIA	RIBO	NIACIN	FOLIC	VIT C
broiler/fryer drumstick w/o skin fried	1 (1.5 oz)	82	26	tr	0.1	2.9	4	0
broiler/fryer drumstick w/o skin roasted	1 (1.5 oz)	76	26	tr	0.1	2.7	4	0
broiler/fryer drumstick w/o skin stewed	1 (1.6 oz)	78	26	tr	0.1	2	4	0
broiler/fryer leg w/ skin batter dipped & fried	1 (5.5 oz)	431	144	0.2	0.3	8.6	14	0
broiler/fryer leg w/ skin floured & fried	1 (3.9 oz)	285	103	0.1	0.3	7.3	9	0
broiler/fryer leg w/ skin roasted	1 (4 oz)	265	154	0.1	0.2	7.1	8	0
broiler/fryer leg w/ skin stewed	1 (4.4 oz)	275	156	0.1	0.2	5.7	8	0
broiler/fryer leg w/o skin fried	1 (3.3 oz)	195	62	0.1	0.2	6.3	8	0
broiler/fryer leg w/o skin roasted	1 (3.3 oz)	182	60	0.1	0.2	6	8	0
broiler/fryer leg w/o skin stewed	1 (3.5 oz)	187	60	0.1	0.2	4.8	8	0
broiler/fryer neck w/ skin stewed	1 (1.3 oz)	94	61	tr	0.1	1.3	1	0
broiler/fryer skin roasted	from ½ chicken (2 oz)	254	146	tr	0.1	3.1	1	0
broiler/fryer skin stewed	from ½ chicken (2.5 oz)	261	143	tr	0.1	2.7	1	0
broiler/fryer thigh w/ skin batter dipped & fried	1 (3 oz)	238	82	0.1	0.2	4.9	8	0
broiler/fryer thigh w/ skin floured & fried	1 (2.2 oz)	162	61	0.1	0.2	4.3	5	0

FOOD	PORTION	CALS	VIT A	THIA	RIBO	NIACIN	FOLIC	VIT C
broiler/fryer thigh w/ skin roasted	1 (2.2 oz)	153	102	tr	0.1	3.9	4	0
broiler/fryer thigh w/ skin stewed	1 (2.4 oz)	158	103	tr	0.1	3.3	4	0
broiler/fryer thigh w/o skin fried	1 (1.8 oz)	113	37	tr	0.1	3.7	4	0
broiler/fryer thigh w/o skin roasted	1 (1.8 oz)	109	34	tr	0.1	3.4	4	0
broiler/fryer thigh w/o skin stewed	1 (1.9 oz)	107	34	tr	0.1	2.9	4	0
broiler/fryer w/ skin fried	½ chicken (16.4 oz)	1347	434	0.5	0.9	32.8	35	0
broiler/fryer w/ skin roasted	½ chicken (10.5 oz)	715	482	0.2	0.5	25.4	16	0
broiler/fryer w/o skin roasted	1 cup (5 oz)	266	74	0.1	0.2	12.8	8	0
broiler/fryer wing w/ skin batter dipped & fried	1 (1.7 oz)	159	55	0.1	0.1	2.6	3	0
broiler/fryer wing w/ skin floured & fried	1 (1.1 oz)	103	40	tr	tr	2.1	1	0
broiler/fryer wing w/ skin roasted	1 (1.2 oz)	99	54	tr	tr	2.3	1	0
broiler/fryer wing w/ skin stewed	1 (1.4 oz)	100	53	tr	tr	1.8	1	0
cornish hen w/ skin roasted	1 hen (8 oz)	595	241	0.2	0.5	13.5	5	1
cornish hen w/skin roasted	½ hen (4 oz)	296	120	0.1	0.2	6.7	3	1
poultry salad sandwich spread	1 tbsp (13 g)	109	18	tr	tr	0.2	1	0

Perdue

FOOD	PORTION	CALS	VIT A	THIA	RIBO	NIACIN	FOLIC	VIT C
Honey Rotisserie Dark Meat	3 oz	200	0	—	—	—	—	2
Honey Rotisserie White Meat	3 oz	140	0	—	—	—	—	0
Seasoned Strips Spicy Fiesta cooked	3 oz	140	300	—	—	—	—	4

FOOD	PORTION	CALS	VIT A	THIA	RIBO	NIACIN	FOLIC	VIT C
CHICKEN DISHES								
boneless breaded & fried w/ barbecue sauce	6 pieces (4.6 oz)	330	342	0.1	0.2	7	28	tr
boneless breaded & fried w/ honey	6 pieces (4 oz)	339	101	tr	0.2	6.8	11	tr
boneless breaded & fried w/ mustard sauce	6 pieces (4.6 oz)	323	110	0.1	0.2	6.9	12	tr
boneless breaded & fried w/ sweet & sour sauce	6 pieces (4.6 oz)	346	242	0.1	0.2	6.9	12	tr
breast & wing breaded & fried	2 pieces (5.7 oz)	494	192	0.1	0.3	12	9	0
chicken & dumplings	¾ cup	256	233	0.1	0.2	4.5	10	4
chicken & noodles	1 cup	365	430	0.1	0.2	4.3	–	tr
chicken a la king	1 cup	470	1130	0.1	0.4	5.4	–	12
chicken cacciatore	¾ cup	394	1586	0.2	0.2	10.3	18	40
chicken pie w/ top crust	1 slice (5.6 oz)	472	800	0.2	0.2	9.3	–	0
drumstick breaded & fried	2 pieces (5.2 oz)	430	222	0.1	0.4	7.2	10	0
groundnut stew hkatenkwan	1 serv (15.7 oz)	576	1535	0.3	0.3	15.8	51	21
jamaican jerk wings	4 wings (9.9 oz)	709	580	0.1	0.3	11.6	10	4
sancocho de pollo dominican chicken stew	1 serv	702	2735	0.3	0.5	23.3	52	49
thigh breaded & fried	2 pieces (5.2 oz)	430	222	0.1	0.4	7.2	10	0
Bumble Bee								
Chicken Salad	1 pkg (3.5 oz)	230	100	–	–	–	–	0
Chicken Skillet Helper								
Stir-Fried Chicken as prep	1 cup	270	300	0.2	0.2	5	60	0

FOOD	PORTION	CALS	VIT A	THIA	RIBO	NIACIN	FOLIC	VIT C
Hamburger Helper								
Reduced Sodium Cheddar Spirals Chicken Recipe as prep	1 cup	240	300	0.3	0.3	4	60	0
Reduced Sodium Italian Herb Chicken Recipe as prep	1 cup	200	200	0.3	0.3	5	60	0
Reduced Sodium Southwestern Beef Chicken Recipe as prep	1 cup	220	200	0.3	0.3	5	60	0
TastyBite								
Chicken Moglai	1 pkg (9.5 oz)	300	200	–	–	–	–	9

CHICKEN SUBSTITUTES
Health Is Wealth

FOOD	PORTION	CALS	VIT A	THIA	RIBO	NIACIN	FOLIC	VIT C
Buffalo Wings	3 pieces (2.2 oz)	100	400	–	–	–	–	2
Chicken-Free Nuggets	3 pieces (2.25 oz)	90	0	–	–	–	–	0
Chicken-Free Patties	1 (3 oz)	120	0	–	–	–	–	0
Quorn								
Cutlets	1 (3.5 oz)	200	0	–	–	–	–	0
Nuggets	3–4 pieces (3 oz)	180	0	–	–	–	–	0
Patties	1 patty (2.6 oz)	160	0	–	–	–	–	0
Tenders	1 cup (3 oz)	90	0	–	–	–	–	0
Yves								
Veggie Chicken Burgers	1 (3 oz)	120	100	0.3	0.2	7	–	5

CHICKPEAS

FOOD	PORTION	CALS	VIT A	THIA	RIBO	NIACIN	FOLIC	VIT C
chickpeas	1 cup	285	58	0.1	0.1	0.3	160	9
cooked	1 cup	269	44	0.2	0.1	0.9	282	2

FOOD	PORTION	CALS	VIT A	THIA	RIBO	NIACIN	FOLIC	VIT C
CHICORY								
greens raw chopped	½ cup	21	3600	0.1	0.1	0.5	–	22
root raw	1 (2.1 oz)	44	4	tr	tr	0.2	–	3
roots raw cut up	½ cup (1.6 oz)	33	3	tr	tr	0.2	–	2
witloof head raw	1 (1.9 oz)	9	15	tr	tr	0.1	20	2
witloof raw	½ cup (1.6 oz)	8	13	tr	tr	0.1	17	1
CHILI								
chili w/ beans	1 cup	286	860	0.1	0.3	0.9	–	4
con carne w/ beans	8.9 oz	254	1663	0.1	1.1	2.3	30	2
dried ancho	1 tsp	3	204	0	tr	0.1	1	0
dried casabel	1 tsp	3	90	0.1	–	–	–	1
dried guajillo	1 tsp	3	165	0	tr	0.1	–	1
dried mulato	1 tsp	3	140	0	tr	0.1	–	1
dried pasilla	1 tsp	3	358	0	tr	0.1	2	0
dried smoked chipotle	1 tsp	3	25	0	tr	0.1	–	0
powder	1 tsp	8	908	tr	tr	0.2	–	2
Carroll Shelby's								
Original Texas Chili Kit	2 tbsp	60	1500	–	–	–	–	0
Del Monte								
Sauce	1 tbsp (0.6 oz)	20	500	–	–	–	–	1
Healthy Choice								
Bowls Chili & Cornbread	1 meal (9.5 oz)	350	750	–	–	–	–	4
Instant India								
Chili Ginger Paste	2 tbsp (1 oz)	90	0	–	–	–	–	0
Lean Cuisine								
Everyday Favorites Three Bean Chili w/ Rice	1 pkg (10 oz)	250	1000	–	–	–	–	18
Marie Callender's								
Chili & Cornbread	1 meal (16 oz)	560	500	–	–	–	–	0

FOOD	PORTION	CALS	VIT A	THIA	RIBO	NIACIN	FOLIC	VIT C
Nature's Entree								
Texas Chili	1 pkg (12 oz)	320	3000	–	–	–	–	2
Wick Fowler's								
2 Alarm Chili Kit	3 tbsp	60	5000	–	–	–	–	0
False Alarm Chili Kit	2 tbsp	50	4500	–	–	–	–	0
Wolf Brand								
Plain	7.5 oz	330	3500	3.5	0.7	4	–	5
Yves								
Veggie Chili	1 pkg (10.5 oz)	230	1600	–	–	–	–	30

CHINESE PRESERVING MELON

FOOD	PORTION	CALS	VIT A	THIA	RIBO	NIACIN	FOLIC	VIT C
cooked	½ cup	11	0	tr	tr	0.3	–	9

CHIPS

FOOD	PORTION	CALS	VIT A	THIA	RIBO	NIACIN	FOLIC	VIT C
barbecue	1 oz	139	62	0.1	0.1	1.3	24	10
barbecue	1 bag (7 oz)	971	430	0.4	0.4	9.3	164	67
corn	1 oz	153	27	tr	tr	0.3	6	0
corn	1 bag (7 oz)	1067	186	0.1	0.3	2.3	40	0
corn barbecue	1 oz	148	173	tr	0.1	0.5	–	1
corn barbecue	1 bag (7 oz)	1036	1210	0.1	0.4	3.3	–	3
potato	1 bag (8 oz)	1217	0	0.4	0.4	8.7	103	71
potato	1 oz	152	0	tr	0.1	1.1	13	9
potato sour cream & onion	1 oz	150	48	0.1	0.1	1.1	18	11
potato sour cream & onion	1 bag (7 oz)	1051	336	0.4	0.4	8	122	74
potato sticks	1 oz	148	0	tr	tr	1.4	11	13
potato sticks	½ cup (0.6 oz)	94	0	tr	tr	0.9	7	9
potato sticks	1 pkg (1 oz)	148	0	tr	tr	1.4	11	13
taro	1 oz	141	0	tr	tr	0.1	–	1
taro	10 (0.8 oz)	115	0	tr	tr	0.1	–	1
tortilla	1 bag (7.5 oz)	1067	418	0.2	0.4	2.7	–	0
tortilla	1 oz	142	56	tr	0.1	0.4	–	0
tortilla nacho	1 oz	141	105	tr	0.1	0.4	4	1
tortilla nacho	1 bag (8 oz)	1131	841	0.3	0.4	3.2	32	4
tortilla nacho light	1 oz	126	108	0.1	0.1	0.1	–	tr
tortilla nacho light	1 bag (6 oz)	757	646	0.4	0.5	0.7	–	tr

FOOD	PORTION	CALS	VIT A	THIA	RIBO	NIACIN	FOLIC	VIT C
tortilla ranch	1 oz	139	73	tr	0.1	0.4	—	tr
tortilla ranch	1 bag (7 oz)	969	507	0.2	0.5	2.9	—	2
Cape Cod								
Potato Golden Russet	1 pkg (0.5 oz)	70	0	—	—	—	—	6
Eden								
Brown Rice Chips	1 oz	150	0	—	—	—	—	0
Sea Vegetable Chips	1 oz	140	0	—	—	—	—	0
GeniSoy								
Soy Crisps	1 oz	110	0	—	—	—	—	0
Soy Crisps Apple Cinnamon Crunch	1 oz	120	100	—	—	—	—	1
Soy Crisps Creamy Ranch	1 oz	110	100	—	—	—	—	1
Soy Crisps Deep Sea Salt	1 oz	110	0	—	—	—	—	0
Soy Crisps Rich Cheddar Cheese	1 oz	110	100	—	—	—	—	0
Soy Crisps Roasted Garlic & Onion	1 oz	100	100	—	—	—	—	1
Soy Crisps Zesty Barbeque	1 oz	110	100	—	—	—	—	1
Husman's								
Deli Style Tortilla	11 chips	150	0	—	—	—	—	0
Potato	18 (1 oz)	160	0	—	—	—	—	9
Potato Sour Cream & Onion	18 (1 oz)	150	0	—	—	—	—	5
Potato Sweet N'Sassy	18 (1 oz)	155	100	—	—	—	—	9
Old Dutch Foods								
Potato	12–15 chips (1 oz)	150	0	0.1	0	1.6	—	9
Potato BBQ	12–15 chips (1 oz)	150	0	tr	0	1.2	—	5
Potato BBQ Ripple	12–15 chips (1 oz)	150	200	tr	0	1.6	—	6
Potato Cajun Ripple	12–15 chips (1 oz)	150	0	tr	tr	—	—	18

FOOD	PORTION	CALS	VIT A	THIA	RIBO	NIACIN	FOLIC	VIT C
Potato Cheddar & Sour Cream Ripple	12–15 chips (1 oz)	160	0	tr	0.1	1.2	—	5
Potato Cheddar & Sour Cream Ripples	12–15 chips (1 oz)	150	0	tr	tr	1.6	—	5
Potato Dill	12–15 chips (1 oz)	140	0	0.1	tr	2	—	9
Potato Dutch Crunch	15–20 chips (1 oz)	130	0	tr	0	1.2	0	6
Potato French Onion Ripple	12–15 chips (1 oz)	150	0	tr	tr	1.6	—	2
Potato Jalapeno & Cheddar Dutch Crunch	15–20 chips (1 oz)	130	0	tr	0	3	16	4
Potato Jalapeno Cheese	12–15 chips (1 oz)	150	0	tr	0.1	1.2	—	6
Potato Mesquite BBQ Dutch Crunch	15–20 chips (1 oz)	130	0	tr	0	1.2	—	5
Potato Onion & Garlic	12–15 chips (1 oz)	140	0	0.1	0	1.6	—	12
Potato Outback Spicy BBQ	12–15 chips (1 oz)	150	0	—	—	—	—	21
Potato Ripples	12–15 chips (1 oz)	150	0	0	0	2	—	4
Potato Salt & Vinegar Dutch Crunch	15–20 chips (1 oz)	130	0	tr	0	1.2	0	5
Potato Sour Cream & Onion	12–15 chips (1 oz)	150	0	0.1	0.1	1.2	—	9
Tortilla Bite Size White Corn	20 chips (1 oz)	150	0	—	—	—	—	0
Tortilla Nacho Cheese	15 chips (1 oz)	150	0	—	—	—	—	0
Tortilla Restaurant Style White	9 chips (1 oz)	140	0	tr	0	0.4	—	0
Tostados White Corn	11 chips (1 oz)	140	0	tr	0	0.4	—	0

FOOD	PORTION	CALS	VIT A	THIA	RIBO	NIACIN	FOLIC	VIT C
Tostados Yellow	11 chips (1 oz)	140	0	0	0	0.4	—	0
Pita-Snax								
Cheddar Cheese	34 (1 oz)	110	0	—	—	—	—	0
Chili & Lime	34 (1 oz)	120	200	—	—	—	—	0
Cinnamon	34 (1 oz)	120	0	—	—	—	—	0
Dill Ranch	34 (1 oz)	120	0	—	—	—	—	0
Garlic	34 (1 oz)	120	200	—	—	—	—	0
Lightly Salted	34 (1 oz)	110	0	—	—	—	—	0
Pringles								
Salt & Vinegar	14 chips (1 oz)	160	100	—	—	—	—	4
Skinny								
BBQ	1½ cups	90	100	—	—	—	—	0
Corn	1½ cups	90	200	—	—	—	—	0
Nacho Cheese	1½ cups	90	200	—	—	—	—	0
Sour Cream & Onion	1½ cups	90	200	—	—	—	—	0
Sticks Garden Veggie	1 oz	140	0	—	—	—	—	4
Sticks Island Lime Chili	1 oz	140	0	—	—	—	—	4
Sticks Maui Wowie	1 oz	140	0	—	—	—	—	4
Sticks Original Spud	1 oz	140	0	—	—	—	—	4
Torengos								
Chips	13 chips (1 oz)	140	0	—	—	—	—	0

CHITTERLINGS

FOOD	PORTION	CALS	VIT A	THIA	RIBO	NIACIN	FOLIC	VIT C
pork cooked	3 oz	258	0	0	0.1	0.1	3	0

CHIVES

FOOD	PORTION	CALS	VIT A	THIA	RIBO	NIACIN	FOLIC	VIT C
freeze-dried	1 tbsp	1	137	tr	tr	tr	—	1
fresh chopped	1 tbsp	1	131	tr	tr	tr	3	2
fresh chopped	1 tsp	0	44	tr	tr	tr	1	1

CHOCOLATE

FOOD	PORTION	CALS	VIT A	THIA	RIBO	NIACIN	FOLIC	VIT C
baking	1 oz	145	10	tr	tr	0.4	—	0
grated unsweetened	1 cup (4.6 oz)	690	129	0.1	0.2	1.5	9	0
milk chocolate	1 cup (6 oz)	862	312	0.1	0.5	0.5	14	1

FOOD	PORTION	CALS	VIT A	THIA	RIBO	NIACIN	FOLIC	VIT C
powder	2–3 heaping tsp	75	4	tr	tr	0.1	–	tr
powder as prep w/ whole milk	9 oz	226	312	0.1	0.4	0.3	12	3
semisweet	60 pieces (1 oz)	136	6	tr	tr	0.1	1	0
semisweet	1 cup (6 oz)	804	35	0.1	0.2	0.7	4	0
squares unsweetened	1 square (1 oz)	148	28	tr	tr	0.3	2	0
Cloud Nine								
Double Dark Chocolate	13 pieces (0.5 oz)	80	0	–	–	–	–	0
Sunspire								
Chocolate Sundrops	47 pieces (1.4 oz)	190	100	–	–	–	–	0
Dark Chocolate Grain Sweetened	13 pieces (0.5 oz)	70	0	–	–	–	–	0
Organic	13 pieces (0.5 oz)	70	0	–	–	–	–	0
Tropical Source								
Espresso Roast Dairy Free	13 pieces (1.5 oz)	70	0	–	–	–	–	0
Semi-Sweet Dairy Free	13 pieces (1.5 oz)	80	0	–	–	–	–	0

CHOCOLATE SYRUP

FOOD	PORTION	CALS	VIT A	THIA	RIBO	NIACIN	FOLIC	VIT C
syrup	1 cup	653	89	tr	0.2	1	12	1
syrup	2 tbsp	82	11	tr	tr	0.1	2	tr
syrup as prep w/ whole milk	9 oz	232	319	0.1	0.4	0.3	14	2

CHUTNEY

FOOD	PORTION	CALS	VIT A	THIA	RIBO	NIACIN	FOLIC	VIT C
apple	1.2 oz	68	5	tr	tr	0.1	–	1
mango	1 tbsp	54	207	0.4	2	5	–	0
Wild Thyme Farms								
Apricot Cranberry Walnut	1 tbsp	15	300	–	–	–	–	5
Pineapple Peach Lime	1 tbsp	14	100	–	–	–	–	5

FOOD	PORTION	CALS	VIT A	THIA	RIBO	NIACIN	FOLIC	VIT C
CILANTRO								
fresh	1 tsp (2 g)	tr	98	0	0	tr	1	1
fresh	1 cup (1.6 oz)	11	2820	tr	0.1	0.6	29	1
CINNAMON								
ground	1 tsp	6	6	tr	tr	tr	–	1
sticks	0.5 oz	39	20	0.1	tr	0.2	–	4
CLOVES								
ground	1 tsp	7	11	tr	tr	tr	–	2
COCOA								
hot cocoa	1 cup	218	318	0.1	0.4	0.4	12	2
mix as prep w/ water	7 oz	103	4	tr	0.2	0.2	tr	1
powder unsweetened	1 tbsp (5 g)	11	1	tr	tr	0.1	2	0
powder unsweetened	1 cup (3 oz)	197	17	0.1	0.2	1.9	27	0
AhiLaska								
Organic	2 tbsp	100	0	–	–	–	–	0
COCONUT								
coconut water	1 tbsp	3	0	tr	tr	tr	–	tr
coconut water	1 cup	46	0	0.1	0.1	0.2	–	6
dried sweetened flaked	7 oz pkg	944	0	0.1	tr	0.6	–	0
dried sweetened flaked	1 cup	351	0	tr	tr	0.2	–	0
dried sweetened shredded	7 oz pkg	997	0	0.1	tr	0.9	–	1
dried sweetened shredded	1 cup	466	0	tr	tr	0.4	–	1
dried unsweetened	1 oz	187	0	tr	tr	0.2	3	tr
fresh	1 piece (1.5 oz)	159	0	tr	tr	0.2	12	2
fresh shredded	1 cup	283	0	0.1	tr	0.4	21	3
COD								
atlantic canned	1 can (11 oz)	327	144	0.3	0.1	7.8	–	1
atlantic canned	3 oz	89	39	0.1	0.1	2.1	–	1

FOOD	PORTION	CALS	VIT A	THIA	RIBO	NIACIN	FOLIC	VIT C
atlantic dried	3 oz	246	120	0.2	0.1	6.4	–	3
atlantic fresh cooked	3 oz	89	39	0.1	0.1	2.1	–	1
atlantic fresh cooked	1 fillet (6.3 oz)	189	83	0.2	0.1	4.5	–	2
COFFEE								
brewed	8 oz	2	0	0	0	0.1	0	0
cafe au lait	1 cup (8 fl oz)	77	230	tr	0.2	0.4	6	1
cafe brulot	1 cup (4.8 fl oz)	48	0	0	0	0.3	tr	0
cappuccino	1 cup (8 fl oz)	77	230	tr	0.2	0.4	6	1
coffee con leche	1 cup (8 fl oz)	77	230	tr	0.2	0.4	6	1
decaffeinated	1 rounded tsp	4	0	0	tr	0.5	0	0
decaffeinated as prep	6 oz	4	0	0	tr	0.5	0	0
espresso	1 cup (3 fl oz)	2	0	0	0	0.2	tr	0
irish coffee	1 serv (9 fl oz)	107	206	tr	tr	0.5	1	0
latte w/ skim milk	13 oz	88	750	0.1	0.3	0.5	13	2
latte w/ whole milk	13 oz	152	460	0.1	0.4	0.5	12	2
mocha	1 mug (9.6 fl oz)	202	655	tr	0.1	0.5	2	tr
COFFEE BEVERAGES								
cappuccino mix as prep	7 oz	62	0	tr	tr	0.3	0	0
mocha mix as prep	7 oz	51	0	tr	tr	0.3	0	0
Chock full o'Nuts								
New York Cappuccino French Vanilla	1 pkg (0.9 oz)	90	0	–	–	–	–	0
New York Cappuccino Hazelnut	1 pkg. (0.9 oz)	90	0	–	–	–	–	0

FOOD	PORTION	CALS	VIT A	THIA	RIBO	NIACIN	FOLIC	VIT C
Silk								
Coffee Soylatte	1 bottle (11 oz)	220	400	–	0.5	–	24	0
COFFEE WHITENERS								
liquid nondairy frzn	1 tbsp (0.5 oz)	20	13	0	0	0	0	0
powder nondairy	1 tsp	11	4	0	tr	0	0	0
Silk								
Creamer	1 tbsp	15	0	–	–	–	–	0
Creamer French Vanilla	1 tbsp	20	0	–	–	–	–	0
Creamer Hazelnut	1 tbsp	15	0	–	–	–	–	0
COLESLAW								
coleslaw w/ dressing	½ cup	42	381	tr	tr	0.2	16	20
vinegar & oil coleslaw	3.5 oz	150	500	0.1	tr	1.6	–	30
COLLARDS								
fresh cooked	½ cup	17	1745	tr	tr	0.2	4	8
frzn chopped cooked	½ cup	31	5084	tr	0.1	0.5	65	23
raw chopped	½ cup	6	599	tr	tr	0.1	2	4
Birds Eye								
Chopped Greens frzn	1 cup	30	2250	–	–	–	–	15
COOKIES								
animal crackers	1 box (2.4 oz)	299	27	0.3	0.2	2.5	22	tr
biscotti with nuts chocolate dipped	1 (1.3 oz)	117	100	–	–	–	–	1
black & white	1 lg (3 oz)	302	465	0.2	0.2	1.6	11	tr
butter	1 (5 g)	23	0	tr	tr	0.2	0	0
chocolate chip	1 box (1.9 oz)	233	52	0	0.2	1.2	16	tr
chocolate chip	1 (0.42 oz)	59	7	tr	tr	0.2	–	0
chocolate chip unbaked	1 oz	126	17	0.1	0.1	0.6	–	0

FOOD	PORTION	CALS	VIT A	THIA	RIBO	NIACIN	FOLIC	VIT C
chocolate w/ creme filling	1 (0.35 oz)	47	0	tr	tr	0.2	0	0
cream cheese	1 (1.1 oz)	141	447	0.1	0.1	0.6	4	0
digestive biscuits plain	2	141	0	tr	tr	0.7	–	0
finikia	1 (1.2 oz)	171	312	0.1	0.1	0.9	6	tr
graham	1 squares (0.24 oz)	30	0	tr	tr	0.3	1	0
graham honey	1 (0.24 oz)	30	0	tr	tr	0.3	1	0
hermits	1 (1 oz)	117	178	0.1	0.1	0.6	5	tr
jumbles coconut	1 (1 oz)	121	264	0.1	0.1	0.4	4	tr
koulourakia butter cookie twist	1 (0.9 oz)	113	278	0.1	0.1	0.6	5	0
ladyfingers	1 (0.38 oz)	40	61	tr	tr	0.2	4	tr
macaroons	1 (0.8 oz)	97	0	tr	tr	tr	1	0
madeleines	1 (0.8 oz)	86	258	tr	0.1	0.3	5	tr
neapolitan tri-color cookie	1 (0.6 oz)	79	154	tr	tr	0.2	4	tr
peanut butter	1 (0.4 oz)	60	6	tr	tr	0.5	–	0
peanut butter dough	1 oz	130	13	0.1	0.1	1.2	–	0
peanut butter soft-type	1 (0.5 oz)	69	0	tr	tr	0.3	1	0
pinenut cookies	1 (1.1 oz)	134	0	0.1	0.1	0.6	7	tr
reginette queen'a biscuit	1 (0.8 oz)	86	129	0.1	0.1	0.8	8	tr
spritz	1 (0.4 oz)	42	66	tr	tr	0.3	2	tr
sugar	1 (0.42 oz)	58	4	tr	tr	0.3	–	0
sugar dough	1 oz	124	10	0.1	tr	0.7	–	0
sugar wafers w/ creme filling sugar free sodium free	1 (0.14 oz)	20	0	tr	tr	0.1	0	0
toll house original	1 (0.8 oz)	105	162	tr	tr	0.3	4	tr
vanilla sandwich	1 (0.35 oz)	48	0	tr	tr	0.3	0	0
zeppole	1 (0.8 oz)	78	8	tr	tr	0.2	3	0
Arnott's								
Raspberry Tartlets	2	100	0	–	–	–	–	0
Cookie Lover's								
Chocolate Chip	1 (0.8 oz)	90	100	–	–	–	–	0

FOOD	PORTION	CALS	VIT A	THIA	RIBO	NIACIN	FOLIC	VIT C
Creme Supremes	2 (0.9 oz)	120	0	–	–	–	–	0
Creme Supremes Mint	2 (0.9 oz)	120	0	–	–	–	–	0
Grahams	2 (1 oz)	100	0	–	–	–	–	0
Grahams Cinnamon	2 (1 oz)	110	0	–	–	–	–	0
Peanut Butter	1 (0.8 oz)	100	100	–	–	–	–	0
Shortbread	1 (0.8 oz)	120	200	–	–	–	–	0
Godiva								
Biscotti Dipped In Milk Chocolate	1 (0.9 oz)	120	100	–	–	–	–	0
Golden Grahams Treats								
Chocolate Chunk	1 bar (0.8 oz)	90	300	0.2	0.2	2	40	6
Honey Graham	1 bar (0.8 oz)	90	300	0.2	0.2	2	40	6
King Size Chocolate Chunk	1 bar (1.6 oz)	190	750	0.4	0.4	5	100	15
King Size Honey Graham	1 bar (1.6 oz)	180	750	0.4	0.4	5	100	15
GoldnBrown								
Fat Free	1 (1.1 oz)	120	0	0.1	0.1	0.8	24	0
Hershey								
Cripsy Rice Snacks Peanut Butter	1 (0.6 oz)	70	100	–	–	–	–	1
LU								
Le Bastogne	2 (0.8 oz)	120	0	–	–	–	–	0
M&M's								
Cookies & Milky Way	1 bar (1.2 oz)	180	0	–	–	–	–	0
Nabisco								
Barnum's Animal Crackers	10 (1 oz)	130	0	–	–	–	–	0
Nonni's								
Biscotti Original	1 (1 oz)	100	200	–	–	–	–	0
Otis Spunkmeyer								
Travel Lite Low Fat Apple Cinnamon	1 (1.3 oz)	130	0	0.1	0.1	0.4	16	0
Travel Lite Low Fat Chocolate Chip	1 (1.3 oz)	130	0	0.1	0.1	0.8	16	0

FOOD	PORTION	CALS	VIT A	THIA	RIBO	NIACIN	FOLIC	VIT C
Travel Lite Low Fat Ginger Spice	1 (1.3 oz)	130	0	0.1	0.1	0.4	16	0
Travel Lite Low Fat Oatmeal Rum Raisin	1 (1.3 oz)	130	0	0.1	tr	0.4	16	0
Parmalat								
Grisbi Lemon	1 (0.6 oz)	90	0	—	—	—	—	0
Grisbi Lemon	1 (0.6 oz)	90	0	—	—	—	—	0
Pepperidge Farm								
Chocolate Chunk Minis Nantauket	1 pkg (1.75 oz)	260	100	—	—	—	—	0
Goldfish Grahams Cinnamon	1 pkg (1.75 oz)	240	0	—	—	—	—	0
Spritzers Cool Key Lime	6 (1.1 oz)	140	0	—	—	—	—	0
Spritzers Ripe Red Raspberry	5 (1.1 oz)	140	0	—	—	—	—	0
Spritzers Zesty Lemon	5 (1.1 oz)	140	0	—	—	—	—	0
Reko								
Pizzelle Maple	5 (1 oz)	150	0	—	—	—	—	0
SnackWell's								
Creme Sandwich	2 (0.9 oz)	105	0	—	—	—	—	0
Tree Of Life								
Fat Free Almond Butter	1 (0.8 oz)	60	0	—	—	—	—	0
Fat Free Carrot Cake	1 (0.8 oz)	60	0	—	—	—	—	0
Fat Free Devil's Food Chocolate	1 (0.8 oz)	70	0	—	—	—	—	0
Fat Free Oatmeal Raisin	1 (0.8 oz)	70	0	—	—	—	—	0
Monster Carob Chip	1 (4.7 oz)	700	0	—	—	—	—	0
Monster Granola	1 (4.7 oz)	700	0	—	—	—	—	0
Monster Macaroon	1 (4.7 oz)	750	0	—	—	—	—	0
Monster Peanut Butter	1 (4.7 oz)	700	0	—	—	—	—	0
Monster Fat Free Carrot Cake	1 cookie (3.8 oz)	240	4000	—	tr	—	—	5

FOOD	PORTION	CALS	VIT A	THIA	RIBO	NIACIN	FOLIC	VIT C
Monster Fat Free Devil's Food Chocolate	1 cookie (3.8 oz)	320	0	—	—	—	—	5
Monster Fat Free Gingerbread	1 cookie (3.8 oz)	320	0	—	—	—	—	5
Monster Fat Free Maple Pecan	1 cookie (3.8 oz)	360	0	—	—	—	—	5
Oatmeal	1 (0.8 oz)	100	100	—	—	—	—	0
Sandwich Royal Vanilla	2 (0.9 oz)	120	0	—	—	—	—	0
Wheat Free Carob	1 (0.8 oz)	100	0	—	—	—	—	0
Wheat Free Maple Walnut	1 (0.8 oz)	100	0	—	—	—	—	0
Wheat Free Oatmeal	1 (0.8 oz)	90	0	—	—	—	—	0
Wheat Free Peanut Butter	1 (0.8 oz)	109	0	—	—	—	—	0

CORIANDER

Instant India

FOOD	PORTION	CALS	VIT A	THIA	RIBO	NIACIN	FOLIC	VIT C
Tomato Coriander Paste	2 tbsp (1 oz)	90	0	—	—	—	—	0

CORN

FOOD	PORTION	CALS	VIT A	THIA	RIBO	NIACIN	FOLIC	VIT C
cooked	½ cup	67	204	0.1	0.1	1.1	19	2
cream style	½ cup	93	124	tr	0.1	1.2	57	6
fritters	1 (1 oz)	62	66	0.1	0.1	0.4	3	1
on-the-cob cooked	1 ear (2.2 oz)	59	133	0.1	tr	1	19	3
on-the-cob w/ butter cooked	1 ear	155	391	0.3	0.1	2.2	44	7
scalloped	½ cup	258	620	0.1	0.1	1.3	12	14
w/ red & green peppers	½ cup	86	265	tr	0.1	1.1	—	10
white cooked	½ cup	89	tr	0.2	0.1	1.3	38	5
white raw	½ cup	66	tr	0.2	tr	1.3	35	5
yellow cooked	1 ear (2.7 oz)	83	167	0.2	0.1	1.2	36	5
yellow cooked	½ cup	89	178	0.2	0.1	1.3	38	5
yellow raw	1 ear (3 oz)	77	253	0.2	0.1	1.5	41	6
yellow raw	½ cup	66	216	0.2	tr	1.3	35	5

FOOD	PORTION	CALS	VIT A	THIA	RIBO	NIACIN	FOLIC	VIT C
Birds Eye								
Cob Big Ear	1 ear	120	200	—	—	—	—	2
Cut	⅓ cup	70	200	—	—	—	—	4
Gold & White Blend	½ cup (3.5 oz)	60	1000	—	—	—	—	12
Del Monte								
Cream Style Golden	½ cup (4.4 oz)	90	0	—	—	—	—	2
Cream Style Golden No Salt Added	½ cup (4.4 oz)	60	0	—	—	—	—	2
Cream Style White	½ cup (4.4 oz)	100	0	—	—	—	—	2
Fiesta	½ cup (4.4 oz)	50	200	—	—	—	—	4
Gold & White Supersweet	½ cup (4.4 oz)	80	0	—	—	—	—	4
Whole Kernel Golden	½ cup (4.4 oz)	90	0	—	—	—	—	4
Whole Kernel Golden Supersweet No Salt Added	½ cup (4.4 oz)	60	0	—	—	—	—	4
Whole Kernel Golden Supersweet No Salt Added	½ cup (4.4 oz)	70	0	—	—	—	—	4
Whole Kernel Golden Supersweet No Sugar	½ cup (4.4 oz)	60	0	—	—	—	—	4
Whole Kernel Golden Supersweet Vacuum Packed	½ cup (3.7 oz)	70	0	—	—	—	—	4
Whole Kernel White Sweet	½ cup (4.4 oz)	60	0	—	—	—	—	4
Fresh Like								
Cut	3.5 oz	85	242	0.1	0.1	1.6	—	5
On The Cob	1 ear (3 in)	96	208	0.1	0.1	1.6	—	6

FOOD	PORTION	CALS	VIT A	THIA	RIBO	NIACIN	FOLIC	VIT C
S&W								
Cream Style	½ cup (4.4 oz)	60	0	—	—	—	—	2
Whole Kernel	⅓ cup (3 oz)	70	0	—	—	—	—	2
Tree Of Life								
Corn	⅔ cup (3.2 oz)	80	0	—	—	—	—	2
Veg-All								
Whole Kernel	½ cup	80	0	—	—	—	—	4
CORNMEAL								
hush puppies	1 (0.75 oz)	74	31	0.1	0.1	0.6	4	0
white	1 cup (4.8 oz)	505	0	1	0.6	6.9	258	0
whole grain	1 cup (4.3 oz)	442	572	0.5	0.2	4.4	31	0
yellow	1 cup (4.8 oz)	505	570	1	0.6	6.9	258	0
yellow self-rising	1 cup (4.3 oz)	407	572	0.8	0.5	6.5	228	0
Aunt Jemima								
Yellow	3 tbsp	102	115	0.1	0.1	1	15	0
Hodgson Mill								
Yellow Organic	¼ cup (1 oz)	100	0	—	—	—	—	0
Yellow Self Rising	¼ cup (1 oz)	90	0	0.3	0.2	2.0	—	0
CORNSTARCH								
cornstarch	1 cup (4.5 oz)	488	0	0	0	0	0	0
COTTAGE CHEESE								
creamed	4 oz	117	184	tr	0.2	0.1	14	tr
creamed	1 cup (7.4 oz)	217	342	tr	0.3	0.3	26	tr
creamed w/ fruit	4 oz	140	139	tr	0.1	0.1	11	tr
dry curd	1 cup (5.1 oz)	123	44	tr	0.2	0.2	21	0
dry curd	4 oz	96	34	tr	0.2	0.2	17	0
lowfat 1%	1 cup (7.9 oz)	164	84	tr	0.4	0.3	28	tr
lowfat 1%	4 oz	82	42	tr	0.2	0.1	14	tr

FOOD	PORTION	CALS	VIT A	THIA	RIBO	NIACIN	FOLIC	VIT C
lowfat 2%	1 cup (7.9 oz)	203	158	0.1	0.4	0.3	30	tr
lowfat 2%	4 oz	101	79	tr	0.2	0.2	15	tr
COUSCOUS								
cooked	1 cup (5.5 oz)	176	0	0.1	tr	0.5	24	0
dry	1 cup (6.1 oz)	650	0	0.3	0.1	6	35	0
COWPEAS								
catjang dried cooked	1 cup (2.9 oz)	200	17	0.3	0.1	1.2	242	1
common canned	1 cup	184	32	0.2	0.2	0.9	123	7
frozen cooked	½ cup	112	64	0.2	0.1	0.6	120	2
leafy tips chopped cooked	1 cup	12	305	0.1	0.1	0.5	—	10
leafy tips raw chopped	1 cup	10	256	0.1	0.1	0.4	—	13
CRAB								
baked	1 (3.8 oz)	160	78	0.3	0.2	4.5	20	3
cake	1 (2 oz)	160	313	0.1	0.1	1.2	10	tr
soft-shell fried	1 (4.4 oz)	334	15	0.1	0	1.8	20	tr
CRACKER CRUMBS								
cracker meal	1 cup (4 oz)	440	0	0.8	0.5	6.6	—	0
graham cracker crumbs	½ cup (4.4 oz)	540	0	0.3	0.4	5.2	18	0
Kellogg's								
Corn Flake Crumbs	2 tbsp (0.4 oz)	40	0	0.2	0.2	1.8	10	0
CRACKERS								
cheese	14 (½ oz)	71	23	0.1	0.1	0.7	4	0
cheese	1 (1 in sq) (1 g)	5	2	tr	tr	tr	0	0
crispbread	3	61	0	tr	tr	0.5	—	0
crispbread rye	1 (0.35 oz)	37	0	tr	tr	0.1	2	0
crispbread rye	3	77	0	0.1	tr	0.7	—	0
melba toast plain	1 (5 g)	19	0	tr	tr	0.2	1	0

FOOD	PORTION	CALS	VIT A	THIA	RIBO	NIACIN	FOLIC	VIT C
melba toast wheat	1 (5 g)	19	0	tr	tr	0.3	1	0
oyster cracker	1 (1 g)	4	0	tr	tr	0.1	tr	0
saltines	1 (3 g)	13	0	tr	tr	0.1	1	0
snack cracker	1 (3 g)	15	0	tr	tr	0.1	0	0
soup cracker	1 (1 g)	4	0	tr	tr	0.1	tr	0
water biscuits	3	92	0	tr	tr	0.7	—	0
wheat w/ cheese filling	1 (0.24 oz)	35	5	tr	tr	0.2	—	tr
wheat thins	1 (2 g)	9	0	tr	tr	0.1	0	0
wheat thins	7 (0.5 oz)	67	0	0.1	tr	0.7	3	0
whole wheat	1 (4 g)	18	tr	tr	tr	0.2	1	0
Dare								
Breton Reduced Fat & Sodium	3 (0.5 oz)	60	0	—	—	—	—	0
Eden								
Nori Nori Rice	15 (1 oz)	110	0	0	0	0	0	0
Gold'n Krackle								
Cheese	½ oz	65	0	—	—	—	—	0
Cheese & Oregano	½ oz	65	0	—	—	—	—	0
Hot & Spicy	½ oz	58	0	—	—	—	—	0
Onion & Garlic	½ oz	58	0	—	—	—	—	0
Plain	½ oz	58	0	—	—	—	—	0
Kashi								
TLC Honey Sesame	15 (1 oz)	130	0	—	—	—	—	0
TLC Natural Ranch	15 (1 oz)	130	0	—	—	—	—	0
TLC Original	15 (1 oz)	130	0	—	—	—	—	0
Keebler								
Harvest Bakery Multigrain	2 (0.6 oz)	70	0	—	—	—	—	0
Toasteds Buttercrisp	5 (0.6 oz)	80	0	—	—	—	—	0
Toasteds Sesame	5 (0.6 oz)	80	0	—	—	—	—	0
Toasteds Wheat	5 (0.6 oz)	80	0	—	—	—	—	0
Pepperidge Farm								
Giant Goldfish Peanut Butter Sandwich	1 pkg (1.4 oz)	190	0	tr	tr	—	—	0

FOOD	PORTION	CALS	VIT A	THIA	RIBO	NIACIN	FOLIC	VIT C
RedOval Farms								
Stoned Wheat Thins Cracked Pepper	4 (0.6 oz)	70	0	–	–	–	–	0
Smucker's								
Snackers Grape	1 pkg (3.3 oz)	410	0	–	–	–	–	1
Snackers Strawberry	1 pkg (3.3 oz)	410	0	–	–	–	–	1
Tree Of Life								
Bite Size Fat Free Cracked Pepper	12 (0.5)	55	0	–	–	–	–	0
Bite Size Fat Free Garden Vegetable	12 (0.5 oz)	55	0	–	–	–	–	0
Bite Size Fat Free Garlic & Herb	12 (0.5 oz)	55	0	–	–	–	–	0
Bite Size Fat Free Toasted Onion	12 (0.5 oz)	55	0	–	–	–	–	0
Oyster	40 (0.5 oz)	60	0	–	–	–	–	0
Saltine Cracked Pepper Fat Free	4 (0.5 oz)	60	0	–	–	–	–	0
Wisecrackers								
Low Fat Poblano Chili & Sweet Onion	4 (0.5 oz)	45	0	–	–	–	–	0

CRANBERRIES

FOOD	PORTION	CALS	VIT A	THIA	RIBO	NIACIN	FOLIC	VIT C
cranberry sauce sweetened	½ cup	209	28	tr	tr	0.1	–	3
fresh chopped	1 cup	54	50	tr	tr	0.1	2	15
Wild Thyme Farms								
Cranberry Sauce	1 tbsp	19	50	–	–	–	–	2

CRANBERRY BEANS

FOOD	PORTION	CALS	VIT A	THIA	RIBO	NIACIN	FOLIC	VIT C
canned	1 cup	216	0	0.1	0.1	1.3	201	2
dried cooked	1 cup	240	0	0.4	0.1	0.9	366	0

CRANBERRY JUICE

FOOD	PORTION	CALS	VIT A	THIA	RIBO	NIACIN	FOLIC	VIT C
cranberry juice cocktail	6 oz	108	7	tr	tr	0.1	1	67
cranberry juice cocktail frzn as prep	6 oz	102	18	tr	tr	tr	0	18

FOOD	PORTION	CALS	VIT A	THIA	RIBO	NIACIN	FOLIC	VIT C
Nantucket Nectars								
Big Cran	8 oz	140	0	–	–	–	–	60
CREAM								
clotted cream	2 tbsp (1 oz)	164	985	tr	0.1	–	2	0
creme fraiche	2 tbsp (1 oz)	100	400	–	–	–	–	0
half & half	1 tbsp (0.5 oz)	20	65	tr	tr	tr	tr	tr
half & half	1 cup (8.5 oz)	315	1050	0.1	0.4	0.2	6	2
heavy whipping	1 tbsp (0.5 oz)	52	220	tr	tr	tr	1	tri
heavy whipping whipped	1 cup (4.1 oz)	411	3499	0.1	0.3	0.1	9	1
light coffee	1 cup (8.4 oz)	496	1728	0.1	0.4	0.1	6	2
light coffee	1 tbsp (0.5 oz)	29	108	tr	tr	tr	tr	tr
light whipping	1 tbsp (0.5 oz)	44	169	tr	tr	tr	1	tr
light whipping cream whipped	1 cup (4.2 oz)	345	2694	0.1	0.3	0.1	9	1
CREAM CHEESE								
cream cheese	1 oz	99	405	tr	0.1	tr	4	0
cream cheese	1 pkg (3 oz)	297	1213	tr	0.2	0.1	11	0
Alpine Lace								
Reduced Fat Roasted Garlic & Herbs	1 tsp (1 oz)	60	400	–	–	–	–	0
Reduced Fat Sundried Tomato & Basil	2 tsp (1 oz)	70	500	–	–	–	–	0
Boar's Head								
Cream Cheese	2 tbsp (1 oz)	100	300	–	–	–	–	0
CREAM OF TARTAR								
cream of tartar	1 tsp	8	0	0	0	0	0	0
CROCODILE								
cooked	3 oz	78	15	0.1	0.2	2.6	–	0

FOOD	PORTION	CALS	VIT A	THIA	RIBO	NIACIN	FOLIC	VIT C
CROISSANT								
w/ egg & cheese	1 (4.5 oz)	368	1001	0.2	0.4	1.5	47	tr
w/ egg cheese & bacon	1 (4.5 oz)	413	472	0.3	0.3	2.2	45	2
w/ egg cheese & ham	1 (5.3 oz)	474	451	0.5	0.3	3.2	46	11
w/ egg cheese & sausage	1 (5.6 oz)	523	422	1	0.3	4	43	tr
Sara Lee								
Broccoli & Cheese	1 (3.7 oz)	280	100	–	–	–	–	0
Ham & Swiss	1 (3.7 oz)	300	100	–	–	–	–	1
CROUTONS								
plain	1 cup (1 oz)	122	0	0.2	0.1	1.6	7	0
CUCUMBER								
cucumber salad	3.5 oz	50	750	tr	tr	1.2	–	9
fresh raw	1 (11 oz)	38	647	0.1	0.1	0.7	38	16
fresh raw sliced	½ cup (1.8 oz)	7	112	tr	tr	0.1	7	3
kimchee	½ cup (1.8 oz)	36	158	tr	tr	0.2	6	6
tzatziki	½ cup (3.4 oz)	72	83	tr	0.1	0.2	10	3
CUMIN								
seed	1 tsp	8	27	tr	tr	0.1	–	tr
CURRANT JUICE								
black currant nectar	7 oz	110	tr	tr	tr	tr	tr	60
red currant nectar	7 oz	108	tr	tr	tr	tr	tr	12
CURRANTS								
black fresh	½ cup	36	129	tr	tr	0.2	–	101
zante dried	½ cup	204	52	0.1	0.1	1.2	7	3
CUSTARD								
baked	½ cup (5 oz)	148	313	tr	0.3	0.1	44	1
flan	½ cup (5.4 oz)	220	314	tr	0.3	0.1	–	1
zabaione	½ cup (57.2 g)	135	485	tr	0.1	tr	24	0
DANDELION GREENS								
fresh cooked	½ cup	17	6084	0.1	0.1	–	–	9
raw chopped	½ cup.	13	3920	0.1	0.1	–	–	10

FOOD	PORTION	CALS	VIT A	THIA	RIBO	NIACIN	FOLIC	VIT C
DANISH PASTRY								
almond	1 (4¼ in) (2.3 oz)	280	34	0.1	0.2	1.5	–	1
apple	1 (4¼ in) (2.5 oz)	264	27	0.2	0.2	1.4	12	3
cheese	1 (3.2 oz)	353	155	0.3	0.2	2.5	55	3
cinnamon	1 (3.1 oz)	349	18	0.3	0.2	2.2	55	3
cinnamon nut	1 (4¼ in) (2.3 oz)	280	34	0.1	0.2	1.5	–	1
fruit	1 (3.3 oz)	335	86	0.3	0.2	1.8	31	2
lemon	1 (4¼ in) (2.5 oz)	264	124	0.2	0.2	1.4	12	3
plain ring	1 (12 oz)	1305	360	1	1	8.5	–	tr
raisin	1 (4¼ in) (2.5 oz)	264	27	0.2	0.2	1.4	12	3
raisin nut	1 (4¼ in) (2.3 oz)	280	34	0.1	0.2	1.5	–	1
raspberry	1 (4¼ in) (2.5 oz)	264	142	0.2	0.2	1.4	12	3
strawberry	1 (4¼ in) (2.5 oz)	264	37	0.2	0.2	1.4	12	3
Morton								
Honey Buns	1 (2.28 oz)	270	0	–	–	–	–	0
Honey Buns Mini	1 (1.3 oz)	160	0	–	–	–	–	0
DATES								
dried chopped	1 cup	489	89	0.2	0.2	3.9	22	0
dried whole	10	228	42	0.1	0.1	1.8	10	0
jujube dried	1 oz	75	5	tr	0.1	0.3	–	4
jujube fresh	1 oz	30	tr	tr	tr	0.2	–	17
jujube preserved in sugar	1 oz	91	2	0.4	–	7	tr	tr
California Redi-Date								
Deglet Noor Dried	5–6 (1.4 oz)	120	0	tr	tr	0.4	8	0
DELI MEATS/COLD CUTS								
braunschweiger pork	1 oz	102	3984	0.1	0.4	2.4	–	3
liver cheese pork	1 oz	86	4957	0.1	0.6	3.3	–	1
Boar's Head								
Bologna Beef	2 oz	150	0	–	–	–	–	0

FOOD	PORTION	CALS	VIT A	THIA	RIBO	NIACIN	FOLIC	VIT C
Bologna Pork & Beef	2 oz	150	0	—	—	—	—	0
Braunschweiger Lite	2 oz	120	11000	—	—	—	—	0
Head Cheese	2 oz	90	0	—	—	—	—	0
Liverwurst Strassburger	2 oz	170	11000	—	—	—	—	0
Olive Loaf	2 oz	130	0	—	—	—	—	0
Pastrami	2 oz	90	0	—	—	—	—	0
Prosciutto	1 oz	60	0	—	—	—	—	0
Salami Genoa	2 oz	180	0	—	—	—	—	0
Salami Hard	1 oz	110	0	—	—	—	—	0
Spiced Ham	2 oz	120	0	—	—	—	—	0

DINNER
Banquet

FOOD	PORTION	CALS	VIT A	THIA	RIBO	NIACIN	FOLIC	VIT C
Beef Patty w/ Country Style Vegetables	1 meal (9.5 oz)	310	300	—	—	—	—	1
Boneless Pork Rib	1 meal (10 oz)	400	0	—	—	—	—	2
Boneless White Fried Chicken	1 meal (8.25 oz)	540	0	—	—	—	—	6
Chicken Parmigiana	1 meal (9.5 oz)	320	100	—	—	—	—	30
Chicken Fingers Meal	1 meal (7.1 oz)	740	0	—	—	—	—	0
Chicken Fried Beef Steak	1 pkg (10 oz)	420	100	—	—	—	—	0
Chicken Nuggets Meal	1 meal (6.75 oz)	430	0	—	—	—	—	6
Extra Helping Boneless Pork Riblet	1 meal (15.25 oz)	720	500	—	—	—	—	0
Extra Helping Fried Beef Steak	1 meal (16 oz)	820	0	—	—	—	—	0
Extra Helping Fried Chicken	1 meal (14.7 oz)	910	0	—	—	—	—	1
Extra Helping Meatloaf	1 meal (16 oz)	610	2000	—	—	—	—	6

FOOD	PORTION	CALS	VIT A	THIA	RIBO	NIACIN	FOLIC	VIT C
Extra Helping Salisbury Steak	1 meal (16.5 oz)	740	0	–	–	–	–	0
Extra Helping Turkey & Gravy w/ Dressing	1 meal (17 oz)	620	0	–	–	–	–	0
Extra Helping White Fried Chicken	1 meal (13 oz)	690	0	–	–	–	–	6
Extra Helping Yankee Pot Roast	1 meal (14.5 oz)	410	750	–	–	–	–	1
Family Size Brown Gravy & Salisbury Steak	1 serv	240	0	–	–	–	–	0
Family Size Brown Gravy & Sliced Beef	1 serv	140	0	–	–	–	–	0
Family Size Chicken & Broccoli Alfredo	1 serv	270	0	–	–	–	–	6
Family Size Country Style Chicken & Dumplings	1 serv	290	0	–	–	–	–	0
Family Size Creamy Broccoli Chicken Cheese & Rice	1 serv	280	0	–	–	–	–	0
Family Size Hearty Beef Stew	1 cup	170	500	–	–	–	–	4
Family Size Homestyle Gravy & Sliced Turkey	2 slices	140	0	–	–	–	–	0
Family Size Mushroom Gravy & Charbroiled Beef Patties	1 patty	250	0	–	–	–	–	0
Family Size Potato Ham & Broccoli Au Gratin	⅔ cup	210	200	–	–	–	–	18

FOOD	PORTION	CALS	VIT A	THIA	RIBO	NIACIN	FOLIC	VIT C
Family Size Savory Gravy & Meatloaf	1 slice	120	0	—	—	—	—	0
Fish Sticks	1 meal (6.6 oz)	290	500	—	—	—	—	4
Grilled Chicken	1 meal (9.9 oz)	330	0	—	—	—	—	5
Honey Roast Turkey Breast	1 meal (9 oz)	270	1500	—	—	—	—	0
Meatloaf	1 meal (9.5 oz)	280	200	—	—	—	—	0
Our Original Fried Chicken	1 meal (9 oz)	470	0	—	—	—	—	1
Pork Cutlet Meal	1 meal (10.25 oz)	420	100	—	—	—	—	0
Salisbury Steak	1 meal (9.5 oz)	380	0	—	—	—	—	0
Sliced Beef	1 meal (9 oz)	270	100	—	—	—	—	1
Turkey	1 meal (9.25 oz)	270	0	—	—	—	—	0
Veal Parmagiana	1 meal (8.75 oz)	330	100	—	—	—	—	42
Western Style Beef Patty	1 meal (9.5 oz)	360	0	—	—	—	—	0
White Meat Fried Chicken	1 meal (8.75 oz)	460	0	—	—	—	—	2
Yankee Pot Roast	1 meal (9.4 oz)	230	750	—	—	—	—	4
Birds Eye								
Easy Recipe Creations Sweet & Sour w/ Pineapple Tidbits	1⅓ cups	200	2000	—	—	—	—	30
Voila! Zesty Garlic Chicken	2 cups (6.2 oz)	260	1250	—	—	—	—	12
Voila! Beef Sirloin Steak And Garlic Potatoes	1 cup	240	2250	—	—	—	—	4
Voila! Chicken Alfredo	1 cup	230	300	—	—	—	—	21

FOOD	PORTION	CALS	VIT A	THIA	RIBO	NIACIN	FOLIC	VIT C
Voila! Garden Herb Chicken	1 cup	310	1500	—	—	—	—	4
Voila! Grilled Salsa Chicken w/ Rice	1 cup	240	300	—	—	—	—	9
Voila! Homestyle Turkey w/ Roasted Potatoes	1 cup	200	1250	—	—	—	—	9
Voila! Teriyaki	2 cups (6.4 oz)	240	1250	—	—	—	—	18
Healthy Choice								
Beef Pepper Steak Oriental	1 meal (9.5 oz)	260	200	—	—	—	—	9
Beef Pot Roast	1 meal (11 oz)	300	1250	—	—	—	—	18
Beef Stroganoff	1 meal (11 oz)	320	200	—	—	—	—	12
Beef Tips Francais	1 meal (9.5 oz)	300	0	—	—	—	—	0
Beef Tips Portabello	1 meal (11.25 oz)	270	500	—	—	—	—	12
Bowls Chicken Teriyaki w/ Rice	1 meal (9.5 oz)	270	2000	—	—	—	—	12
Bowls Country Chicken Bake	1 meal (9.5 oz)	230	1000	—	—	—	—	2
Bowls Fiesta Chicken	1 meal (9.5 oz)	220	100	—	—	—	—	0
Bowls Garlic Lemon Chicken w/ Rice	1 meal (9.5 oz)	300	2000	—	—	—	—	15
Bowls Roasted Potatoes w/ Ham	1 meal (8.5 oz)	210	100	—	—	—	—	24
Bowls Southwestern Chicken & Pasta	1 meal (9.5 oz)	320	400	—	—	—	—	24
Bowls Turkey Divan	1 meal (9.5 oz)	250	300	—	—	—	—	9
Charbroiled Beef Patty	1 meal (11 oz)	310	1000	—	—	—	—	0
Chicken Cantonese	1 meal (10.75)	280	3000	—	—	—	—	6

FOOD	PORTION	CALS	VIT A	THIA	RIBO	NIACIN	FOLIC	VIT C
Chicken Parmigiana	1 meal (11.5 oz)	330	3000	—	—	—	—	9
Chicken & Vegetables Marsala	1 meal (11.5 oz)	240	500	—	—	—	—	4
Chicken Broccoli Alfredo	1 meal (11.5 oz)	300	100	—	—	—	—	12
Chicken Dijon	1 meal (11 oz)	270	4500	—	—	—	—	18
Chicken Teriyaki	1 meal (11 oz)	270	1000	—	—	—	—	12
Country Breaded Chicken	1 meal (10.25 oz)	350	500	—	—	—	—	0
Country Glazed Chicken Breast	1 meal (8.5 oz)	250	0	—	—	—	—	0
Country Herb Chicken	1 meal (12.15 oz)	320	1250	—	—	—	—	0
Country Inn Roast Turkey	1 meal (10 oz)	250	500	—	—	—	—	0
Garlic Chicken Milano	1 meal (9.5 oz)	260	500	—	—	—	—	18
Grilled Chicken Sonoma	1 meal (9 oz)	230	1000	—	—	—	—	12
Grilled Chicken w/ Mashed Potatoes	1 meal (8 oz)	180	200	—	—	—	—	1
Herb Baked Fish	1 meal (10.9 oz)	340	3000	—	—	—	—	0
Herb Breaded Pork Patty	1 meal (8 oz)	280	500	—	—	—	—	5
Homestyle Chicken & Pasta	1 meal (9 oz)	270	1500	—	—	—	—	4
Honey Glazed Chicken	1 meal (10 oz)	270	1000	—	—	—	—	6
Honey Mustard Chicken	1 meal (9.5 oz)	290	1000	—	—	—	—	0
Lemon Pepper Fish	1 meal (10.7 oz)	320	500	—	—	—	—	30
Mandarin Chicken	1 meal (10 oz)	280	1500	—	—	—	—	15

FOOD	PORTION	CALS	VIT A	THIA	RIBO	NIACIN	FOLIC	VIT C
Mesquite Beef w/ Barbecue Sauce	1 meal (11 oz)	320	1250	—	—	—	—	9
Mesquite Chicken Barbecue	1 meal (10.5 oz)	310	1250	—	—	—	—	9
Oriental Style Chicken & Vegetable Stir Fry	1 meal (11.9)	360	1250	—	—	—	—	5
Oven Roasted Beef	1 meal (10.15 oz)	280	0	—	—	—	—	12
Roast Turkey Breast	1 meal (8.5 oz)	220	2250	—	—	—	—	1
Roasted Chicken	1 meal (11 oz)	230	2500	—	—	—	—	4
Sesame Chicken	1 meal (10.8 oz)	360	3000	—	—	—	—	6
Shrimp & Vegetables	1 meal (11.8 oz)	270	1000	—	—	—	—	30
Sweet & Sour Chicken	1 meal (11 oz)	360	2000	—	—	—	—	15
Traditional Meatloaf	1 meal (12 oz)	330	750	—	—	—	—	42
Tradtional Breast Of Turkey	1 meal (10.5 oz)	290	400	—	—	—	—	36
Tradtional Salisbury Steak	1 meal (11.5 oz)	330	1000	—	—	—	—	12
Tuna Casserole	1 meal (8 oz)	240	0	—	—	—	—	0
Kid Cuisine								
Circus Show Corn Dog	1 meal (8.8 oz)	490	0	—	—	—	—	12
Cosmic Chicken Nuggets	1 meal (9.1 oz)	500	0	—	—	—	—	0
Futuristic Fish Sticks	1 meal (8.25 oz)	410	0	—	—	—	—	0
Game Time Taco Roll Up	1 meal (7.35 oz)	420	0	—	—	—	—	0
High Flying Fried Chicken	1 meal (10.1 oz)	440	0	—	—	—	—	0

FOOD	PORTION	CALS	VIT A	THIA	RIBO	NIACIN	FOLIC	VIT C
Parachuting Pork Ribettes	1 meal (7.55 oz)	390	0	—	—	—	—	0
Lean Cuisine								
Cafe Classics Baked Chicken	1 pkg (8.6 oz)	240	300	—	—	—	—	0
Cafe Classics Baked Fish	1 pkg (9 oz)	290	0	—	—	—	—	9
Cafe Classics Beef Peppercorn	1 pkg (8.75 oz)	260	200	—	—	—	—	5
Cafe Classics Beef Portobello	1 pkg (9 oz)	220	0	—	—	—	—	0
Cafe Classics Beef Pot Roast	1 pkg (9 oz)	210	1000	—	—	—	—	2
Cafe Classics Chicken Carbonara	1 pkg (9 oz)	280	400	—	—	—	—	12
Cafe Classics Chicken Medallions w/ Creamy Cheese Sauce	1 pkg (9.37 oz)	300	1500	—	—	—	—	12
Cafe Classics Chicken Mediterranean	1 pkg (10.5 oz)	260	500	—	—	—	—	5
Cafe Classics Chicken & Vegetables	1 pkg (10.5 oz)	240	1500	—	—	—	—	4
Cafe Classics Chicken In Peanut Sauce	1 pkg (9 oz)	260	500	—	—	—	—	6
Cafe Classics Chicken In Wine Sauce	1 pkg (8.1 oz)	220	1250	—	—	—	—	1
Cafe Classics Chicken L'Orange	1 pkg (9 oz)	230	2250	—	—	—	—	9
Cafe Classics Chicken Parmesan	1 pkg (10.9 oz)	300	500	—	—	—	—	9
Cafe Classics Chicken Piccata	1 pkg (9 oz)	300	300	—	—	—	—	12

FOOD	PORTION	CALS	VIT A	THIA	RIBO	NIACIN	FOLIC	VIT C
Cafe Classics Chicken w/ Basil Cream Sauce	1 pkg (8.5 oz)	260	500	—	—	—	—	5
Cafe Classics Country Vegetables & Beef	1 pkg (9 oz)	210	1000	—	—	—	—	6
Cafe Classics Fiesta Chicken	1 pkg (9.25 oz)	270	400	—	—	—	—	24
Cafe Classics Glazed Chicken	1 pkg (8.5 oz)	240	100	—	—	—	—	4
Cafe Classics Glazed Turkey Tenderloins	1 pkg (9 oz)	260	4500	—	—	—	—	0
Cafe Classics Grilled Chicken	1 pkg (9.4 oz)	250	300	—	—	—	—	18
Cafe Classics Herb Roasted Chicken	1 pkg (8 oz)	190	400	—	—	—	—	27
Cafe Classics Honey Mustard Chicken	1 pkg (8 oz)	270	750	—	—	—	—	6
Cafe Classics Honey Roasted Chicken	1 pkg (8.5 oz)	270	500	—	—	—	—	9
Cafe Classics Honey Roasted Pork	1 serv (9.5 oz)	250	500	—	—	—	—	15
Cafe Classics Meatloaf w/ Whipped Potatoes	1 pkg (9.4 oz)	260	100	—	—	—	—	0
Cafe Classics Oriental Beef	1 pkg (9.25 oz)	210	1000	—	—	—	—	4
Cafe Classics Oven Roasted Beef	1 pkg (9.25 oz)	260	300	—	—	—	—	15
Cafe Classics Roasted Turkey Breast	1 pkg (9.75 oz)	270	0	—	—	—	—	54

FOOD	PORTION	CALS	VIT A	THIA	RIBO	NIACIN	FOLIC	VIT C
Cafe Classics Salisbury Steak	1 pkg (9.5 oz)	280	200	–	–	–	–	0
Cafe Classics Southern Beef Tips	1 pkg (8.75 oz)	270	200	–	–	–	–	4
Everday Favorites Vegetable Lasagna	1 pkg (10.5 oz)	260	2500	–	–	–	–	9
Everyday Favorites Chicken Florentine	1 pkg (8 oz)	220	2500	–	–	–	–	0
Everyday Favorites Chicken Chow Mein	1 pkg (9 oz)	240	1000	–	–	–	–	0
Everyday Favorites Homestyle Turkey	1 pkg (9.4 oz)	240	2250	–	–	–	–	1
Everyday Favorites Hunan Beef & Broccoli	1 pkg (8.5 oz)	240	100	–	–	–	–	6
Everyday Favorites Mandarin Chicken	1 pkg (9 oz)	260	2500	–	–	–	–	18
Everyday Favorites Roasted Chicken	1 pkg (8.1 oz)	260	2250	–	–	–	–	1
Everyday Favorites Stuffed Cabbage	1 pkg (9.5 oz)	210	100	–	–	–	–	4
Everyday Favorites Swedish Meatballs	1 pkg (9.1 oz)	290	0	–	–	–	–	0
Hearty Portions Cheese & Spinach Manicotti	1 serv	370	4500	–	–	–	–	48
Hearty Portions Chicken & Barbecue Sauce	1 serv	370	500	–	–	–	–	12
Hearty Portions Homestyle Beef Stroganoff	1 serv	350	2500	–	–	–	–	12

FOOD	PORTION	CALS	VIT A	THIA	RIBO	NIACIN	FOLIC	VIT C
Hearty Portions Jumbo Rigatoni w/ Meatballs	1 serv	440	1000	—	—	—	—	24
Hearty Portions Oriental Glazed Chicken	1 serv	370	2250	—	—	—	—	27
Hearty Portions Roasted Chicken w/ Mushrooms	1 serv	330	1000	—	—	—	—	48
Skillet Sensations Beef Teriyaki & Rice	1 serv	280	2000	—	—	—	—	18
Skillet Sensations Chicken Primavera	1 serv	320	4500	—	—	—	—	51
Skillet Sensations Chicken Oriental	1 serv	280	4500	—	—	—	—	24
Skillet Sensations Fiesta Beef & Rice	1 serv	300	500	—	—	—	—	30
Skillet Sensations Garlic Chicken	1 serv	340	1000	—	—	—	—	54
Skillet Sensations Herb Chicken & Roasted Potatoes	1 serv	270	3250	—	—	—	—	18
Skillet Sensations Roasted Turkey	1 serv	220	4500	—	—	—	—	60
Skillet Sensations Savory Beef & Vegetables	1 serv	290	5000	—	—	—	—	9
Skillet Sensations Three Cheese Chicken	1 serv	370	3500	—	—	—	—	3
Luzianne								
Cajun Creole Dirty Rice	1 serv	160	300	—	—	—	—	0
Cajun Creole Etouffee	1 serv	200	400	—	—	—	—	2
Cajun Creole Gumbo	1 serv	160	200	—	—	—	—	2

FOOD	PORTION	CALS	VIT A	THIA	RIBO	NIACIN	FOLIC	VIT C
Cajun Creole Jambalaya	1 serv	200	1000	–	–	–	–	2
Marie Callender's								
Beef Stroganoff w/ Noodles	1 meal (13 oz)	600	200	–	–	–	–	0
Beef Tips In Mushroom Sauce	1 meal (13 oz)	430	300	–	–	–	–	9
Breaded Chicken Parmigiana	1 meal (16 oz)	860	1000	–	–	–	–	4
Breaded Fish w/ Mac & Cheese	1 meal (12 oz)	550	1500	–	–	–	–	24
Cheesy Rice w/ Chicken & Broccoli	1 meal (12 oz)	390	500	–	–	–	–	30
Chicken & Dumplings	1 meal (14 oz)	390	2500	–	–	–	–	5
Chicken & Noodles	1 meal (13 oz)	520	4000	–	–	–	–	9
Chicken Cordon Bleu	1 meal (13 oz)	610	2250	–	–	–	–	18
Chicken Fried Beef Steak & Gravy	1 meal (15 oz)	650	750	–	–	–	–	24
Chicken Teriyaki	1 meal (13 oz)	510	3500	–	–	–	–	42
Country Fried Chicken & Gravy	1 meal (16 oz)	620	0	–	–	–	–	4
Country Fried Pork Chop	1 meal (15 oz)	540	5000	–	–	–	–	6
Escalloped Noodles & Chicken	1 meal (13 oz)	740	750	–	–	–	–	0
Glazed Chicken	1 meal (13 oz)	490	2250	–	–	–	–	2
Grilled Southwestern Style Chicken	1 meal (14 oz)	410	0	–	–	–	–	4
Grilled Chicken & Mashed Potatoes	1 meal (10 oz)	340	0	–	–	–	–	0

FOOD	PORTION	CALS	VIT A	THIA	RIBO	NIACIN	FOLIC	VIT C
Grilled Chicken Breast & Rice Pilaf	1 meal (11.75 oz)	360	2250	–	–	–	–	1
Grilled Chicken In Mushroom Sauce	1 meal (14 oz)	480	500	–	–	–	–	54
Grilled Turkey Breast & Rice Pilaf	1 meal (11.75 oz)	310	750	–	–	–	–	0
Herb Roasted Chicken & Mashed Potatoes	1 meal (14 oz)	580	750	–	–	–	–	36
Homestyle Turkey & Noodles	1 meal (12 oz)	600	100	–	–	–	–	0
Honey Roasted Chicken	1 meal (14 oz)	440	0	–	–	–	–	12
Honey Smoked Ham Steak w/ Macroni & Cheese	1 meal (14 oz)	490	2000	–	–	–	–	12
Meatloaf & Gravy w/ Mashed Potatoes	1 meal (14 oz)	540	1250	–	–	–	–	0
Old Fashioned Beef Pot Roast & Gravy	1 meal (15 oz)	500	3500	–	–	–	–	0
Roast Beef	1 meal (14.5 oz)	390	0	–	–	–	–	12
Sirloin Salisbury Steak & Gravy	1 meal (14 oz)	550	400	–	–	–	–	4
Skillet Meal Au Gratin Potatoes	⅔ cup (5 oz)	190	0	–	–	–	–	4
Skillet Meal Beef Pot Roast	½ pkg	290	3000	–	–	–	–	0
Skillet Meal Beef Stroganoff	½ pkg	310	3000	–	–	–	–	0
Skillet Meal Chicken & Rice w/ Broccoli & Cheese	½ pkg	440	1000	–	–	–	–	18

FOOD	PORTION	CALS	VIT A	THIA	RIBO	NIACIN	FOLIC	VIT C
Skillet Meal Chicken Teriyaki	½ pkg	340	2000	—	—	—	—	12
Skillet Meal Herb Chicken	½ pkg	290	1250	—	—	—	—	12
Skillet Meal Roasted Chicken & Vegetables	½ pkg	260	2250	—	—	—	—	12
Skillet Meal White & Wild Rice In Cheese Sauce	1 cup	300	0	—	—	—	—	12
Swedish Meatballs	1 meal (12.5 oz)	520	100	—	—	—	—	0
Sweet & Sour Chicken	1 meal (14 oz)	570	2500	—	—	—	—	0
Turkey w/ Gravy & Dressing	1 meal (14 oz)	500	400	—	—	—	—	24
Morton								
Breaded Chicken Pattie	1 meal (6.75 oz)	290	3000	—	—	—	—	0
Chicken Nuggets	1 meal (7 oz)	340	2000	—	—	—	—	2
Chili Gravy w/ Beef Enchilada & Tamale	1 meal (10 oz)	270	500	—	—	—	—	6
Fried Chicken	1 meal (9 oz)	470	2250	—	—	—	—	6
Veal Parmagiana w/ Tomato Sauce	1 meal (8.75 oz)	290	2250	—	—	—	—	18
Nature's Choice								
Broccoli Parmesan Alfredo	1 pkg (12 oz)	270	1250	—	—	—	—	36
Nature's Entree								
Tuscany White Bean	1 pkg (12 oz)	330	6000	—	—	—	—	9
Patio								
Ranchera	1 pkg (13 oz)	470	500	—	—	—	—	1

FOOD	PORTION	CALS	VIT A	THIA	RIBO	NIACIN	FOLIC	VIT C
Swanson								
Chicken Parmigiana w/ Spaghetti	1 pkg (11 oz)	380	6500	–	–	–	–	24
Weight Watchers								
Smart Ones Swedish Meatballs	1 pkg (9 oz)	280	200	–	–	–	–	1
DOCK								
fresh cooked	3½ oz	20	3474	tr	0.1	0.4	–	26
DRINK MIXERS								
whiskey sour mix	2 oz	55	14	tr	tr	0	0	2
DUCK								
w/ skin roasted	1 cup (4.9 oz)	472	294	0.2	0.4	6.8	8	0
w/o skin roasted	1 cup (4.9 oz)	281	108	0.4	0.7	7.1	14	0
DURIAN								
fresh	3.5 oz	141	tr	0.5	0.4	1.2	–	42
EGG								
duck	1 (2.5 oz)	130	930	0.1	0.3	0.1	56	0
fresh	1	75	317	tr	0.3	tr	23	0
hard cooked	1	77	280	tr	0.3	tr	22	0
hard cooked chopped	1 cup	210	762	0.1	0.7	0.1	60	0
poached	1	74	316	tr	0.2	tr	18	0
quail	1 (9 g)	14	27	tr	0.1	tr	–	0
EGG DISHES								
deviled	2 halves	145	285	tr	0.2	tr	25	0
omelette plain	1 serv (3.5 oz)	172	1125	0.1	0.4	0.1	30	0
salad	½ cup	307	578	0.1	0.3	0	49	0
scrambled plain	2 (3.3 oz)	199	836	0.1	0.5	0.2	53	3
scrambled w/ whole milk & margarine	1 serv	365	1500	0.1	1	0.2	66	1
sunny side up	1	91	394	tr	0.2	tr	18	0

FOOD	PORTION	CALS	VIT A	THIA	RIBO	NIACIN	FOLIC	VIT C
EGG ROLLS								
egg roll wrapper fresh	1	83	4	0.1	0.1	1.5	5	0
EGG SUBSTITUTES								
liquid	1½ oz	40	1015	0.1	0.1	0.1	–	0
liquid	1 cup (8.8 oz)	211	5422	0.3	0.8	0.3	–	0
Egg Beaters								
Egg Substitute	¼ cup	30	750	0.2	0.8	–	60	0
Second Nature								
No Cholesterol	2 fl oz	60	400	0.1	0.3	0	32	0
No Fat	2 fl oz	40	600	0.1	0.3	2.4	32	0
No Fat With Garden Vegetables	2.5 fl oz	40	600	0.1	0.3	2.4	32	0
EGGNOG								
eggnog	1 cup	342	894	0.1	0.5	0.3	2	4
eggnog	1 qt	1368	3576	0.3	1.9	1.1	9	15
EGGPLANT								
cubed cooked	1 cup	28	63	0.1	tr	0.6	14	1
iman bayildi eggplant w/ onion & tomato	1 serv (15.6 oz)	345	497	0.2	0.1	1.8	59	29
indian eggplant runi	1 serv	180	378	0.1	0.1	1.5	13	15
papoutsakis little shoes	1 serv (15.5 oz)	245	461	0.2	0.2	3.8	37	12
slices grilled	4 (7 oz)	38	20	0.1	0.1	1.0	–	6
ELDERBERRIES								
fresh	1 cup	105	870	0.1	0.1	0.7	–	52
EMU								
cooked	3 oz	130	9	0.4	–	–	–	tr
ENDIVE								
raw chopped	½ cup	4	513	tr	tr	0.1	36	2

FOOD	PORTION	CALS	VIT A	THIA	RIBO	NIACIN	FOLIC	VIT C
ENERGY BARS								
AllGoode Organics								
Amazin' Peanut Raisin	1 bar	210	0	0.2	–	3	40	0
Cashew Almond Passion	1 bar	210	0	0.2	–	–	–	5
Honey Nut Harvest	1 bar	210	0	0.3	–	–	–	0
Nutty Chocolate Apricot	1 bar	200	3000	–	0.2	–	–	12
Back To Nature								
10th Tee Chocolate Fudge	1 bar	200	1500	0.5	0.5	8	120	18
10th Tee Peanut Honey	1 bar	260	1250	–	–	5	100	15
1st Tee Chocolate Peanut	1 bar	290	2000	0.7	0.7	8	160	60
1st Tee Oatmeal Raisin	1 bar	280	2000	0.6	0.7	8	160	60
Balance								
Oasis Strawberry Cheesecake	1 bar (1.69 oz)	180	2250	0.5	0.6	7	140	60
BeneFit								
Nutrition Bar	1 bar (2 oz)	240	1750	0.5	0.6	7	140	21
Better Bar								
Chocolate Coated Caramel Pecan	1 bar (1.8 oz)	180	1000	0.3	0.3	4	80	12
Chocolate Coated Peanut	1 bar (1.8 oz)	180	1000	0.3	0.3	4	80	12
Yogurt Coated Raspberry	1 bar (1.8 oz)	180	1000	0.3	0.3	4	80	12
Breakthru								
Organic Chocolate Fudge	1 bar (2.1 oz)	230	2500	0.9	0.9	10	200	30
Organic Cinnamon Crunch	1 bar (2.1 oz)	220	2500	0.9	0.9	10	200	30
Organic Honey Graham	1 bar (2.1 oz)	220	2500	0.9	0.9	10	200	30
Organic Mocha Fudge	1 bar (2.1 oz)	230	2500	0.9	0.9	10	200	30

FOOD	PORTION	CALS	VIT A	THIA	RIBO	NIACIN	FOLIC	VIT C
Centrum								
Energy Chocolate Nougat	1 (1.98 oz)	220	1250	0.2	0.4	6	40	1
Energy Chocolate Peanut Butter	1 (1.98 oz)	220	1250	0.2	0.4	6	40	1
Clif Bar								
Apricot	1 bar (2.4 oz)	220	1500	0.4	0.3	3	80	60
Carrot Cake	1 bar (2.4 oz)	240	5000	0.4	0.3	4	80	60
Chocolate Brownie	1 bar (2.4 oz)	240	1500	0.4	0.3	4	80	60
Chocolate Almond Fudge	1 bar (2.4 oz)	230	1500	0.4	0.3	4	80	60
Chocolate Chip	1 bar (2.4 oz)	240	1500	0.4	0.3	3	80	60
Chocolate Chip Peanut Crunch	1 bar (2.4 oz)	240	1250	0.4	0.3	6	8	60
Cookies'N Cream	1 bar (2.4 oz)	230	1500	0.4	0.3	3	80	60
Cranberry Apple Cherry	1 bar (2.4 oz)	220	1500	0.4	0.3	3	80	60
Crunchy Peanut Butter	1 bar (2.4 oz)	240	1500	0.5	0.3	6	80	60
GingerSnap	1 bar (2.4 oz)	230	1500	0.4	0.3	4	80	60
DrSoy								
Double Chocolate	1 bar (1.76 oz)	180	5000	1.5	1.7	20	400	60
Gatorade								
GatorBar	1 bar (1.17 oz)	110	750	0.5	0.6	7	120	42
GeniSoy								
Soy Protein Artic Frost Crispy Chocolate Mint	1 bar (2.2 oz)	230	1250	0.4	0.4	5	400	15
Soy Protein Dutch Crunch Sour Apple Crisp	1 bar (2.2 oz)	230	1250	0.4	0.4	5	400	15

FOOD	PORTION	CALS	VIT A	THIA	RIBO	NIACIN	FOLIC	VIT C
Soy Protein Fair Trade Arabica Cafe Mocha Fudge	1 bar (2.2 oz)	220	1250	0.4	0.4	5	400	15
Soy Protein New York Style Blueberry Cheesecake	1 bar (2.2 oz)	220	1250	0.4	0.4	5	400	15
Soy Protein Obsession Fudge Cookies & Cream	1 bar (2.2 oz)	230	1250	0.4	0.4	5	400	15
Soy Protein Pure Golden Honey Creamy Peanut Yogurt	1 bar (2.2 oz)	230	1250	0.4	0.4	4	400	15
Soy Protein Southern Style Chunky Peanut Butter Fudge	1 bar (2.2 oz)	240	1250	0.4	0.4	5	400	15
Soy Protein Ultimate Chocolate Fudge Brownie	1 bar (2.2 oz)	230	1250	0.4	0.4	5	400	15
Xtreme Carrot Cake Quake	1 bar (1.6 oz)	190	1250	0.4	0.4	5	100	15
Xtreme Peanut Butter Fix	1 bar (1.6 oz)	200	1250	0.4	0.4	5	100	15
Xtreme Raspberry Rush	1 bar (1.6 oz)	190	1250	0.4	0.4	5	100	15
Xtreme Rocky Roadtrip	1 bar (1.6 oz)	190	1250	0.4	0.4	5	100	15
Jenny Craig								
Meal Bar Chocolate Peanut	1 bar (2 oz)	220	5000	0.6	0.5	9	100	60
Meal Bar Lemon Meringue	1 bar (2 oz)	210	5000	0.6	0.5	9	100	60
Meal Bar Milk Chocolate	1 bar (2 oz)	210	5000	0.6	0.5	9	100	60
Meal Bar Oatmeal Raisin	1 bar (1.97 oz)	210	5000	0.6	0.5	9	100	60

FOOD	PORTION	CALS	VIT A	THIA	RIBO	NIACIN	FOLIC	VIT C
Meal Bar Yogurt Peanut	1 bar (2 oz)	220	5000	0.6	0.5	9	100	60
Lean Body For Her								
Chocolate Honey Peanut	1 bar (1.76 oz)	190	2500	0.8	0.9	10	200	30
Luna								
Chai Tea	1 bar (1.7 oz)	180	1250	1.5	1.7	20	400	60
Chocolate Pecan Pie	1 bar (1.7 oz)	180	1250	1.5	1.7	20	400	60
LemonZest	1 bar (1.7 oz)	180	1250	1.5	1.7	20	140	60
Nutz Over Chocolate	1 bar (1.7 oz)	180	1250	1.5	1.7	20	400	60
S'Mores	1 bar (1.7 oz)	180	1250	1.5	1.7	20	400	60
Sesame Raisin Crunch	1 bar (1.7 oz)	170	1250	1.5	1.7	20	400	60
Toasted Nuts 'n Cranberry	1 bar (1.7 oz)	170	1250	1.5	1.7	20	400	60
Tropical Crisp	1 bar (1.7 oz)	180	1250	1.5	1.7	20	400	60
Met-Rx								
Big 100 Gram Bar Peanut Butter	1 bar (3.5 oz)	340	4500	0.9	1	20	400	60
Source/One Chocolate Cheesecake	1 bar (2.1 oz)	160	2250	1.5	1.7	20	400	78
Nutribar								
Chocolate Covered Belgian Chocolate	1 bar (2.3 oz)	252	2000	0.6	0.6	7	140	15
Chocolate Covered Caramel	1 bar (2.3 oz)	261	2000	0.6	0.6	7	140	15
Chocolate Covered Chocolate Fudge	1 bar (2.3 oz)	267	2000	0.6	0.6	7	140	15
Chocolate Covered Hazelnut	1 bar (2.3 oz)	261	2000	0.6	0.6	7	140	15
Chocolate Covered Mocha Almond	1 bar (2.3 oz)	261	2000	0.6	0.6	7	140	15

FOOD	PORTION	CALS	VIT A	THIA	RIBO	NIACIN	FOLIC	VIT C
Chocolate Covered Peanut	1 bar (2.3 oz)	262	2000	0.6	0.6	7	140	15
Yogurt Covered Peach Apricot	1 bar (2.3 oz)	261	2000	0.6	0.6	7	140	15
Yogurt Covered Raspberry	1 bar (2.3 oz)	261	2000	0.6	0.6	7	140	15
Yogurt Covered Wildberry	1 bar (2.3 oz)	261	2000	0.6	0.6	7	140	15
Odwalla Bar!								
Peanut Crunch	1 bar (2.2 oz)	260	0	–	–	–	400	60
PermaLean								
Protein Crunch Chocoholic Chocolate	1 bar (1.8 oz)	170	1000	1.5	1.7	20	400	90
Protein Crunch Chocolate Raspberry	1 bar (1.8 oz)	180	5000	1.5	1.7	20	400	90
Protein Crunch Stark Raving Peanutz	1 bar (1.8 oz)	180	5000	1.5	1.7	20	400	90
PowerBar								
Apple Cinnamon	1 bar (2.3 oz)	230	0	1.5	1.7	20	400	60
Banana	1 bar (2.3 oz)	230	0	1.5	1.7	20	400	60
Chocolate	1 bar (2.3 oz)	230	0	1.5	1.7	20	400	60
Essentials Chocolate	1 bar (1.9 oz)	180	0	0.8	0.9	10	200	60
Harvest Blueberry	1 bar (2.3 oz)	240	0	0.8	0.9	10	200	60
Malt-Nut	1 bar (2.3 oz)	230	0	1.5	1.7	20	400	60
Mocha	1 bar (2.3 oz)	230	0	1.5	1.7	20	400	60
Oatmeal Raisin	1 bar (2.3 oz)	230	0	1.5	1.7	20	400	60
Peanut Butter	1 bar (2.3 oz)	230	0	1.5	1.7	20	400	60

FOOD	PORTION	CALS	VIT A	THIA	RIBO	NIACIN	FOLIC	VIT C
Pria Chocolate Honey Graham	1 bar (1 oz)	110	750	0.5	0.5	6	240	36
Pria Double Chocolate Cookie	1 bar (1 oz)	110	750	0.5	0.5	6	240	36
Pria French Vanilla Crisp	1 bar (1 oz)	110	750	0.5	0.5	6	240	36
Vanilla Crisp	1 bar (2.3 oz)	230	0	1.5	1.7	20	400	60
Wild Berry	1 bar (2.3 oz)	230	0	1.5	1.7	20	400	60
Slim-Fast								
Crispy Peanut Caramel	1 bar	120	500	0.2	0.3	3	60	6
Dutch Chocolate	1 bar	140	1250	0.4	0.4	5	40	15
Meal On-The-Go Apple Cobbler	1 bar	220	1750	0.5	0.6	7	120	21
Meal On-The-Go Chocolate Cookie Dough	1 bar	220	1750	0.5	0.6	7	120	21
Meal On-The-Go Honey Peanut	1 bar	220	1750	0.5	0.6	7	120	21
Meal On-The-Go Milk Chocolate Peanut	1 bar	220	1750	0.5	0.6	7	120	21
Meal On-The-Go Oatmeal Raisin	1 bar	220	1750	0.5	0.6	7	120	21
Meal On-The-Go Rich Chocolate Brownie	1 bar	220	1750	0.5	0.6	7	120	21
Meal On-The-Go Toasted Oat & Spice	1 bar	220	1750	0.5	0.6	7	120	21
Peanut Butter	1 bar	150	1250	0.4	0.4	5	40	15
Peanut Butter Crunch	1 bar	130	750	0.2	0.3	3	60	9
Rich Chewy Caramel	1 bar	120	750	0.2	0.3	3	60	60
Sweet Success								
Chewy Chocolate Brownie	1 bar (1.2 oz)	120	750	0.2	0.3	3.0	60	9

FOOD	PORTION	CALS	VIT A	THIA	RIBO	NIACIN	FOLIC	VIT C
ZonePerfect								
Honey Peanut	1 bar (1.8 oz)	200	2500	0.8	0.9	20	160	120
ENERGY DRINKS								
Gatorade								
GatorPro	1 can (11 fl oz)	360	1250	0.8	0.8	9	180	60
GeniSoy								
Soy Protein Shake Chocolate	1 scoop (1.2 oz)	120	1250	0.4	0.4	5	100	15
Soy Protein Shake Vanilla	1 scoop (1.2 oz)	130	1250	0.4	0.4	5	100	15
Soy Protein Shake Strawberry Banana	1 scoop	130	1250	0.4	0.4	5	100	15
Hansen's								
Healthy Start Tropical Orange Vitamix Blend	8 oz	110	5000	1.5	1.7	20	–	60
Healthy Pleasures								
Chocolate Irish Cream	1 bottle (10.5 oz)	260	1750	0.4	0.9	5	140	30
Kashi								
GoLean Shake Man	1 pkg (2.5 oz)	260	2500	0.8	0.9	10	200	30
GoLean Shake Woman	1 pkg (2.5 oz)	250	2500	0.8	0.9	10	200	30
Pounds Off								
Dark Chocolate Ectasy	1 can (11 oz)	200	1750	0.7	1.2	7	140	27
French Vanilla	1 can (11 oz)	220	1750	0.7	1.2	7	140	27
Slim-Fast								
Chocolate as prep w/ fat free milk	1 serv	190	1250	0.5	0.5	7	120	21
Chocolate Malt as prep w/ fat free milk	1 serv	190	1250	0.5	0.5	7	120	21

FOOD	PORTION	CALS	VIT A	THIA	RIBO	NIACIN	FOLIC	VIT C
JumpStart Chocolate as prep w/ fat free milk	1 serv	240	1250	0.5	0.6	7	160	24
JumpStart Vanilla as prep w/ fat free milk	1 serv	240	1250	0.5	0.6	7	160	24
Strawberry as prep w/ fat free milk	1 serv	190	1250	0.5	0.5	7	120	21
Vanilla as prep w/ fat free milk	1 serv	190	1250	0.5	0.5	7	120	21
Sweet Success								
Creamy Milk Chocolate	1 can	200	1250	0.4	0.4	5	100	15
Creamy Milk Chocolate as prep w/ skim milk	1 serv	180	1250	0.4	0.4	5	100	15

ENGLISH MUFFIN

FOOD	PORTION	CALS	VIT A	THIA	RIBO	NIACIN	FOLIC	VIT C
w/ butter	1 (2.2 oz)	189	136	0.3	0.3	2.6	57	1
w/ cheese & sausage	1 (4 oz)	393	380	0.7	0.3	4.1	67	1
w/ egg cheese & canadian bacon	1 (4.8 oz)	289	586	0.5	0.4	3.3	44	2
w/ egg cheese & sausage	1 (5.8 oz)	487	660	0.8	0.5	4.5	54	2
whole wheat	1	134	0	0.2	0.1	2.3	–	0
Pepperidge Farm								
Original	1	130	0	0.2	0.2	0.4	32	0

EPAZOTE

FOOD	PORTION	CALS	VIT A	THIA	RIBO	NIACIN	FOLIC	VIT C
fresh	1 tbsp (1 g)	tr	tr	0	0	tr	2	0
fresh sprig	1 (2 g)	1	1	0	tr	tr	4	tr

EPPAW

FOOD	PORTION	CALS	VIT A	THIA	RIBO	NIACIN	FOLIC	VIT C
raw	½ cup	75	0	0.1	0.1	0.2	–	7

FALAFEL

FOOD	PORTION	CALS	VIT A	THIA	RIBO	NIACIN	FOLIC	VIT C
falafel	1 (1.2 oz)	57	2	tr	tr	0.2	13	tr

FOOD	PORTION	CALS	VIT A	THIA	RIBO	NIACIN	FOLIC	VIT C
FAT								
beef cooked	1 oz	193	0	0	0	0.4	1	0
duck	1 tbsp (13 g)	115	0	0	0	0	0	0
pork backfat	1 oz	230	4	tr	tr	0.3	tr	tr
pork cooked	1 oz	178	4	0.1	tr	0.7	1	0
FEIJOA								
fresh	1 (1.75 oz)	25	0	tr	tr	0.1	19	7
puree	1 cup	119	0	tr	0.1	0.7	93	32
FENNEL								
leaves	1 oz	7	1119	0.1	tr	0.1	29	27
FIDDLEHEAD FERNS								
fresh	3.5 oz	34	3676	tr	0.2	5	–	27
FIGS								
canned in heavy syrup	3	75	31	tr	tr	0.4	–	1
canned in light syrup	3	58	32	tr	tr	0.4	–	1
dried california	½ cup (3.5 oz)	200	100	0.1	0.1	0.4	24	2
dried cooked	½ cup	140	207	tr	0.1	0.8	1	6
fresh	1 med	50	71	tr	tr	0.2	–	1
FIREWEED								
leaves chopped	1 cup (0.8 oz)	24	828	tr	tr	1.1	26	tr
FISH								
fish cake	1 (4.7 oz)	166	140	0.1	0.2	7.9	–	5
kedgeree	5.6 oz	242	640	0.1	0.2	5.8	–	0
mousse	1 serv (3.5 oz)	185	170	tr	0.2	4	–	tr
stew	1 cup (7.9 oz)	157	160	0.1	0.1	3.7	–	11
FLOUNDER								
battered & fried	3.2 oz	211	35	0.1	0.1	1.9	51	0
breaded & fried	3.2 oz	211	35	0.1	0.1	1.9	51	0

FOOD	PORTION	CALS	VIT A	THIA	RIBO	NIACIN	FOLIC	VIT C
FLOUR								
buckwheat whole groat	1 cup (4.2 oz)	402	0	0.5	0.2	7.4	65	0
corn masa	1 cup (4 oz)	416	552	1.6	0.9	11.2	213	0
peanut defatted	1 cup	196	0	0.4	0.3	16.2	149	0
potato	1 cup (6.3 oz)	628	0	0.8	0.3	6.1	–	34
rice brown	1 cup (5.5 oz)	574	0	0.7	0.1	10	25	0
rice white	1 cup (5.5 oz)	578	0	0.2	0	4.1	6	0
rye dark	1 cup (4.5 oz)	415	0	0.4	0.3	5.5	77	0
rye light	1 cup (3.6 oz)	374	0	0.3	0.1	0.8	22	0
triticale whole grain	1 cup (4.6 oz)	439	0	0.5	0.2	3.7	96	0
white bread	1 cup (4.8 oz)	495	0	1.1	0.7	10.3	211	0
white cake unsifted	1 cup (4.8 oz)	496	0	1.2	0.6	9.3	211	0
white self-rising	1 cup (4.4 oz)	443	0	0.8	0.5	7.3	193	0
white unbleached	1 cup (4.4 oz)	455	0	1	0.6	7.4	193	0
whole wheat	1 cup (4.2 oz)	407	0	0.5	0.3	7.6	53	0
Gold Medal								
All Purpose	¼ cup (1 oz)	100	0	0.2	0.1	1.6	40	0
Better For Bread	¼ cup (1 oz)	100	0	0.2	0.1	1.6	40	0
Self Rising	¼ cup (1 oz)	100	0	0.2	0.1	1.6	40	0
Unbleached	¼ cup (1 oz)	100	0	0.2	0.1	1.6	40	0
La Pina								
Flour	¼ cup (1 oz)	100	0	0.2	0.1	1.6	100	0
FRENCH BEANS								
dried cooked	1 cup	228	5	0.2	0.1	1	132	2
FRENCH TOAST								
plain	1 slice	151	298	0.1	0.2	1.1	15	tr
sticks	5 (4.9 oz)	513	45	0.2	0.3	3	82	0

FOOD	PORTION	CALS	VIT A	THIA	RIBO	NIACIN	FOLIC	VIT C
w/ butter	2 slices (4.7 oz)	356	473	0.6	0.5	3.9	73	tr
FROG'S LEGS								
as prep w/ seasoned flour & fried	1 (0.8)	70	0	tr	0.1	0.3	tr	0
FRUIT DRINKS								
fruit punch	6 fl oz	87	26	tr	tr	tr	2	55
pineapple & orange drink	8 fl oz	125	1320	0.1	tr	0.5	27	56
Fresh Samantha								
Banana Strawberry	1 cup (8 oz)	130	0	0.1	0.1	0.4	24	30
Carrot Orange	1 cup (8 oz)	100	17500	0.3	0.1	0.8	40	72
Desperately Seeking C	1 cup (8 oz)	110	5000	0.1	0.1	0.8	40	600
Protein Blast	1 cup (8 oz)	160	200	0.2	0.1	0.4	32	48
Super Juice	1 cup (8 oz)	140	100	0.2	0.1	1	40	48
The Big Bang	1 cup (8 oz)	100	200	0.1	tr	0.4	24	21
Hansen's								
Juice Slam Wild Berry	1 box	120	1250	0.4	0.4	5	—	15
Smoothie Energy Island Blast	1 can	170	5000	—	0.9	—	—	60
FRUIT MIXED								
fruit cocktail in heavy syrup	½ cup	93	262	tr	tr	0.5	—	2
fruit cocktail juice pack	½ cup	56	378	tr	tr	0.5	—	3
fruit cocktail water pack	½ cup	40	305	tr	tr	0.4	—	3
fruit salad in heavy syrup	½ cup	94	646	tr	tr	0.4	—	3
fruit salad in light syrup	½ cup	73	541	tr	tr	0.4	—	3
fruit salad juice pack	½ cup	62	744	tr	tr	0.4	—	4
fruit salad water pack	½ cup	37	536	tr	tr	0.5	—	2

FOOD	PORTION	CALS	VIT A	THIA	RIBO	NIACIN	FOLIC	VIT C
FRUIT SNACKS								
fruit leather	1 bar (0.8 oz)	81	27	tr	tr	tr	—	16
fruit leather rolls	1 sm (0.5 oz)	49	16	tr	tr	tr	—	1
GARLIC								
clove	1	4	0	tr	tr	tr	tr	1
fresh chopped	1 tsp	4	0	tr	tr	tr	0	1
GELATIN								
low calorie	½ cup	8	0	0	0	0	0	0
GIBLETS								
capon simmered	1 cup (5 oz)	238	19236	0.1	1.5	6	601	13
chicken floured & fried	1 cup (5 oz)	402	17298	0.1	2.2	15.9	550	13
chicken simmered	1 cup (5 oz)	228	10774	0.1	1.4	5.9	545	12
turkey simmered	1 cup (5 oz)	243	8753	0.1	1.3	6.5	501	3
GINGER								
root fresh	5 slices	8	0	tr	tr	0.1	—	1
root fresh sliced	¼ cup	17	0	tr	tr	0.2	—	1
Eden								
Pickled w/ Shiso Leaves	1 tbsp	15	0	0	0	0	0	0
GINKGO NUTS								
dried	1 oz	99	310	0.1	0.1	3.3	—	8
GINSENG								
dried	1 oz	90	0	0.1	0.1	0.3	—	2
fresh	1 oz	28	0	tr	tr	0.2	—	4
GIZZARDS								
chicken simmered	1 cup (5 oz)	222	273	tr	0.4	5.8	77	2
turkey simmered	1 cup (5 oz)	236	268	tr	0.5	4.5	75	2
GOOSE								
w/ skin roasted	6.6 oz	574	131	0.1	0.6	7.8	4	0
GOOSEBERRIES								
canned in light syrup	½ cup	93	174	tr	0.1	0.2	4	13
fresh	1 cup	67	435	0.1	tr	0.5	—	42

FOOD	PORTION	CALS	VIT A	THIA	RIBO	NIACIN	FOLIC	VIT C
GRAPE JUICE								
bottled	1 cup	155	20	0.1	0.1	0.7	7	tr
grape drink	6 oz	84	2	tr	tr	tr	1	64
GRAPE LEAVES								
canned	1 (4 g)	3	210	0	tr	0.2	3	0
GRAPEFRUIT								
pink	½	37	318	tr	tr	0.2	15	47
pink sections	1 cup	69	595	0.1	tr	0.4	28	88
red	½	37	318	tr	tr	0.2	15	47
red sections	1 cup	69	595	0.1	tr	0.4	28	88
unsweetened	1 cup	93	18	0.1	tr	0.6	26	72
water pack	½ cup	44	0	tr	tr	0.3	11	27
white	½	39	12	tr	tr	0.3	12	39
white sections	1 cup	76	23	0.1	tr	0.6	23	77
GRAPEFRUIT JUICE								
sweetened	1 cup	116	0	0.1	0.1	0.8	26	67
Fresh Samantha								
Juice	1 cup (8 oz)	90	0	0.1	0	0	24	72
GRAPES								
fresh	10	36	35	tr	tr	0.2	2	5
thompson seedless in heavy syrup	½ cup	94	81	tr	tr	0.2	–	1
thompson seedless water pack	½ cup	48	81	tr	tr	0.2	–	1
GRAVY								
au jus	1 cup	38	0	tr	0.1	1.9	–	2
beef	1 cup	124	0	0.1	0.1	1.5	–	0
chicken	1 cup	189	880	tr	0.1	1.1	–	0
mushroom	1 cup	120	0	0.1	0.2	1.6	–	0
turkey	1 cup	122	0	tr	0.2	3.1	–	0
Bovril								
Extract	1 heaping tsp	9	0	0.5	0.4	4.3	–	0
Marmite								
Extract	1 heaping tsp	9	0	0.2	0.6	3.4	–	0

FOOD	PORTION	CALS	VIT A	THIA	RIBO	NIACIN	FOLIC	VIT C
GREAT NORTHERN BEANS								
cooked	1 cup	210	2	0.3	0.1	1.2	181	2
Eden								
Organic	½ cup (4.6 oz)	110	0	tr	0.1	0	25	0
GREEN BEANS								
cooked	½ cup	18	359	tr	0.1	0.3	–	6
italian	½ cup	13	237	tr	tr	0.1	22	3
raw	½ cup	17	368	tr	0.1	0.4	20	9
Fresh Like								
Cut	3.5 oz	29	534	0.1	0.1	0.4	–	11
French Cut	3.5 oz	29	459	0.1	0.1	0.4	–	9
GROUNDCHERRIES								
fresh	½ cup	37	504	0.1	tr	2	–	8
GUAVA								
fresh	1	45	713	tr	tr	1.1	–	165
guava sauce	½ cup	43	337	tr	tr	0.5	–	174
HADDOCK								
breaded & fried	1 piece (3.5 oz)	187	50	tr	0.1	4	3	0
HAM								
canned extra lean roasted	3 oz	116	0	0.9	0.2	4.2	4	0
center slice country style lean roasted	4 oz	220	0	0.6	0.3	4.4	6	0
patty cooked	1 patty (2 oz)	203	0	0.2	0.1	1.9	2	0
prosciutto	1 oz	55	0	0.2	0.1	1.1	1	0
steak boneless extra lean	1 (2 oz)	69	0	0.5	0.1	2.9	2	18
Alpine Lace								
Boneless Cooked 98% Fat Free	2 slices (2 oz)	60	0	–	–	–	–	0
Honey Ham 98% Fat Free	2 slices (2 oz)	60	0	–	–	–	–	0
Smoked Virginia 98% Fat Free	2 slices (2 oz)	60	0	–	–	–	–	0

FOOD	PORTION	CALS	VIT A	THIA	RIBO	NIACIN	FOLIC	VIT C
Boar's Head								
Black Forest Smoked	2 oz	60	0	–	–	–	–	0
Cappy	2 oz	60	0	–	–	–	–	0
Deluxe	2 oz	60	0	–	–	–	–	0
Deluxe Lowered Sodium	2 oz	50	0	–	–	–	–	0
Maple Glazed Honey	2 oz	60	0	–	–	–	–	0
Pepper	2 oz	60	0	–	–	–	–	0
Rosemary & Sundried Tomato	2 oz	70	0	–	–	–	–	0
Sweet Slice Smoked	3 oz	100	0	–	–	–	–	0
Virgina	2 oz	60	0	–	–	–	–	0
Virginia Smoked	2 oz	60	0	–	–	–	–	0
Hillshire								
Deli Select Honey Ham	6 slices (2 oz)	60	0	–	–	–	–	4

HAM DISHES

FOOD	PORTION	CALS	VIT A	THIA	RIBO	NIACIN	FOLIC	VIT C
croquettes	1 (3.1 oz)	217	206	0.3	0.2	2.1	11	tr
salad	½ cup	287	253	0.3	0.2	2.2	22	1

HAM SUBSTITUTES

FOOD	PORTION	CALS	VIT A	THIA	RIBO	NIACIN	FOLIC	VIT C
Yves								
Veggie Ham Deli Slices	1 serv (2.2 oz)	80	0	0.6	–	–	–	0

HAMBURGER

FOOD	PORTION	CALS	VIT A	THIA	RIBO	NIACIN	FOLIC	VIT C
double patty w/ bun	1 reg	544	0	0.3	0.4	0.3	38	0
double patty w/ cheese & bun	1 reg	457	332	0.3	0.4	6	29	0
double patty w/ cheese & double bun	1 reg	461	276	0.3	0.4	6	36	0
double patty w/ cheese ketchup mayonnaise onion pickle tomato & bun	1 reg	416	398	0.4	0.3	8.1	23	2

FOOD	PORTION	CALS	VIT A	THIA	RIBO	NIACIN	FOLIC	VIT C
double patty w/ ketchup mayonnaise onion pickle tomato & bun	1 reg	649	371	0.6	0.4	8.3	34	3
double patty w/ ketchup cheese mayonnaise mustard pickle tomato & bun	1 lg	706	348	0.4	0.5	7.2	48	tr
double patty w/ ketchup mustard mayonnaise onion pickle tomato & bun	1 lg	540	102	0.4	0.4	7.6	27	1
double patty w/ ketchup mustard onion pickle & bun	1 reg	576	53	0.4	0.4	6.7	45	1
single patty w/ bacon ketchup cheese mustard onion pickle & bun	1 lg	609	406	0.3	0.4	6.6	33	2
single patty w/ bun	1 lg	400	0	0.3	0.3	6.2	32	0
single patty w/ bun	1 reg	275	0	0.3	0.3	3.7	25	0
single patty w/ cheese & bun	1 lg	608	615	0.5	0.6	11.2	38	0
single patty w/ cheese & bun	1 reg	320	153	0.4	0.4	3.7	26	0
single patty w/ ketchup cheese ham mayonnaise pickle tomato & bun	1 lg	745	505	0.5	0.6	9.2	50	7
single patty w/ ketchup mustard mayonnaise onion pickle tomato & bun	1 reg	279	82	0.2	0.2	3.7	18	2
triple patty w/ cheese & bun	1 lg	769	359	0.6	0.6	11.5	51	3

FOOD	PORTION	CALS	VIT A	THIA	RIBO	NIACIN	FOLIC	VIT C
triple patty w/ ketchup mustard pickle & bun	1 lg	693	158	0.3	0.6	11	31	1
Kid Cuisine								
Buckaroo Beef Patty Sandwich w/ Cheese	1 meal (8.5 oz)	410	100	–	–	–	–	0

HAMBURGER SUBSTITUTES

Harmony Farms

FOOD	PORTION	CALS	VIT A	THIA	RIBO	NIACIN	FOLIC	VIT C
Soy Burger Onion	1 (2.5 oz)	90	0	–	–	–	–	0
Soy Burgers Garlic	1 (2.5 oz)	110	0	–	–	–	–	0
Soy Burgers Mushroom	1 (2.5 oz)	110	0	–	–	–	–	0
Soy Burgers Original	1 (2.5 oz)	110	0	–	–	–	–	0
V'dora								
Vegetable BurgerLites	1 (3.3 oz)	58	3250	–	–	–	–	35
Yves								
Black Bean & Mushroom Burgers	1 (3 oz)	100	0	–	–	–	–	0
Garden Vegetable Patties	1 (3 oz)	90	1250	–	–	–	–	0
Veggie Burger	1 (3 oz)	119	100	0.3	0.2	6	–	1

HAZELNUTS

FOOD	PORTION	CALS	VIT A	THIA	RIBO	NIACIN	FOLIC	VIT C
dried	1 oz	179	19	0.1	tr	0.3	20	tr

HEART

FOOD	PORTION	CALS	VIT A	THIA	RIBO	NIACIN	FOLIC	VIT C
beef simmered	3 oz	148	0	0.1	1.3	3.5	2	1
chicken simmered	1 cup (5 oz)	268	41	0.1	1.1	4.1	116	3
lamb braised	3 oz	158	0	0.4	1	3.7	2	6
pork braised	1 cup	215	32	0.8	2.5	8.8	6	3
pork braised	1	191	28	0.7	2.2	7.8	5	3
turkey simmered	1 cup (5 oz)	257	40	0.1	1.3	4.7	114	3

HEARTS OF PALM

FOOD	PORTION	CALS	VIT A	THIA	RIBO	NIACIN	FOLIC	VIT C
canned	1 cup (5.1 oz)	41	0	tr	0.1	0.6	57	12
canned	1 (1.2 oz)	9	0	tr	tr	0.1	13	3

FOOD	PORTION	CALS	VIT A	THIA	RIBO	NIACIN	FOLIC	VIT C
HERBS/SPICES								
curry powder	1 tsp	6	20	tr	tr	0.1	–	tr
garam masala	1 tsp	8	2	0.7	8	7	0	0
poultry seasoning	1 tsp	5	39	tr	tr	tr	–	tr
pumpkin pie spice	1 tsp	6	4	tr	tr	tr	–	tr
Eden								
Furikake Seasoning	½ tsp	5	1	–	–	–	–	0
Instant India								
Curry Paste Cilantro Garlic	2 tbsp (1 oz)	110	0	–	–	–	–	0
Curry Paste Ginger Garlic	2 tbsp (1 oz)	90	0	–	–	–	–	0
HERRING								
atlantic kippered	1 fillet (1.4 oz)	87	51	0.1	0.1	1.8	–	tr
atlantic cooked	1 fillet (5 oz)	290	146	0.2	0.4	5.9	–	1
atlantic cooked	3 oz	172	87	0.1	0.3	3.5	–	1
atlantic raw	3 oz	134	80	0.1	0.2	2.7	–	1
fried	1 serv (3.5 oz)	233	225	tr	0.2	3.5	10	0
smoked	3.5 oz	210	65	0.1	0.2	6.5	10	0
HOMINY								
white	1 cup (5.6 oz)	482	176	tr	tr	0.1	2	0
HONEY								
honey	1 cup (11.9 oz)	1031	0	0	0.1	0.4	5	2
honey	1 tbsp (0.7 oz)	64	0	0	tr	tr	0	tr
HONEYDEW								
cubed	1 cup	60	68	0.1	tr	1	–	42
wedge	⅒	46	52	0.1	tr	0.8	–	32
Chiquita								
Wedge	⅒ melon (4.7 oz)	50	100	–	–	–	–	27
HORSERADISH								
japanese wasabi	¼ tsp	1	tr	1	0	0	tr	1
wasabi root raw	1 (5.9 oz)	184	78	0.2	0.2	1.3	30	71

FOOD	PORTION	CALS	VIT A	THIA	RIBO	NIACIN	FOLIC	VIT C
wasabi root raw sliced	1 cup (4.6 oz)	142	60	0.2	0.2	1	23	71
Boar's Head								
Horseradish	1 tsp (5 g)	5	0	–	–	–	–	0
Eden								
Wasabi Powder	1 tsp	10	13	–	–	–	–	1

HOT DOG

FOOD	PORTION	CALS	VIT A	THIA	RIBO	NIACIN	FOLIC	VIT C
corndog	1	460	207	0.3	0.7	4.2	60	0
w/ bun chili	1	297	58	0.2	0.4	3.7	50	3
w/ bun plain	1	242	0	0.2	0.3	3.7	30	tr
Boar's Head								
Beef	1 (2 oz)	160	300	–	–	–	–	0
Beef Lite	1 (1.6 oz)	90	100	–	–	–	–	0
Pork & Beef	1 (2 oz)	150	0	–	–	–	–	0
Health Is Wealth								
Uncured Chicken	1 (1.5 oz)	100	100	–	–	–	–	1
Healthy Choice								
Beef Low Fat	1 (1.8 oz)	70	0	–	–	–	–	2
Low Fat Turkey Pork Beef	1 (1.4 oz)	60	0	–	–	–	–	4
Kid Cuisine								
Mystical Mini Corn Dogs	4 pieces	230	0	–	–	–	–	0

HOT DOG SUBSTITUTES

FOOD	PORTION	CALS	VIT A	THIA	RIBO	NIACIN	FOLIC	VIT C
Yves								
Good Dog	1 (1.8 oz)	70	0	0.3	0.3	4	–	0
Tofu Dogs	1 (1.3 oz)	45	0	0.2	–	–	–	1
Veggie Dogs	1 (1.6 oz)	60	0	0.2	–	–	–	0
Veggie Dogs Chili	1 (1.6 oz)	50	0	0.2	–	–	–	0
Veggie Dogs Jumbo	1 (2.7 oz)	100	0	0.4	–	–	–	0
Veggie Dogs Jumbo Hot N' Spicy	1 (2.7 oz)	106	200	0.1	–	–	–	1

HUMMUS

FOOD	PORTION	CALS	VIT A	THIA	RIBO	NIACIN	FOLIC	VIT C
hummus	⅓ cup	140	20	0.1	tr	0.3	49	6
hummus	1 cup	420	61	0.2	0.1	1	146	19

ICE CREAM AND FROZEN DESSERT

FOOD	PORTION	CALS	VIT A	THIA	RIBO	NIACIN	FOLIC	VIT C
chocolate	½ cup (4 fl oz)	143	275	tr	0.1	0.1	10	1
cone vanilla light soft serve	1 (4.6 oz)	164	211	0	0.3	0.3	5	1
dixie cup chocolate	1 (3.5 fl oz)	125	241	tr	0.1	0.1	9	tr
dixie cup strawberry	1 (3.5 fl oz)	112	185	tr	0.1	0.1	7	5
dixie cup vanilla	1 (3.5 fl oz)	116	237	tr	0.1	0.1	3	tr
gelato chocolate hazelnut	½ cup (5.3 oz)	370	76	0.2	0.2	0.5	35	1
gelato vanilla	½ cup (3 oz)	211	191	tr	0.1	tr	15	tr
strawberry	½ cup (4 fl oz)	127	211	tr	0.2	0.1	8	5
sundae caramel	1 (5.4 oz)	303	263	0	0.3	1	12	3
sundae hot fudge	1 (5.4 oz)	284	221	0	0.3	1.1	9	2
sundae strawberry	1 (5.4 oz)	269	222	0	0.3	0.9	18	2
vanilla	½ cup (4 fl oz)	132	270	tr	0.2	0.1	3	tr
vanilla soft serve	½ cup	111	90	tr	0.2	0.1	6	1
Better Than Ice Creme								
Soy Vanilla as prep	½ cup	110	0	–	–	–	–	0
Edy's								
Dreamery Banana Split	½ cup	240	100	–	–	–	–	5
Dreamery Black Raspberry Avalanche	½ cup	270	750	–	–	–	–	0
Dreamery Caramel Toffee Bar Heaven	½ cup	290	750	–	–	–	–	0
Dreamery Cashew Praline Parfait	½ cup	280	750	–	–	–	–	0
Dreamery Chocolate Truffle Explosion	½ cup	280	500	–	–	–	–	0
Dreamery Chocolate Peanut Butter Chunk	½ cup	310	500	–	–	–	–	0
Dreamery Coney Island Waffle Cone	½ cup	310	500	–	–	–	–	0

FOOD	PORTION	CALS	VIT A	THIA	RIBO	NIACIN	FOLIC	VIT C
Dreamery Cool Mint	½ cup	300	750	—	—	—	—	0
Dreamery Deep Dish Apple Pie	½ cup	280	750	—	—	—	—	0
Dreamery Dulce De Leche	½ cup	270	750	—	—	—	—	0
Dreamery Grandma's Cookie Dough	½ cup	300	1000	—	—	—	—	0
Dreamery Harvest Peach	½ cup	230	750	—	—	—	—	8
Dreamery New York Strawberry Cheesecake	½ cup	260	750	—	—	—	—	4
Dreamery Nothing But Chocolate	½ cup	280	500	—	—	—	—	0
Dreamery Nuts About Malt	½ cup	290	750	—	—	—	—	0
Dreamery Raspberry Brownie A La Mode	½ cup	270	500	—	—	—	—	0
Dreamery Raspberry Brownie A La Mode	½ cup	130	500	—	—	—	—	0
Dreamery Strawberry Fields	½ cup	220	500	—	—	—	—	6
Dreamery Tiramisu	½ cup	260	750	—	—	—	—	0
Dreamery Vanilla	½ cup	260	750	—	—	—	—	0
Häagen-Dazs								
Bars Chocolate & Almonds	1 (3.7 oz)	380	500	—	—	—	—	0
Bars Chocolate & Dark Chocolate	1 (3.6 oz)	350	500	—	—	—	—	0

FOOD	PORTION	CALS	VIT A	THIA	RIBO	NIACIN	FOLIC	VIT C
Bars Chocolate Peanut Butter Swirl	1 (3 oz)	320	400	—	—	—	—	0
Bars Coffee & Almond Crunch	1 (3.7 oz)	370	500	—	—	—	—	0
Bars Cookies & Cream Crunch	1 (3.6 oz)	370	500	—	—	—	—	0
Bars Dulce De Leche Caramel	1 (3.7 oz)	370	500	—	—	—	—	0
Bars Tropical Coconut	1 (3.5 oz)	340	500	—	—	—	—	2
Bars Vanilla & Almonds	1 (3.7 oz)	380	500	—	—	—	—	0
Bars Vanilla & Dark Chocolate	1 (3.6 oz)	350	500	—	—	—	—	0
Bars Vanilla & Milk Chocolate	1 (3.5 oz)	340	500	—	—	—	—	0
Butter Pecan	½ cup	310	500	—	—	—	—	0
Cherry Vanilla	½ cup	240	400	—	—	—	—	1
Chocolate	½ cup	270	500	—	—	—	—	0
Chocolate Chocolate Fudge	½ cup	290	500	—	—	—	—	0
Chocolate Chocolate Chip	½ cup	300	500	—	—	—	—	0
Coffee	½ cup	270	750	—	—	—	—	0
Coffee Mocha Chip	½ cup	290	500	—	—	—	—	0
Cookie Dough Chip	½ cup	310	500	—	—	—	—	0
Cookies & Cream	½ cup	270	500	—	—	—	—	0
Creme Caramel Pecan	½ cup	320	500	—	—	—	—	0
Dulce De Leche Caramel	½ cup	290	500	—	—	—	—	0
Low Fat Chocolate	½ cup	170	300	—	—	—	—	0
Low Fat Coffee Fudge	½ cup	170	300	—	—	—	—	0
Low Fat Strawberry	½ cup	150	300	—	—	—	—	5
Low Fat Vanilla	½ cup	170	300	—	—	—	—	0
Macadamia Brittle	½ cup	300	500	—	—	—	—	0
Mango	½ cup	250	1000	—	—	—	—	5

FOOD	PORTION	CALS	VIT A	THIA	RIBO	NIACIN	FOLIC	VIT C
Mint Chip	½ cup	300	500	–	–	–	–	0
Pineapple Coconut	½ cup	230	500	–	–	–	–	0
Pistachio	½ cup	290	750	–	–	–	–	0
Rum Raisin	½ cup	270	500	–	–	–	–	0
Strawberry	½ cup	250	500	–	–	–	–	6
Vanilla	½ cup	270	750	–	–	–	–	0
Vanilla Chocolate Chip	½ cup	310	500	–	–	–	–	0
Vanilla Fudge	½ cup	290	500	–	–	–	–	0
Vanilla Swiss Almond	½ cup	300	500	–	–	–	–	0
Healthy Choice								
Butter Pecan Crunch	½ cup	120	200	–	–	–	–	0
Cappuccino Chocolate Chunk	½ cup	120	200	–	–	–	–	0
Cappuccino Mocha Crunch	½ cup	120	300	–	–	–	–	0
Cherry Chocolate Chunk	½ cup	110	200	–	–	–	–	0
Chocolate Chocolate Chunk	½ cup	120	200	–	–	–	–	0
Coconut Cream Pie	½ cup	120	200	–	–	–	–	0
Cookies 'N Cream	½ cup	120	200	–	–	–	–	0
Cookies Creme De Mint	½ cup	130	200	–	–	–	–	0
Fudge Brownie	½ cup	120	200	–	–	–	–	0
Mint Chocolate Chip	½ cup	120	200	–	–	–	–	0
Old Fashioned Blueberry Hill	½ cup	120	200	–	–	–	–	0
Old Fashioned Butterscotch Blonde	½ cup	140	100	–	–	–	–	0
Old Fashioned Cherry Vanilla	½ cup	120	0	–	–	–	–	0
Old Fashioned Strawberry	½ cup	110	200	–	–	–	–	4
Peanut Butter Cup	½ cup	110	200	–	–	–	–	0

FOOD	PORTION	CALS	VIT A	THIA	RIBO	NIACIN	FOLIC	VIT C
Praline & Caramel	½ cup	130	200	—	—	—	—	0
Praline Caramel Cluster	½ cup	130	200	—	—	—	—	0
Rocky Road	½ cup	140	200	—	—	—	—	0
Turtle Fudge Cake	½ cup	130	200	—	—	—	—	0
Vanilla	½ cup	100	300	—	—	—	—	0
Vanilla Bean	½ cup	110	300	—	—	—	—	0
Wild Raspberry Truffle	½ cup	120	200	—	—	—	—	0
Klondike								
Choco Taco Fudge Grande	1 bar (3.2 oz)	310	100	—	—	—	—	0
Oreo Ice Cream Cookie Sandwich	1 (2.6 oz)	240	200	—	—	—	—	0
Silhouette								
The Skinny Cow Low Fat Ice Cream Sandwich Vanilla	1	130	0	—	—	—	—	0
Turkey Hill								
Black Cherry	½ cup	140	300	—	—	—	—	0
Butter Pecan	½ cup	170	300	—	—	—	—	0
Cookies 'N Cream	½ cup	160	300	—	—	—	—	0
Light Butter Pecan	½ cup	130	300	—	—	—	—	0
Light Choco Mint Chip	½ cup	140	300	—	—	—	—	0
Light Vanilla & Chocolate	½ cup	110	300	—	—	—	—	0
Light Vanilla Bean	½ cup	110	300	—	—	—	—	0
Neapolitan	½ cup	150	300	—	—	—	—	0
Rocky Road	½ cup	170	200	—	—	—	—	0
Tin Roof Sundae	½ cup	160	200	—	—	—	—	0
Vanilla & Chocolate	½ cup	150	300	—	—	—	—	0
Vanilla Bean	½ cup	140	300	—	—	—	—	0

ICE CREAM CONES AND CUPS

FOOD	PORTION	CALS	VIT A	THIA	RIBO	NIACIN	FOLIC	VIT C
sugar cone	1	40	0	0.1	tr	0.5	1	0
wafer cone	1	17	0	tr	tr	0.2	0	0

FOOD	PORTION	CALS	VIT A	THIA	RIBO	NIACIN	FOLIC	VIT C
ICE CREAM TOPPINGS								
pineapple	2 tbsp (1.5 oz)	106	9	tr	tr	tr	1	25
pineapple	1 cup (11.5 oz)	861	72	0.1	tr	0.3	9	199
strawberry	1 cup (11.5 oz)	863	61	tr	0.1	0.8	5	85
strawberry	2 tbsp (1.5 oz)	107	9	tr	tr	0.1	1	11
ICED TEA								
instant unsweetened lemon flavor as prep w/ water	8 oz	4	0	0	tr	0.1	—	0
ICES AND ICE POPS								
fruit & juice bar	1 (3 fl oz)	75	27	tr	tr	0.1	5	1
ice coconut pineapple	½ cup (4 fl oz)	109	0	—	—	—	—	13
ice fruit w/ Equal	1 bar (1.7 oz)	12	0	0	0	0.1	0	0
ice lime	½ cup (4 fl oz)	75	0	—	—	—	—	1
ice pop	1 (2 fl oz)	42	0	0	0	0	—	0
Cold Fusion								
Protein Juice Bar All Flavors	1 bar (3.8 oz)	130	5000	—	—	—	—	60
Edy's								
Fruit Bars Strawberry	1 (3 oz)	80	0	—	—	—	—	15
Sorbet Coconut	½ cup	140	0	—	—	—	—	0
Sorbet Lemon	½ cup	140	0	—	—	—	—	9
Sorbet Mandarin Orange	½ cup	130	300	—	—	—	—	2
Sorbet Peach	½ cup	130	200	—	—	—	—	18
Sorbet Raspberry	½ cup	130	0	—	—	—	—	9
Sorbet Strawberry	½ cup	120	0	—	—	—	—	18
Häagen-Dazs								
Sorbet Chocolate	½ cup	120	0	—	tr	—	—	0
Sorbet Mango	½ cup	120	750	—	—	—	—	2

FOOD	PORTION	CALS	VIT A	THIA	RIBO	NIACIN	FOLIC	VIT C
Sorbet Orange	½ cup	120	100	–	–	–	–	15
Sorbet Orchard Peach	½ cup	130	200	–	–	–	–	4
Sorbet Raspberry	½ cup	120	0	–	–	–	–	2
Sorbet Strawberry	½ cup	120	0	–	–	–	–	12
Sorbet Zesty Lemon	½ cup	120	0	–	–	–	–	4
Sorbet Bar Chocolate	1 (2.7 oz)	80	0	–	–	–	–	0
Sorbet Bars Raspberry & Vanilla Yogurt	1 (2.5 oz)	90	0	–	–	–	–	1
Sorbet Bars Strawberry & Vanilla Ice Cream	1 (2.5 oz)	110	200	–	–	–	–	5

JACKFRUIT

FOOD	PORTION	CALS	VIT A	THIA	RIBO	NIACIN	FOLIC	VIT C
fresh	3.5 oz	70	tr	tr	0.1	0.6	–	9

JAM/JELLY/PRESERVES

FOOD	PORTION	CALS	VIT A	THIA	RIBO	NIACIN	FOLIC	VIT C
apple butter	1 tbsp (0.6 oz)	33	0	tr	tr	tr	–	tr
apple jelly	1 pkg (0.5 oz)	38	2	0	–	tr	0	tr
apple jelly	1 tbsp (0.7 oz)	52	3	0	–	tr	0	tr
cherry jam	0.5 oz	36	0	–	–	–	–	tr
orange marmalade	1 tbsp (0.7 oz)	49	9	tr	–	tr	7	1
strawberry jam	1 tbsp (0.7 oz)	48	2	0	–	tr	7	2
strawberry preserve	1 tbsp (0.7 oz)	48	2	0	–	tr	7	2
Eden								
Cherry Butter	1 tbsp	35	200	–	–	–	–	0
Organic Apple Butter	1 tbsp	20	0	0	0	0	0	0
Wild Thyme Farms								
Fruit Spreads Mango Apricot	1 tsp	7	100	–	–	–	–	1

FOOD	PORTION	CALS	VIT A	THIA	RIBO	NIACIN	FOLIC	VIT C
JAVA PLUM								
fresh	3	5	0	tr	tr	tr	--	1
fresh	1 cup	82	5	tr	tr	0.4	--	19
JUTE								
cooked	1 cup	32	4511	0.1	0.2	0.8	90	29
KALE								
chopped cooked	½ cup	21	4810	tr	tr	0.3	9	27
frzn chopped cooked	½ cup	20	4130	tr	0.1	0.4	9	16
raw chopped	½ cup	21	3026	tr	tr	0.3	10	41
scotch chopped cooked	½ cup	18	1296	tr	tr	0.5	9	34
KETCHUP								
ketchup	1 tbsp	16	152	tr	tr	0.2	2	2
ketchup	1 pkg (0.2 oz)	6	61	tr	tr	0.1	1	1
Del Monte								
Ketchup	1 tbsp (0.5 oz)	15	100	--	--	--	--	1
Muir Glen								
Organic	1 tbsp (0.6 oz)	15	100	--	--	--	--	1
Tree Of Life								
Ketchup	1 tbsp (0.5 oz)	10	400	--	--	--	--	6
KIDNEY								
beef simmered	3 oz	122	1055	0.2	3.5	5.1	83	1
lamb braised	3 oz	117	387	0.3	1.8	5.1	69	10
pork cooked	1 cup	211	364	0.6	2.2	8.1	57	9
pork cooked	3 oz	128	221	0.3	1.4	4.9	35	9
veal braised	3 oz	139	569	0.2	1.7	3.9	18	7
KIDNEY BEANS								
california red cooked	1 cup	219	5	0.2	0.1	1	131	2
cooked	1 cup	225	0	0.3	0.1	1	229	2
red cooked	1 cup	225	0	0.3	0.1	1	229	2

FOOD	PORTION	CALS	VIT A	THIA	RIBO	NIACIN	FOLIC	VIT C
Eden								
Organic Cannellini	½ cup (4.6 oz)	100	0	0.7	0.1	–	0	0
KIWIS								
fresh	1 med	46	133	tr	tr	0.4	–	75
KNISH								
potato	1 lg (7 oz)	332	225	0.4	0.4	3.4	35	8
potato	1 med (3.5 oz)	166	113	0.2	0.2	1.7	17	4
KOHLRABI								
raw sliced	½ cup	19	25	tr	tr	0.3	–	43
sliced cooked	½ cup	24	29	tr	tr	0.3	–	44
KRILL								
fresh	1 oz	22	210	tr	0.1	0.5	–	1
KUMQUATS								
fresh	1	12	57	tr	tr	–	–	7
LAMB DISHES								
curry	¾ cup	345	145	0.2	0.3	7.8	16	3
moussaka	5.6 oz	312	330	0.1	0.2	5.4	–	6
stew	¾ cup	124	4265	0.1	0.2	2.4	37	20
LAMBSQUARTERS								
chopped cooked	½ cup	29	8730	0.1	0.2	0.8	–	33
LEEKS								
chopped cooked	¼ cup	8	12	tr	tr	0.1	6	1
cooked	1 (4.4 oz)	38	57	tr	tr	0.2	30	5
freeze dried	1 tbsp	1	1	tr	tr	tr	1	tr
raw	1 (4.4 oz)	76	110	0.1	tr	0.5	80	15
raw chopped	¼ cup	16	25	tr	tr	0.1	17	3
LEMON								
fresh	1 med	22	32	0.1	tr	0.2	–	83
peel	1 tbsp	0	3	tr	tr	tr	–	8
wedge	1	5	8	tr	tr	0.1	–	21
LEMON CURD								
lemon curd made w/ egg	2 tsp	29	70	0	tr	0.1	–	1

FOOD	PORTION	CALS	VIT A	THIA	RIBO	NIACIN	FOLIC	VIT C
lemon curd made w/ starch	2 tsp	28	5	0	0	0	–	0
LEMON GRASS								
fresh	1 cup (2.4 oz)	66	7	tr	0.1	0.7	50	tr
fresh	1 tbsp (5 g)	5	1	0	tr	0.1	4	tr
LEMON JUICE								
bottled	1 tbsp	3	2	tr	tr	tr	2	4
fresh	1 tbsp	4	3	tr	tr	tr	2	7
frzn	1 tbsp	3	2	tr	tr	tr	1	5
LEMONADE								
as prep w/ water	1 cup	100	53	tr	0.1	tr	6	10
powder as prep w/ water	9 fl oz	113	0	0	tr	0	0	34
powder w/ equal	1 pitcher (67 oz)	40	0	0	0	0	0	47
LENTILS								
dried cooked	1 cup	231	15	0.3	0.1	2.1	358	3
yemiser selatta eithopian lentil salad	1 serv (3 oz)	115	89	0.1	tr	0.1	73	56
Shiloh Farms								
Organic Green not prep	¼ cup (1.6 oz)	150	0	–	–	–	–	0
Tasty Bite								
Bengal Lentils	½ pkg (5 oz)	190	0	–	–	–	–	0
Jodhpur Lentils	½ pkg (5 oz)	190	0	–	–	–	–	0
Madras Lentils	½ pkg (5 oz)	130	0	–	–	–	–	0
LETTUCE								
arugula	½ cup (0.4 oz)	3	235	0	tr	tr	10	2
bibb	1 head (6 oz)	21	1581	0.1	0.1	0.5	119	13
boston	2 leaves	2	146	tr	tr	tr	11	1
boston	1 head (6 oz)	21	1581	0.1	0.1	0.5	119	13
cornsalad field salad	1 cup (1.9 oz)	7	1790	tr	tr	0.2	80	19
iceberg	1 leaf	3	66	tr	tr	tr	11	1
iceberg	1 head (19 oz)	70	1779	0.2	0.2	1	302	21

FOOD	PORTION	CALS	VIT A	THIA	RIBO	NIACIN	FOLIC	VIT C
looseleaf shredded	½ cup	5	532	tr	tr	0.1	—	5
romaine shredded	½ cup	4	728	tr	tr	0.1	38	7
LILY ROOT								
dried	1 oz	89	25	tr	tr	0.7	—	5
fresh	1 oz	32	3	tr	tr	0.1	—	6
LIMA BEANS								
baby cooked	1 cup	229	0	0.3	0.1	1.2	273	0
cooked	½ cup	94	150	0.1	0.1	0.7	—	5
fordhook cooked	½ cup	85	162	0.1	0.1	0.9	—	11
large cooked	1 cup	217	0	0.3	0.1	0.8	156	0
Birds Eye								
Baby	½ cup	130	100	—	—	—	—	15
Fordhook	½ cup	100	100	—	—	—	—	15
Del Monte								
Green	½ cup (4.4 oz)	80	100	—	—	—	—	5
Eden								
Organic Baby	½ cup (4.6 oz)	100	0	0.4	0.1	0	8	0
Fresh Like								
Baby	3.5 oz	138	231	0.1	0.1	1.1	—	19
S&W								
Small Green	½ cup (4.4 oz)	80	100	—	—	—	—	5
Veg-All								
Baby Green	½ cup	90	0	—	—	—	—	0
LIME								
fresh	1	20	7	tr	tr	0.1	6	20
LIME JUICE								
bottled	1 tbsp	3	3	tr	tr	tr	1	1
fresh	1 tbsp	4	2	tr	tr	tr	—	5
LIQUOR/LIQUEUR								
aquavit	1 oz	65	0	—	—	—	—	0
bloody mary	5 oz	116	508	0.1	tr	0.6	20	20
bourbon & soda	4 oz	105	0	tr	0	tr	0	0
coffee liqueur	1½ oz	174	0	tr	tr	0.1	0	0

FOOD	PORTION	CALS	VIT A	THIA	RIBO	NIACIN	FOLIC	VIT C
cognac	1 oz	67	0	0	0	0	—	0
cosmopolitan	1 (4 oz)	213	tr	tr	tr	tr	1	13
daiquiri	2 oz	111	2	tr	tr	tr	1	1
gin	1½ oz	110	0	0	0	0	0	0
gin & tonic	7.5 oz	171	2	tr	0	tr	1	1
long island ice tea	1 serv (7.5 oz)	159	1	tr	tr	tr	1	5
manhattan	2 oz	128	0	tr	tr	0.1	tr	0
pina colada	4½ oz	262	3	tr	tr	0.2	14	7
rum	1½ oz	97	0	tr	0	0	0	0
screwdriver	7 oz	174	133	0.1	tr	0.3	75	67
sloe gin fizz	2½ oz	132	5	0	0	tr	tr	11
tequila sunrise	5½ oz	189	166	0.1	tr	0.3	—	13
tom collins	7½ oz	121	2	tr	tr	tr	2	4
vodka	1½ oz	97	0	tr	tr	0	0	0
whiskey	1½ oz	105	0	tr	0	tr	0	0
whiskey sour	3 oz	123	7	0.2	tr	0.1	5	11

LIVER

FOOD	PORTION	CALS	VIT A	THIA	RIBO	NIACIN	FOLIC	VIT C
beef braised	3 oz	137	30327	0.2	3.5	9.1	184	19
beef pan-fried	3 oz	184	30689	0.2	3.5	12.3	187	19
chicken stewed	1 cup (5 oz)	219	22925	0.2	2.4	6.2	1077	22
lamb braised	3 oz	187	21203	0.2	3.4	10.3	62	3
lamb fried	3 oz	202	22098	0.3	3.9	14.2	340	11
pork braised	3 oz	140	5297	0.2	1.9	7.2	139	20
turkey simmered	1 cup (5 oz)	237	17614	0.1	2	8.3	932	3
veal braised	3 oz	140	22851	0.1	1.7	7.2	645	26
veal fried	3 oz	208	15978	0.2	2.9	14.4	272	18

LOGANBERRIES

FOOD	PORTION	CALS	VIT A	THIA	RIBO	NIACIN	FOLIC	VIT C
frzn	1 cup	80	52	0.1	0.1	1.2	38	23

LOTUS

FOOD	PORTION	CALS	VIT A	THIA	RIBO	NIACIN	FOLIC	VIT C
root raw sliced	10 slices	45	0	0.1	0.2	0.3	—	36
root sliced cooked	10 slices	59	0	0.1	tr	0.3	—	24
seeds dried	1 oz	94	14	0.2	tr	0.5	—	0
Eden								
Root	1 serv (0.3 oz)	35	0	0	0	0	0	0

LYCHEES

FOOD	PORTION	CALS	VIT A	THIA	RIBO	NIACIN	FOLIC	VIT C
fresh	1	6	0	tr	tr	0.1	—	7

FOOD	PORTION	CALS	VIT A	THIA	RIBO	NIACIN	FOLIC	VIT C
MACADAMIA NUTS								
oil roasted	1 oz	204	3	0.1	tr	0.6	–	0
Hawaiian Host								
Chocolate Covered	1 piece (0.5 oz)	53	0	–	–	–	–	0
MACKEREL								
atlantic	3.5 oz	296	350	0.1	0.4	10	1	0
atlantic raw	3 oz	174	140	0.2	0.3	7.7	–	tr
jack	1 cup	296	825	0.1	0.4	11.7	10	2
jack	1 can (12.7 oz)	563	1567	0.1	0.8	22.3	19	3
Eden								
Bonito Flakes	2 tbsp	4	0	–	–	–	–	0
MALANGA								
fresh	½ cup	137	0	–	–	–	–	8
MALTED MILK								
chocolate as prep w/ milk	1 cup	229	326	0.1	0.4	0.6	16	3
chocolate flavor powder	3 heaping tsp (¾ oz)	79	19	tr	tr	0.4	4	tr
natural flavor as prep w/ milk	1 cup	237	369	0.2	0.6	1.3	22	3
natural flavor powder	3 heaping tsp (¾ oz)	87	61	0.1	0.2	1.1	10	1
MAMMY-APPLE								
fresh	1	431	1946	0.2	0.3	3.4	–	118
MANGO								
fresh	1	135	8060	0.1	0.1	1.2	–	57
Del Monte								
In Extra Light Syrup	½ cup (4.4 oz)	100	750	–	–	–	–	42
MANGO JUICE								
Fresh Samantha								
Mango Mama	1 cup (8 oz)	120	2250	0.2	0.1	0.8	32	30
MARGARINE								
squeeze	1 tsp	34	155	tr	tr	tr	tr	tr

FOOD	PORTION	CALS	VIT A	THIA	RIBO	NIACIN	FOLIC	VIT C
stick corn	1 stick (4 oz)	815	3750	tr	tr	tr	1	tr
stick corn	1 tsp	34	155	0	tr	tr	tr	tr
tub corn	1 tsp	34	155	0	tr	tr	tr	tr
tub diet	1 tsp	17	159	0	tr	tr	tr	tr
MARLIN								
raw	3 oz	110	20	0.1	0.1	3.8	—	1
MARSHMALLOW								
marshmallow	1 reg (0.3 oz)	23	0	0	0	tr	0	0
marshmallow	1 cup (1.6 oz)	146	0	0	0	tr	—	0
MATZO								
plain	1 (1 oz)	112	0	0.1	0.1	1.1	4	0
whole wheat	1 (1 oz)	99	0	0.1	0.1	1.5	10	0
Manischewitz								
Matzo Meal	¼ cup (1 oz)	130	0	—	—	—	—	0
MEAT SUBSTITUTES								
Quorn								
Grounds	⅔ cup (3 oz)	80	0	—	—	—	—	0
Yves								
Veggie Bologna	4 slices (2.2 oz)	70	0	0.3	tr	—	—	0
Veggie Ground Italian	⅓ cup (2 oz)	60	0	0.2	0.1	3	—	0
Veggie Ground Round Italian	⅓ cup (1.9 oz)	60	0	0.2	0.1	3	—	0
Veggie Ground Round Original	2 oz	60	0	0.2	0.1	3	—	0
Veggie Pizza Pepperoni Slices	1 serv (1.7 oz)	70	0	0.3	—	—	—	0
Veggie Salami Deli Slices	1 serv (2.2 oz)	90	200	0.3	—	—	—	0
MELON								
melon balls frzn	1 cup	55	3096	0.3	tr	1.1	45	11
Sunfresh								
Melon Salad In Extra Light Syrup	½ cup (4.5 oz)	45	400	—	—	—	—	30

FOOD	PORTION	CALS	VIT A	THIA	RIBO	NIACIN	FOLIC	VIT C
MILK								
1%	1 cup	102	500	0.1	0.4	0.2	12	2
1%	1 qt	409	2000	0.4	1.6	0.8	50	9
2%	1 cup	121	500	0.1	0.4	0.2	12	2
2%	1 qt	485	2000	0.4	1.6	0.8	50	9
buttermilk	1 cup	99	81	0.1	0.4	0.1	–	2
buttermilk	1 tbsp	25	14	tr	0.1	0.1	3	tr
buttermilk	1 qt	396	323	0.3	1.5	0.6	–	10
condensed sweetened	1 oz	123	125	tr	0.2	0.1	4	1
condensed sweetened	1 cup	982	1004	0.3	1.3	0.6	34	8
evaporated	½ cup	169	306	0.1	0.4	0.2	10	2
evaporated skim	½ cup	99	500	0.1	0.4	0.2	11	2
goat	1 cup	168	451	0.1	0.3	0.7	1	3
goat	1 qt	672	1806	0.5	1.3	2.7	6	13
human	1 cup	171	593	tr	0.1	0.4	13	12
indian buffalo	1 cup	236	434	0.1	0.3	0.2	14	5
mare	7 oz	98	tr	tr	tr	0.2	–	30
nonfat	1 cup	86	500	0.1	0.3	0.2	13	2
nonfat	1 qt	342	2000	0.4	1.4	0.9	51	10
nonfat instantized	1 pkg (3.2 oz)	244	2157	0.4	1.6	0.8	45	5
sheep	1 cup	264	360	0.2	0.9	1	–	10
whole	1 cup	150	307	0.1	0.4	0.2	12	2
Lactaid								
1%	8 fl oz	102	500	0.1	0.4	0.2	12	2
Nonfat	8 fl oz	86	500	0.1	0.3	0.2	13	2
NutraBalance								
LactaCare	1 pkg (8 oz)	500	1026	0.6	0.8	6.2	120	20
Turkey Hill								
Cool Moos 2% Reduced Fat	1 cup	130	750	–	–	–	–	1
Cool Moos Whole Milk	1 cup	160	300	–	–	–	–	2
MILK DRINKS								
chocolate milk	1 cup	208	302	0.1	0.4	0.3	12	2
chocolate milk	1 qt	833	1210	0.4	1.6	1.3	47	9

FOOD	PORTION	CALS	VIT A	THIA	RIBO	NIACIN	FOLIC	VIT C
chocolate milk 1%	1 cup	158	500	0.1	0.4	0.3	12	2
chocolate milk 1%	1 qt	630	2000	0.4	1.7	1.3	48	9
chocolate milk 2%	1 cup	179	500	0.1	0.4	0.3	12	2
strawberry flavor mix as prep w/ whole milk	9 oz	234	308	0.1	0.4	0.2	12	2
Lactaid								
Chocolate Milk 1%	8 fl oz	158	500	0.1	0.4	0.3	12	2
Turkey Hill								
Cool Moos Chocolate 1% Lowfat	1 cup	180	500	–	–	–	–	1
Cool Moos Orange Cream 1% Lowfat	1 cup	190	2000	–	–	–	–	36
Cool Moos Strawberry 1% Lowfat	1 cup	160	500	–	–	–	–	2
Cool Moos Vanilla 1% Lowfat	1 cup	160	500	–	–	–	–	2

MILK SUBSTITUTES

FOOD	PORTION	CALS	VIT A	THIA	RIBO	NIACIN	FOLIC	VIT C
imitation milk	1 cup	150	0	tr	0.2	0	0	0
imitation milk	1 qt	600	0	0.1	0.9	0	0	0
8th Continent								
Soymilk Low Fat Chocolate	1 bottle (8 oz)	140	500	–	0.4	–	–	0
Soymilk Low Fat Original	1 bottle (8 oz)	80	500	–	0.4	–	–	0
Soymilk Low Fat Vanilla	1 bottle (8 oz)	90	500	–	0.4	–	–	0
Better Than Milk								
Rice Original	2 tbsp (0.66 oz)	78	500	–	–	–	–	6
Rice Original Light	2 tbsp (0.66 oz)	66	0	–	–	–	–	0
Rice Vanilla	2 tbsp (0.66 oz)	78	500	–	–	–	–	6
Rice Vanilla Light	2 tbsp (0.66 oz)	66	0	–	–	–	–	0

FOOD	PORTION	CALS	VIT A	THIA	RIBO	NIACIN	FOLIC	VIT C
Soy Carob	2 tbsp (1 oz)	90	500	–	–	–	–	6
Soy Chocolate	2 tbsp (1.1 oz)	112	500	–	–	–	–	6
Soy Light	2 tbsp (0.66 oz)	73	500	–	–	–	–	6
Soy Original	2 tbsp (0.8 oz)	100	0	–	–	–	–	0
Soy Vanilla	2 tbsp (0.7 oz)	77	500	–	–	–	–	6
EdenBlend								
Organic	8 oz	120	0	0.1	0.1	0.4	28	0
Edensoy								
Organic Light	8 oz	93	0	0.1	0.1	0.9	48	0
Organic Light Vanilla	8 oz	120	0	0.1	0.1	1.7	69	0
Galaxy								
Veggie Milk Chocolate	1 cup (8 oz)	150	1250	–	0.1	–	100	5
Veggie Milk Original	1 cup (8 oz)	110	1250	–	0.1	–	100	5
Hansen's								
Soy Smoothie Lemon Chiffon	8 oz	150	5000	–	–	–	–	60
Soy Smoothie Orange Dream	8 oz	150	5000	–	–	–	–	60
Harmony House								
Enriched Rice Beverage	1 cup (8 oz)	90	500	–	–	–	–	15
Enriched Soy Beverage	1 cup (8 oz)	90	0	–	–	–	–	0
Original Soy Beverage	1 cup (8 oz)	90	0	–	–	–	–	0
Silk								
Chocolate	1 cup	140	500	–	0.1	–	24	0
Organic Plain	1 cup	100	500	–	0.5	–	24	0
Vanilla	1 bottle (11 oz)	140	750	–	0.7	–	32	0
Soy Dream								
Carob	8 oz	210	0	0.2	0.1	0.8	60	0
Chocolate Enriched	8 oz	210	500	0.2	0.1	0.8	60	0

FOOD	PORTION	CALS	VIT A	THIA	RIBO	NIACIN	FOLIC	VIT C
Original	8 oz	140	0	0.2	0.1	0.8	80	0
Original Enriched	8 oz	140	500	0.2	0.1	0.8	80	0
Vanilla	8 oz	170	0	0.2	0.1	1.2	80	0
Vanilla Enriched	8 oz	140	500	0.2	0.1	1.2	80	0
Tree Of Life								
Original Rice Beverage	1 cup	90	0	—	—	—	—	0
Vegelicious								
Milk	8 fl oz	100	500	0.2	0.2	2.0	40	6
Vitamite								
Non-Dairy	1 cup (8 oz)	110	500	0.2	0.3	—	—	0
Vitasoy								
1% Low Fat Vanilla Delight	8 oz	90	500	—	—	—	—	0
Carob Supreme	8 fl oz	150	0	—	—	—	—	0
Creamy Unsweetened	8 oz	80	500	—	—	—	—	0
Creamy Original	8 fl oz	110	0	—	—	—	—	0
Enriched Light Original	8 fl oz	60	500	—	—	—	—	0
Enriched Light Vanilla	8 fl oz	90	500	—	—	—	—	0
Green Tea Soymilk	8 oz	130	0	—	—	—	—	0
Original Creamy	8 fl oz	110	500	—	—	—	—	0
Original Light	8 fl oz	60	500	—	—	—	—	0
Rich Chocolate	8 fl oz	160	500	—	—	—	—	0
Rich Cocoa	8 fl oz	150	0	—	—	—	—	0
Vanilla Light	8 fl oz	90	0	—	—	—	—	0
Vanilla Delite	8 fl oz	120	0	—	—	—	—	0
White Wave								
Mocha	1 cup	140	300	—	0.4	—	—	0

MILKSHAKE

FOOD	PORTION	CALS	VIT A	THIA	RIBO	NIACIN	FOLIC	VIT C
chocolate	10 oz	360	263	0.2	0.7	0.5	10	1
strawberry	10 oz	319	340	0.1	0.6	0.5	9	2
thick shake chocolate	10.6 oz	356	258	0.1	0.7	0.4	15	0
thick shake vanilla	11 oz	350	357	0.1	0.6	0.5	21	0
vanilla	10 oz	314	368	0.1	0.5	0.5	9	2

FOOD	PORTION	CALS	VIT A	THIA	RIBO	NIACIN	FOLIC	VIT C
MILLET								
cooked	1 cup (6.1 oz)	207	0	0.2	0.1	2.3	33	0
MISO								
dried	1 oz	86	0	tr	tr	0.6	–	0
miso	½ cup	284	120	0.1	0.3	1.1	46	0
Eden								
Organic Genmai	1 tbsp	25	0	tr	0.3	0	0	0
Tekka	1 tsp	5	4	–	–	–	–	0
MOTH BEANS								
dried cooked	1 cup	207	17	0.2	tr	1.2	–	2
MOUSSE								
Sara Lee								
Chocolate	⅓ pkg (4.3 oz)	400	200	–	–	–	–	0
MUFFIN								
corn	1 (1.75 oz)	160	105	0.1	0.1	1.1	6	tr
raisin bran lowfat	1 (4 oz)	270	0	0.2	–	–	–	0
toaster type blueberry	1	103	105	0.1	0.1	0.7	–	0
toaster type corn	1	114	32	0.1	0.1	0.8	–	0
toaster type wheat bran w/ raisins	1 (1.3 oz)	106	64	0.1	0.1	0.9	–	0
wheat bran as prep	1 (1¼ oz)	138	51	0.1	0.1	1.4	–	0
Hodgson Mill								
Bran	¼ cup (1.3 oz)	130	0	–	–	–	–	0
Cornbread	¼ cup (1.3 oz)	130	0	–	–	–	–	0
Otis Spunkmeyer								
Apple Cinnamon	1 (2 oz)	220	0	–	–	–	–	1
Low Fat Wild Blueberry	1 (2.25 oz)	200	0	–	–	–	–	0
Mayport Cheese Streusel	½ muffin (2 oz)	220	100	0.1	0.1	0.8	32	0
Mayport Harvest Bran	1 (2.25 oz)	240	0	2	0.1	1.2	32	0

FOOD	PORTION	CALS	VIT A	THIA	RIBO	NIACIN	FOLIC	VIT C
Mayport Low Fat Apple Cinnamon	1 (4 oz)	380	100	0.2	0.3	1.6	60	0
Mayport Low Fat Banana Nut	1 (4 oz)	350	100	0.2	0.3	1.6	60	0
Mayport Low Fat Chocolate Chocolate Chip	1 (4 oz)	370	100	0.2	0.3	1.6	60	0
MULBERRIES								
fresh	1 cup	61	35	tr	0.1	0.9	–	51
MUNG BEANS								
dried cooked	1 cup	213	48	0.3	0.1	1.2	321	2
MUNGO BEANS								
dried cooked	1 cup	190	56	0.3	0.1	2.7	170	2
MUSHROOMS								
chanterelle	3.5 oz	12	1	–	–	–	–	3
cloud ear	1 (5 g)	13	0	0	tr	0.3	2	0
cloud ears	1 cup (1 oz)	80	0	0	0.2	1.8	11	0
enoki raw	1 (4 in)	2	0	tr	tr	0.2	1	1
oyster raw	1 lg (5.2 oz)	55	71	0.1	0.5	5.3	70	0
oyster raw	1 sm (0.5 oz)	6	7	tr	0.1	0.5	7	0
portabella	1 serv (2 oz)	14	0	tr	0.1	1.3	6	0
raw	1 (½ oz)	5	0	tr	0.1	0.7	4	1
raw sliced	½ cup	9	0	tr	0.2	1.4	7	1
shitake cooked	4 (2.5 oz)	40	0	tr	0.1	1.1	–	tr
sliced cooked	½ cup	21	0	0.1	0.1	3.5	14	3
straw	1 piece (6 g)	2	0	0	0	tr	2	0
straw	1 cup (6.4 oz)	58	0	tr	0.1	0.4	69	0
tree ear	½ cup (0.4 oz)	36	8	0.1	tr	0.4	19	0
whole cooked	1 (0.4 oz)	3	0	tr	tr	0.5	2	1
MUSTARD								
yellow ready-to-use	1 tsp	5	0	0	0	0	–	0
Boar's Head								
Delicatessen Style	1 tsp (5 g)	0	0	–	–	–	–	0
Honey	1 tsp (5 g)	10	0	–	–	–	–	0

FOOD	PORTION	CALS	VIT A	THIA	RIBO	NIACIN	FOLIC	VIT C
Eden								
Organic Stone Ground	1 tsp	0	0	0	0	0	0	0
Luzianne								
Creole Mustard	1 tbsp	10	0	–	–	–	–	0
MUSTARD GREENS								
fresh chopped cooked	½ cup	11	2122	tr	tr	0.3	–	18
frozen chopped cooked	½ cup	14	3352	tr	tr	0.2	–	10
Birds Eye								
Chopped	1 cup	30	2250	–	–	–	–	15
NATTO								
natto	½ cup	187	0	0.1	0.2	0	–	11
NAVY BEANS								
cooked	1 cup	259	3	0.4	0.1	1	255	2
NECTARINE								
fresh	1	67	1001	tr	0.1	1.3	5	7
NEUFCHATEL								
neufchatel	1 oz	74	321	tr	0.1	tr	3	0
neufchatel	1 pkg (3 oz)	221	964	tr	0.2	0.1	10	0
NOODLE DISHES								
noodle pudding	½ cup	132	260	0.1	0.1	0.5	8	1
Annie Chun								
Chow Mein Noodles w/ Garlic Black Bean Sauce	1 serv	230	0	–	–	–	–	5
Japanese Soba Noodles w/ Soy Ginger Sauce	1 serv	210	0	–	–	–	–	2
Kraft								
Noodle Classics Cheddar Cheese as prep	1 cup (7.4 oz)	400	750	0.3	0.2	3	40	0
Noodle Classics Savory Chicken as prep	1 cup (8.5 oz)	340	200	0.3	0.2	3	40	0

FOOD	PORTION	CALS	VIT A	THIA	RIBO	NIACIN	FOLIC	VIT C
Lipton								
Noodles & Sauce Alfredo Broccoli as prep	1 cup (2.2 oz)	340	500	0.6	0.4	4	100	5
Noodles & Sauce Alfredo as prep	1 cup (2.2 oz)	330	500	0.6	0.3	4	100	0
Noodles & Sauce Beef as prep	1 cup (2.1 oz)	280	300	0.6	0.3	4	100	0
Noodles & Sauce Butter as prep	1 cup (2.2 oz)	310	400	0.6	0.3	4	100	0
Noodles & Sauce Butter & Herb as prep	1 cup (2.2 oz)	300	200	0.6	0.3	4	100	0
Noodles & Sauce Chicken Broccoli as prep	1 cup (2.1 oz)	310	400	0.6	0.4	4	100	4
Noodles & Sauce Chicken Tetrazzini as prep	1 cup (2 oz)	300	500	0.6	0.3	4	100	0
Noodles & Sauce Chicken as prep	1 cup (2.1 oz)	290	500	0.7	0.3	5	100	0
Noodles & Sauce Creamy Chicken as prep	1 cup (2.1 oz)	320	1000	0.6	0.3	4	100	0
Noodles & Sauce Parmesan as prep	1 cup (2.1 oz)	330	500	0.6	0.3	4	100	2
Noodles & Sauce Sour Cream & Chives as prep	1 cup (2.2 oz)	310	400	0.6	0.3	4	100	1
Noodles & Sauce Stroganoff as prep	1 cup (2 oz)	300	500	0.6	0.3	4	100	0
NOODLES								
cellophane	1 cup	492	0	0.2	0	0.3	–	0
chow mein	1 cup (1.6 oz)	237	39	0.2	0.2	2.6	39	0
egg cooked	1 cup (5.6 oz)	213	32	0.3	0.1	2.4	102	0

FOOD	PORTION	CALS	VIT A	THIA	RIBO	NIACIN	FOLIC	VIT C
japanese soba cooked	1 cup (4 oz)	113	0	0.1	tr	0.6	8	0
japanese somen cooked	1 cup (6.2 oz)	231	0	tr	0.1	0.2	4	0
korean acorn noodles not prep	2 oz	195	0	0.5	0	2.2	—	0
rice cooked	1 cup (6.2 oz)	192	0	tr	tr	0.1	5	0
spinach/egg cooked	1 cup (5.6 oz)	211	165	0.4	0.2	2.4	102	0
Annie Chun								
Chow Mein	2 oz	200	0	—	—	—	—	0
Rice	2 oz	210	0	—	—	—	—	0
Rice Hunan	2 oz	210	0	—	—	—	—	0
Rice Pad Thai	2 oz	210	0	—	—	—	—	0
Rice Pad Thai Basil	2 oz	210	0	—	—	—	—	0
Azumaya								
Spinach	1 cup	210	0	—	—	—	—	0
Thin Cut	1 cup	210	0	—	—	—	—	0
Wide Cut	1 cup	210	0	—	—	—	—	0
Eden								
Kudzu	2 oz	200	0	0	0	0	0	0
Golden Grain								
Egg	2 oz	210	0	0.6	0.3	4.5	27	0
Hodgson Mill								
Four Color Veggie Egg	2 oz	200	0	0.6	0.3	4.0	—	0
Whole Wheat Egg	2 oz	190	100	0.3	0.1	1.6	—	0
Manischewitz								
Fine Yolk Free	1½ cups	210	0	0.5	0.2	3	120	0
Fine Egg	1½ cups	220	0	0.5	0.2	3	120	0
Nasoya								
Chinese	1 cup	210	0	—	—	—	—	0
Japanese	1 cup	210	0	—	—	—	—	0
Spinach	1 cup	210	0	—	tr	—	—	0

NOPALES

FOOD	PORTION	CALS	VIT A	THIA	RIBO	NIACIN	FOLIC	VIT C
cooked	1 cup (5.2 oz)	23	685	tr	0.1	0.4	4	8

FOOD	PORTION	CALS	VIT A	THIA	RIBO	NIACIN	FOLIC	VIT C
NUTRITION SUPPLEMENTS								
Enlive!								
Drink All Flavors	1 box (8.1 oz)	300	1250	–	–	–	–	24
Ensure								
Supplement All Flavors	1 can (8 fl oz)	250	1250	0.4	0.4	5	100	30
GeniSoy								
Soy Natural Protein Powder	1 scoop (1 oz)	100	1250	0.4	0.4	5	100	15
Glucerna								
Shakes All Flavors	1 can (8 oz)	220	1750	–	–	–	–	60
Met-Rx								
Lite	1 pkg (1.6 oz)	170	2500	0.8	0.9	10	200	30
Original	1 pkg (2.5 oz)	250	4500	0.9	1	20	400	60
Protein Shake	1 can	200	2250	0.5	0.5	10	200	78
Ultra	1 pkg (2.6 oz)	250	2500	0.8	0.9	10	200	30
Nestle								
Additions	2⅓ tsp (0.7 oz)	100	0	–	–	–	–	0
NutraBalance								
EggPro	1 tbsp (7.5 g)	30	0	tr	0.2	tr	tr	0
Nutribar								
Shake Chocolate Supreme as prep w/ 2% milk	1 serv (10 oz) (4.6 oz)	262	1750	0.5	0.6	7.6	140	13
Shake Vanilla as prep w/ 2% milk	1 (10 oz)	259	1750	0.5	0.6	7.6	140	13
PermaLean								
Protein Powder Bodacious Berry	1 scoop (1 oz)	104	tr	–	–	–	–	tr
Protein Powder Chocoholic Chocolate	1 scoop (1 oz)	104	tr	–	–	–	–	tr
Pounds Off								
All Flavors	1 bar (2.1 oz)	210	5000	1.5	1.7	20	400	60

FOOD	PORTION	CALS	VIT A	THIA	RIBO	NIACIN	FOLIC	VIT C
NUTS MIXED								
dry roasted w/ peanuts	1 oz	169	4	0.1	0.1	1.3	14	tr
mixed nuts chocolate covered	¼ cup (1.5 oz)	240	100	–	–	–	–	0
oil roasted w/ peanuts	1 oz	175	6	0.1	0.1	1.4	24	tr
oil roasted w/o peanuts	1 oz	175	6	0.1	0.1	0.6	16	tr
Maranatha								
Cashew Macadamia Butter	2 tbsp	210	0	–	–	–	–	0
Tamari Organic	¼ cup	160	0	–	–	–	–	0
Tamari Roasted	¼ cup	160	0	–	–	–	–	0
OHELOBERRIES								
fresh	1 cup	39	1162	tr	0.1	0.4	–	8
OIL								
Eden								
Olive Spanish Extra Virgin	1 tbsp	120	0	0	0	0	0	0
OKRA								
sliced cooked	1 pkg (10 oz)	94	1311	0.3	0.3	2	371	31
sliced cooked	½ cup	25	460	0.1	tr	0.7	37	13
sliced cooked	8 pods	27	489	0.1	tr	0.7	39	14
Birds Eye								
Cut	¾ cup	25	100	–	–	–	–	2
Whole	9 pods	25	100	–	–	–	–	2
OLIVES								
green	4 med	15	40	tr	tr	tr	–	0
green	3 extra lg	15	40	tr	tr	tr	–	0
green olive tapenade	1 tbsp	25	200	–	–	–	–	2
ripe	1 sm	4	13	0	0	0	0	0
ripe	1 lg	5	18	0	0	.0	0	0
ripe	1 colossal	12	53	–	–	0	–	tr
ripe	1 jumbo	7	29	–	–	0	–	tr

FOOD	PORTION	CALS	VIT A	THIA	RIBO	NIACIN	FOLIC	VIT C
Vlasic								
Ripe Colossal Pitted	2 (0.6 oz)	20	0	–	–	–	–	0
Ripe Jumbo Pitted	3 (0.6 oz)	25	0	–	–	–	–	0
Ripe Large Pitted	4 (0.5 oz)	25	0	–	–	–	–	0
Ripe Medium Pitted	5 (0.5 oz)	25	0	–	–	–	–	0
Ripe Sliced	¼ cup (0.5 oz)	25	0	–	–	–	–	0
Ripe Small Pitted	6 (0.5 oz)	25	0	–	–	–	–	0
ONION								
chopped cooked	1 tbsp	4	5	tr	tr	tr	0	tr
chopped cooked	½ cup	30	36	tr	tr	0.1	14	3
flakes	1 tbsp	16	0	tr	tr	0.1	8	4
fried	½ cup (7.5 oz)	176	540	0.1	0.1	0.4	–	20
raw chopped	1 tbsp	4	0	tr	tr	tr	2	1
raw chopped	½ cup	30	0	tr	tr	0.1	15	5
rings	7 (2.5 oz)	285	158	0.2	0.1	2.5	9	1
scallions raw chopped	1 tbsp	2	23	tr	tr	tr	4	1
scallions raw sliced	½ cup	16	193	tr	tr	0.3	32	9
whole cooked	3½ oz	28	21	tr	tr	0.1	13	5
Antioch Farms								
Vidalia	1 med	60	tr	tr	tr	tr	tr	12
Birds Eye								
Diced	⅔ cup	30	0	–	–	–	–	0
Pearl Onions In Real Cream Sauce	½ cup	60	0	–	–	–	–	0
Small Whole	17	30	0	–	–	–	–	6
Boar's Head								
Sweet Vidalia In Sauce	1 tbsp	10	0	–	–	–	–	1
ORANGE								
california navel	1	65	256	0.1	0.1	0.4	47	80
california valencia	1	59	278	0.1	tr	0.3	47	59
florida	1	69	302	0.2	0.1	0.6	26	68
peel	1 tbsp	6	25	tr	tr	0.1	–	8
sections	1 cup	85	369	0.2	0.1	0.5	55	96

FOOD	PORTION	CALS	VIT A	THIA	RIBO	NIACIN	FOLIC	VIT C
Del Monte								
Mandarin In Light Syrup	½ cup (4.5 oz)	80	0	–	–	–	–	4
ORANGE JUICE								
canned	1 cup	104	432	0.1	0.1	0.8	–	86
chilled	1 cup	110	194	0.3	0.1	0.7	45	82
fresh	1 cup	111	496	0.2	0.1	1	–	124
frzn as prep	1 cup	112	194	0.2	tr	0.5	109	97
mandarin orange	7 oz	94	tr	0.2	tr	0.4	–	64
orange drink	6 oz	94	33	tr	tr	0.1	–	64
Fresh Samantha								
Juice	1 cup (8 oz)	100	400	0.2	0	0	40	72
OYSTERS								
breaded & fried	6 (4.9 oz)	368	363	0.3	0.4	4.4	13	4
stew	1 cup	278	892	0.2	0.5	2.6	14	4
PANCAKE/WAFFLE SYRUP								
low calorie	1 tbsp	12	0	0	0	0	0	0
pancake syrup	1 cup (11 oz)	903	0	–	–	–	0	0
pancake syrup	1 tbsp (0.7 oz)	57	0	–	–	–	0	0
pancake syrup light	1 oz	46	0	–	–	–	0	0
pancake syrup w/ butter	1 tbsp (0.7 oz)	59	12	–	–	–	0	0
pancake syrup w/ butter	1 cup (11 oz)	933	193	–	–	–	0	0
PANCAKES								
blueberry	1 (4 in diam)	84	76	0.1	0.1	0.6	5	1
buckwheat	1 (4 in diam)	62	70	0.1	0.2	0.4	–	tr
plain	1 (4 in diam)	86	75	0.1	0.1	0.6	5	tr
potato	1 (4 in diam)	78	27	tr	0.1	0.3	7	4
w/ butter & syrup	2 (8.1 oz)	520	281	0.4	0.6	3.4	30	4
whole wheat	1 (4 in diam)	92	99	0.1	0.2	1	–	tr
Bisquick								
Shake 'N Pour Blueberry as prep	3	210	0	0.2	0.2	1.2	40	0

FOOD	PORTION	CALS	VIT A	THIA	RIBO	NIACIN	FOLIC	VIT C
Bruce								
Sweet Potato Pancakes	2	210	750	–	–	–	40	5
Eggo								
Buttermilk	3 (4.1 oz)	270	1000	0.3	0.3	4	60	0
Hodgson Mill								
Buckwheat	⅓ cup (1.8 oz)	160	0	–	–	–	–	0
PAPAYA								
fresh	1	117	6122	0.1	0.1	1	–	188
fresh cubed	1 cup	54	2819	tr	tr	0.5	–	87
Sunfresh								
In Extra Light Syrup	½ cup (4.5 oz)	70	300	–	–	–	–	5
PAPAYA JUICE								
nectar	1 cup	142	277	tr	tr	0.4	5	8
PAPRIKA								
paprika	1 tsp	6	1273	tr	tr	0.3	–	1
PARSLEY								
dry	1 tsp	1	70	tr	tr	tr	–	tr
dry	1 tbsp	1	253	tr	tr	tr	6	1
fresh chopped	½ cup	11	1560	tr	tr	0.4	46	40
PARSNIPS								
fresh cooked	1 (5.6 oz)	130	0	0.1	0.1	1.2	93	21
fresh sliced cooked	½ cup	63	0	0.1	tr	0.6	45	10
PASSION FRUIT								
purple fresh	1	18	126	–	tr	0.3	–	5
PASSION FRUIT JUICE								
purple	1 cup	126	1771	–	0.3	3.6	–	74
yellow	1 cup	149	5953	–	0.2	5.5	–	45
PASTA								
cooked	2 oz	75	11	0.1	0.1	0.6	36	0
corn cooked	1 cup (4.9 oz)	176	80	0.1	0	0.8	8	0
elbows cooked	1 cup (4.9 oz)	197	0	0.3	0.1	2.3	98	0

FOOD	PORTION	CALS	VIT A	THIA	RIBO	NIACIN	FOLIC	VIT C
shells small cooked	1 cup (4 oz)	162	0	0.2	0.1	1.9	81	0
spaghetti cooked	1 cup (4.9 oz)	197	0	0.3	0.1	2.3	98	0
spinach spaghetti cooked	1 cup (4.9 oz)	182	213	0.1	0.1	2.1	17	0
spinach cooked	2 oz	74	59	0.1	0.1	0.6	36	0
spirals cooked	1 cup (4.7 oz)	189	0	0.3	0.1	2.2	94	0
vegetable cooked	1 cup (4.7 oz)	172	71	0.2	0.1	1.4	87	0
whole wheat cooked	1 cup (4.9 oz)	174	0	0.2	0.1	1	7	0
whole wheat spaghetti cooked	1 cup (4.9 oz)	174	0	0.2	0.1	1	7	0
Barilla								
Conchiglie Rigate	1 cup (2 oz)	200	0	0.5	0.3	3	120	0
Pennette Rigate	1⅓ cups (2 oz)	200	0	4.3	0.3	3	120	0
Tortelloni Porcini Mushroom	¾ cup	240	0	–	–	–	–	0
Tortelloni Ricotta & Asparagus	¾ cup	240	100	–	–	–	–	0
Tortelloni Ricotta & Spinach	¾ cup	220	300	–	–	–	–	0
Cuore								
Capellini cooked	1⅓ cup (2 oz)	190	0	0.5	0.3	3	120	0
Fusilli cooked	1⅓ cup (2 oz)	190	0	0.5	0.3	3	120	0
Tortiglioni cooked	1⅓ cup (2 oz)	190	0	0.5	0.3	3	120	0
Di Giorno								
Angel's Hair	1 cup	160	0	0.4	0.2	3	40	0
Beef & Roasted Garlic Tortellini	1 cup	340	0	0.8	0.3	4	60	0
Fettuccine	1 cup	200	0	0.5	0.2	4	60	0
Four Cheese Raviolo	1 cup	350	400	0.6	0.4	3	60	0
Herb Linguine	1 cup	200	0	0.5	0.3	4	60	0
Italian Sausage Ravioli In Green Bell Pepper Pasta	1¼ cup	350	200	0.9	0.4	4	60	0

FOOD	PORTION	CALS	VIT A	THIA	RIBO	NIACIN	FOLIC	VIT C
Lemon Chicken Tortellini In Cracked Black Pepper Pasta	1 cup	270	100	0.7	0.3	5	40	0
Light Cheese Ravioli	1 cup	280	400	0.6	0.4	3	60	0
Linguine	1 cup	200	0	0.5	0.3	4	60	0
Mozzarella Garlic Tortelloni	1 cup	300	200	0.6	0.3	4	60	0
Pesto Tortelloni	1 cup	320	200	0.9	0.4	4	60	0
Portabello Mushroom Tortelloni	1 cup	310	300	0.8	0.3	4	60	0
Red Bell Pepper Fettuccine	1 cup	200	300	0.5	0.2	4	60	2
Spinach Fettuccine	1 cup	190	200	0.5	0.3	4	60	0
Sun-Dried Tomato Ravioli	1⅓ cup	380	750	0.9	0.4	4	60	1
Three Cheese Tortellini	¾ cup	250	100	0.5	0.3	2	40	0
Duc Amici								
Pasta Lite Low Carb Fusilli	2 oz	160	0	—	—	—	—	0
Eden								
Organic Extra Fine	2 oz	210	200	0.2	0.1	1.6	—	0
Organic Gemelli	2 oz	210	0	0.2	0.1	3	21	0
Organic Pesto Gemelli	2 oz	210	100	0.1	tr	1.6	18	0
Organic Ribbons Saffron	2 oz	210	200	0.2	0.1	1.6	9	0
Organic Spaghetti Semolina	2 oz	200	100	0.1	tr	1.6	9	0
Organic Spaghetti 50% Whole Grain	2 oz	210	0	0.2	0.1	3	18	0
Organic Spirals Kamut Vegetable	2 oz	210	200	0.2	0.1	0	24	0
Organic Spirals Sesame Rice	2 oz	200	0	0.3	0.1	8	16	0
Organic Spirals Mixed Grain	2 oz	210	0	0.1	0.1	2	32	0

FOOD	PORTION	CALS	VIT A	THIA	RIBO	NIACIN	FOLIC	VIT C
Organic Spirals Spinach	2 oz	210	0	0.2	0.1	3	18	0
Organic Vegetable Alphabets	2 oz	200	0	0.1	tr	1.6	9	0
Spirals Rye	2 oz	200	0	0.4	0.2	4	130	1
Hodgson Mill								
Four Color Veggie Bows	2 oz	200	0	0.6	0.3	4.0	120	0
Four Color Veggie Rotini Spirals	2 oz	200	0	0.6	0.3	4.0	120	0
Four Color Veggie Wagon Wheels	2 oz	200	0	0.6	0.3	4	120	0
Pastamania! Durum Wheat Fettuccine	2 oz	200	0	—	—	—	—	0
Pastamania! Fettuccine Garlic & Parsley	2 oz	200	0	—	—	—	—	0
Pastamania! Fettuccine w/ Jerusalem Artichoke	2 oz	210	0	—	—	—	—	0
Pastamania! Fettucinne w/ Mushroom	2 oz	210	0	—	—	—	—	0
Pastamania! Fusilli Tre Colore w/ Tomato & Spinach	2 oz	200	0	0.5	0.2	3	—	0
Pastamania! Pesto Fettuccine	2 oz	200	0	—	—	—	—	0
Pastamania! Sea Shell Mix	2 oz	200	0	0.6	0.3	4	—	0
Pastamania! Spinach Fettuccine	2 oz	200	0	—	—	—	—	0
Pastamania! Thin Linguine	2 oz	200	0	—	—	—	—	0

FOOD	PORTION	CALS	VIT A	THIA	RIBO	NIACIN	FOLIC	VIT C
Pastamania! Tomato Spinach & Durum Wheat	2 oz	210	200	–	–	–	–	0
Spaghetti Whole Wheat	2 oz	190	0	0.3	0.1	2.0	–	0
Real Torino								
Tirali not prep	1 cup (2 oz)	210	0	0.5	0.2	3	140	0

PASTA DINNERS

FOOD	PORTION	CALS	VIT A	THIA	RIBO	NIACIN	FOLIC	VIT C
lasagna	1 piece (2.5 in x 2.5 in)	374	1315	0.2	0.3	2.3	11	13
macaroni & cheese	1 cup	230	260	0.1	0.2	1	–	tr
manicotti	¾ cup (6.4 oz)	273	2613	0.2	0.2	3.1	17	12
rigatoni w/ sausage sauce	¾ cup	260	999	0.3	0.2	3.2	8	16
spaghetti w/ meatballs & cheese	1 cup	407	2724	0.3	0.3	4.9	22	45
Annie's Homegrown								
Mac & Cheese Meals	1 pkg	230	100	0.5	0.2	3	100	0
Banquet								
Chicken Pasta Primavera	1 meal (9.5 oz)	320	2500	–	–	–	–	0
Family Size Egg Noodles w/ Beef & Brown Gravy	1 serv	150	0	–	–	–	–	0
Family Size Lasagna w/ Meat Sauce	1 cup	270	300	–	–	–	–	54
Family Size Macaroni & Cheese	1 cup	230	100	–	–	–	–	0
Fettuccine Alfredo	1 meal (9.5 oz)	350	200	–	–	–	–	6
Homestyle Noodles & Chicken	1 meal (12 oz)	390	3500	–	–	–	–	0

FOOD	PORTION	CALS	VIT A	THIA	RIBO	NIACIN	FOLIC	VIT C
Lasagna w/ Meat Sauce	1 meal (9.5 oz)	260	750	—	—	—	—	1
Macaroni & Cheese	1 meal (12 oz)	420	0	—	—	—	—	0
Birds Eye								
Easy Recipe Creations Basil Herb Primavera	2¼ cup	260	1500	—	—	—	—	24
Easy Recipe Creations Tortellini Parmigiana	2¼ cups	240	2500	—	—	—	—	36
Pasta Secrets Italian Pesto	2⅓ cups	240	1500	—	—	—	—	18
Pasta Secrets Primavera	2⅓ cups	230	2000	—	—	—	—	30
Pasta Secrets Ranch	2⅓ cups	300	3000	—	—	—	—	4
Pasta Secrets Three Cheese	2 cups	230	1750	—	—	—	—	21
Pasta Secrets White Cheddar	2 cups	240	1250	—	—	—	—	21
Pasta Secrets Zesty Garlic	2 cups	240	1750	—	—	—	—	15
Chef Boyardee								
99% Fat Free Beef Ravioli	1 cup (8.6 oz)	210	750	—	—	—	—	0
99% Fat Free Cheese Ravioli	1 cup (8.8 oz)	210	500	—	—	—	—	1
Beef Ravioli	1 cup (8.6 oz)	230	750	—	—	—	—	0
Beefaroni	1 cup (8.7 oz)	260	300	—	—	—	—	0
Mini Ravioli	1 cup (8.8 oz)	252	500	—	—	—	—	0
Spaghetti & Meat Balls	1 cup (8.4 oz)	240	300	—	—	—	—	0
Franco-American								
Beef Raviolios	1 can (7.7 oz)	250	440	—	—	—	—	0
Beefy Mac	1 can (7.5 oz)	228	454	—	—	—	—	1

FOOD	PORTION	CALS	VIT A	THIA	RIBO	NIACIN	FOLIC	VIT C
Elbow Macaroni & Cheese	1 can (7.5 oz)	187	967	–	–	–	–	0
Spaghetti 'N Beef	1 can (7.5 oz)	226	130	–	–	–	–	0
Spaghetti w/ Meatballs	1 can (7.2 oz)	249	0	–	–	–	–	0
Hamburger Helper								
Ravioli as prep	1 cup	280	400	0.3	0.3	5	60	0
Ravioli w/ White Cheese Topping as prep	1 cup	310	400	0.3	0.3	4	60	0
Healthy Choice								
Beef Macaroni	1 meal (8.5 oz)	220	500	–	–	–	–	54
Bowls Cheese & Chicken Tortellini	1 meal (8.7 oz)	250	1500	–	–	–	–	36
Breaded Chicken Breast Stips w/ Macaroni & Cheese	1 meal (8 oz)	270	0	–	–	–	–	1
Cheese Ravioli Parmigiana	1 meal (9 oz)	260	750	–	–	–	–	0
Chicken Fettuccine Alfredo	1 meal (8.5 oz)	280	0	–	–	–	–	2
Fettuccine Alfredo	1 meal (8 oz)	240	0	–	–	–	–	0
Lasagna Roma	1 meal (13.5 oz)	420	500	–	–	–	–	6
Macaroni & Cheese	1 meal (9 oz)	240	0	–	–	–	–	0
Manicotti w/ Three Cheeses	1 meal (11 oz)	300	750	–	–	–	–	0
Spaghetti & Sauce w/ Seasoned Beef	1 meal (10 oz)	260	500	–	–	–	–	15
Stuffed Pasta Shells	1 meal (10.35 oz)	370	500	–	–	–	–	5
Hodgson Mill								
Macaroni & Cheese Whole Wheat	1 serv	250	0	–	–	–	–	0

FOOD	PORTION	CALS	VIT A	THIA	RIBO	NIACIN	FOLIC	VIT C
It's Pasta Anytime								
Penne With Tomato Italian Sausage Sauce	1 pkg (15.25 oz)	540	750	–	–	–	–	9
Kid Cuisine								
Magical Macaroni & Cheese	1 meal (10.6 oz)	440	800	–	–	–	–	0
Kraft								
Deluxe Macaroni & Cheese Four Cheese Blend as prep	1 cup (6.2 oz)	320	500	0.4	0.3	3	60	0
Deluxe Macaroni & Cheese Original as prep	1 cup (6.1 oz)	320	500	0.4	0.3	3	60	0
Light Deluxe Macaroni & Cheese as prep	1 cup (6.5 oz)	290	200	0.4	0.3	3	60	0
Macaroni & Cheese All Shapes as prep	1 cup (6.9 oz)	410	750	0.4	0.3	3	60	0
Macaroni & Cheese Original as prep	1 cup (6.9 oz)	410	750	0.4	0.3	3	60	0
Macaroni & Cheese Original as prep light recipe	1 cup (6.4 oz)	290	200	0.4	0.3	3	60	0
Premium Macaroni & Cheese Cheesy Alfredo as prep	1 cup (6.9 oz)	410	750	0.4	0.3	3	60	0
Premium Macaroni & Cheese Mild White Cheddar as prep	1 cup (6.8 oz)	410	1000	0.4	0.3	3	60	0
Premium Macaroni & Cheese Thick 'N Creamy as prep	1 cup (7.6 oz)	420	750	0.4	0.3	3	60	0

FOOD	PORTION	CALS	VIT A	THIA	RIBO	NIACIN	FOLIC	VIT C
Premium Macaroni & Cheese Three Cheese as prep	1 cup (6.9 oz)	410	750	0.4	0.3	3	60	0
Spaghetti Classics Mild Italian as prep	1 cup (9.1 oz)	240	500	0.3	0.2	3	40	9
Spaghetti Classics Tangy Italian as prep	1 cup (8.9 oz)	240	500	0.3	0.2	3	40	9
Spaghetti Classics Zesty Cheese as prep	1 cup (8.6 oz)	240	500	0.3	0.2	3	40	9
Spaghetti Classics w/ Meat Sauce as prep	1 cup (8.2 oz)	330	750	0.3	0.2	3	40	4
Lean Cuisine								
Cafe Classics Bow Tie Pasta & Chicken	1 pkg (9.5 oz)	220	1250	—	—	—	—	15
Cafe Classics Cheese Lasagna w/ Chicken Scaloppini	1 pkg (10 oz)	270	500	—	—	—	—	6
Cafe Classics Shrimp & Angel Hair Pasta	1 pkg (10 oz)	240	2500	—	—	—	—	18
Everyday Favorites	1 pkg (10 oz)	270	2250	—	—	—	—	9
Everyday Favorites Alfredo Pasta Primavera	1 pkg (10 oz)	290	400	—	—	—	—	12
Everyday Favorites Angel Hair Pasta	1 pkg (10 oz)	240	1000	—	—	—	—	15
Everyday Favorites Cheese Cannelloni	1 pkg (9.1 oz)	230	500	—	—	—	—	4
Everyday Favorites Cheese Ravioli	1 pkg (8.5 oz)	260	500	—	—	—	—	5
Everyday Favorites Chicken Lasagna	1 pkg (10 oz)	280	2000	—	—	—	—	2

FOOD	PORTION	CALS	VIT A	THIA	RIBO	NIACIN	FOLIC	VIT C
Everyday Favorites Classic Cheese Lasagna	1 pkg (11.5 oz)	290	750	—	—	—	—	9
Everyday Favorites Fettucini Alfredo	1 pkg (9.25 oz)	280	0	—	—	—	—	0
Everyday Favorites Fettucini Primavera	1 pkg (10 oz)	270	2000	—	—	—	—	0
Everyday Favorites Lasagna w/ Meat Sauce	1 pkg (10.5 oz)	300	500	—	—	—	—	12
Everyday Favorites Macaroni & Cheese	1 pkg (10 oz)	290	0	—	—	—	—	0
Everyday Favorites Macaroni & Beef	1 pkg (10 oz)	270	400	—	—	—	—	0
Everyday Favorites Penne Pasta	1 pkg (10 oz)	260	500	—	—	—	—	6
Everyday Favorites Spaghetti w/ Meat Sauce	1 pkg (11.5 oz)	290	500	—	—	—	—	9
Everyday Favorites Spaghetti w/ Meatballs	1 pkg (9.5 oz)	270	300	—	—	—	—	6
Everyday Favorites	1 pkg (9.25 oz)	270	0	—	—	—	—	0
Family Style Favorites Five Cheese Lasagna	1 serv (8 oz)	210	400	—	—	—	—	1
Skillet Sensations Chicken Alfredo	1 serv	280	750	—	—	—	—	48
Lipton								
Pasta & Sauce Angel Hair Chicken Broccoli as prep	1 cup	260	300	0.5	0.3	3	100	4
Pasta & Sauce Angel Hair Parmesan as prep	1 cup	280	400	0.5	0.3	3	100	0

FOOD	PORTION	CALS	VIT A	THIA	RIBO	NIACIN	FOLIC	VIT C
Pasta & Sauce Bow Tie Chicken Primavera as prep	1 cup	290	1000	0.6	0.3	3	100	1
Pasta & Sauce Bow Tie Italian Cheese as prep	1 cup	300	400	0.5	0.3	3	100	0
Pasta & Sauce Butter & Herbs as prep	1 cup	270	0	0.5	0.2	3	100	0
Pasta & Sauce Cheddar Broccoli as prep	1 cup	340	500	0.6	0.3	4	120	4
Pasta & Sauce Chicken Herb Parmesan as prep	1 cup	80	400	0.7	0.3	4	100	0
Pasta & Sauce Chicken Stir-Fry as prep	1 cup	270	750	0.7	0.3	4	100	1
Pasta & Sauce Creamy Garlic as prep	1 cup	350	500	0.6	0.3	4	100	0
Pasta & Sauce Creamy Mushroom as prep	1 cup	320	400	0.7	0.3	5	100	0
Pasta & Sauce Garlic & Butter Linguine as prep	1 cup	260	300	0.5	0.3	2	100	0
Pasta & Sauce Mild Cheddar Cheese as prep	1 cup	290	400	0.5	0.3	3	100	0
Pasta & Sauce Roasted Garlic Chicken as prep	1 cup	290	400	0.5	0.3	4	100	0
Pasta & Sauce Roasted Garlic & Olive Oil w/ Tomato as prep	1 cup	270	500	0.6	0.3	3	100	2

FOOD	PORTION	CALS	VIT A	THIA	RIBO	NIACIN	FOLIC	VIT C
Pasta & Sauce Rotini Primavera as prep	1 cup	320	750	0.6	0.3	4	100	4
Pasta & Sauce Savory Herb w/ Garlic as prep	1 cup	280	300	0.7	0.3	4	100	0
Pasta & Sauce Three Cheese Rotini as prep	1 cup	320	400	0.5	0.3	4	100	0
Marie Callender's								
Cheese Ravioli In Marinara Sauce w/ Spirals & Garlic Bread	1 meal (16 oz)	750	1000	–	–	–	–	0
Extra Cheese Lasagna	1 meal (15 oz)	590	2250	–	–	–	–	0
Fettuccine Alfredo & Garlic Bread	1 meal (14 oz)	920	200	–	–	–	–	0
Fettuccine Alfredo Supreme	1 meal (13 oz)	450	200	–	–	–	–	1
Fettuccine Primavera w/ Tortellini	1 meal (14 oz)	750	2250	–	–	–	–	6
Fettuccine w/ Broccoli & Chicken	1 meal (13 oz)	710	500	–	–	–	–	9
Lasagna w/ Meat Sauce	1 meal (15 oz)	630	1000	–	–	–	–	0
Macaroni & Cheese	1 meal (12 oz)	540	100	–	–	–	–	0
Skillet Meal Chicken Alfredo	½ pkg	490	2500	–	–	–	–	30
Skillet Meal Penne Pasta & Meatballs	½ pkg	600	1000	–	–	–	–	0
Skillet Meal Rigatoni Vegetables In Cheese Sauce	1 cup	290	0	–	–	–	–	4

FOOD	PORTION	CALS	VIT A	THIA	RIBO	NIACIN	FOLIC	VIT C
Spaghetti w/ Meat Sauce & Garlic Bread	1 meal (17 oz)	670	750	—	—	—	—	0
Stuffed Pasta Trio	1 meal (10.5 oz)	380	750	—	—	—	—	1
Morton								
Macaroni & Cheese	1 serv (8 oz)	240	200	—	—	—	—	0
Spaghetti w/ Meat Sauce	1 meal (8.5 oz)	200	500	—	—	—	—	0
Quorn								
Fettuccine Alfredo	1 pkg (10.5 oz)	360	1250	—	—	—	—	21
Lasagna	1 pkg (10.5 oz)	360	750	—	—	—	—	9
Velveeta								
Rotini & Cheese w/ Broccoli as prep	1 cup (7.2 oz)	400	750	0.4	0.3	3	60	4
Shells & Cheese Bacon as prep	1 cup (6.8 oz)	360	500	0.4	0.3	3	60	0
Shells & Cheese Original as prep	1 cup (6.6 oz)	360	500	0.4	0.3	3	60	0
Shells & Cheese Salsa as prep	1 cup (7.5 oz)	380	750	0.4	0.3	3	60	0
Yves								
Veggie Lasagna	1 pkg (10.5 oz)	300	0	—	—	—	—	9
Veggie Macaroni	1 pkg (10.5 oz)	230	300	—	—	—	—	9
Veggie Penne	1 pkg (10.5 oz)	220	400	—	—	—	—	15

PASTA SALAD

FOOD	PORTION	CALS	VIT A	THIA	RIBO	NIACIN	FOLIC	VIT C
Italian style pasta salad	3.5 oz	140	300	0.2	0.1	3	—	9
Kraft								
Herb & Garlic as prep	¾ cup (4.9 oz)	280	500	0.2	0.1	1.2	40	2

FOOD	PORTION	CALS	VIT A	THIA	RIBO	NIACIN	FOLIC	VIT C
Pasta Salad Classic Ranch w/ Bacon as prep	¾ cup (4.7 oz)	350	400	0.2	0.1	1.2	40	0
Pasta Salad Creamy Ceasar as prep	¾ cup (4.8 oz)	340	200	0.2	0.1	1.2	40	4
Pasta Salad Garden Primavera as prep	¾ cup (5 oz)	240	300	0.2	0.1	1.2	40	4
Pasta Salad Italian 97% Fat Free as prep	¾ cup (4.9 oz)	190	300	0.2	0.1	1.2	40	4
Pasta Salad Parmesan Peppercorn as prep	¾ cup (4.9 oz)	360	500	0.2	0.1	1.2	40	1

PATE

FOOD	PORTION	CALS	VIT A	THIA	RIBO	NIACIN	FOLIC	VIT C
liver canned	1 tbsp (13 g)	41	429	tr	0.1	0.4	8	0
pate foie gras	1 oz	127	1357	tr	0.2	–	162	1
pork pate	1 oz	107	6000	tr	0.2	1.1	29	tr

PEACH

FOOD	PORTION	CALS	VIT A	THIA	RIBO	NIACIN	FOLIC	VIT C
halves dried	1 cup	383	3461	tr	0.3	7	–	8
halves in heavy syrup	1 half	60	269	tr	tr	0.5	3	2
halves in light syrup	1 half	44	286	tr	tr	0.5	3	2
halves juice pack	1 half	34	294	tr	tr	0.4	–	3
halves water pack	1 half	18	410	tr	tr	0.4	3	2
peach	1	37	465	tr	tr	0.9	3	6
sliced	1 cup	73	910	tr	0.1	1.7	6	11
spiced in heavy syrup	1 fruit	66	279	tr	tr	0.5	–	5
spiced in heavy syrup	1 cup	180	768	tr	0.1	1.3	–	13

Chiquita

FOOD	PORTION	CALS	VIT A	THIA	RIBO	NIACIN	FOLIC	VIT C
Peach	1 med (3.4 oz)	40	100	–	–	–	–	6

FOOD	PORTION	CALS	VIT A	THIA	RIBO	NIACIN	FOLIC	VIT C
Del Monte								
Fruit Cup Diced Extra Light Syrup	1 pkg (4 oz)	50	200	–	–	–	–	12
Fruit Cup Diced In Heavy Syrup	1 serv (4 oz)	80	200	–	–	–	–	12
Fruit Cup Fruit Naturals Diced	1 pkg (4 oz)	50	200	–	–	–	–	12
Fruit Pleasures Raspberry Flavor	½ cup (4.5 oz)	80	100	–	–	–	–	4
Fruit To Go Banana Berry Peaches	1 pkg (4 oz)	70	200	–	–	–	–	60
Fruitrageous Peachy Pie	1 pkg (4 oz)	80	400	–	–	–	–	12
Fruitrageous Wild Raspberry Flavor	1 pkg (4 oz)	80	100	–	–	–	–	12
Halves Ginger Flavor	½ cup (4.5 oz)	90	0	–	–	–	–	2
Halves In Extra Light Syrup	½ cup (4.4 oz)	60	300	–	–	–	–	5
Halves In Heavy Syrup	½ cup (4.5 oz)	100	100	–	–	–	–	1
Halves Melba In Heavy Syrup	½ cup (4.5 oz)	100	300	–	–	–	–	5
Slice Fruit Natural	½ cup (4.4 oz)	60	300	–	–	–	–	5
Sliced In Extra Light Syrup	½ cup (4.4 oz)	60	100	–	–	–	–	1
Sliced In Heavy Syrup	½ cup (4.5 oz)	100	100	–	–	–	–	1
Sliced Natural Raspberry Flavor	½ cup (4.4 oz)	80	100	–	–	–	–	4
Sliced Natural Harvest Spice Flavor	½ cup (4.5 oz)	80	400	–	–	–	–	4
Whole Spiced In Heavy Syrup	½ cup (4.2 oz)	100	300	–	–	–	–	5

FOOD	PORTION	CALS	VIT A	THIA	RIBO	NIACIN	FOLIC	VIT C
PEACH JUICE								
nectar	1 cup	134	643	tr	tr	0.7	–	13
PEANUT BUTTER								
chunky	1 cup	1520	0	0.3	0.3	35.3	237	0
chunky	2 tbsp	188	0	tr	tr	4.4	29	0
smooth	1 cup	1517	0	0.4	0.3	33.8	202	0
smooth	2 tbsp	188	0	tr	tr	4.2	25	0
Maranatha								
Salted	2 tbsp	190	0	–	–	–	–	0
Peanut Wonder								
Regular	2 tbsp	100	0	–	–	–	–	5
Skippy								
Creamy	2 tbsp	190	0	–	–	4	–	0
Tropical Source								
Chips Dairy Free	13 pieces (1.5 oz)	80	0	–	–	–	–	0
PEANUTS								
chocolate coated	10 (1.4 oz)	208	0	tr	0.1	1.7	3	0
chocolate coated	1 cup (5.2 oz)	773	0	0.2	0.3	6.3	12	0
cooked	½ cup	102	0	0.1	tr	1.7	24	0
dry roasted	1 cup	855	0	0.6	0.1	19.7	212	0
Planters								
Reduced Fat Honey Roasted	⅓ cup (1 oz)	130	0	–	–	3	60	0
PEAR								
asian	1 (4.3 oz)	51	0	tr	tr	0.3	10	2
halves dried	10	459	6	tr	0.3	2.4	–	12
halves dried	1 cup	472	6	tr	0.3	2.5	–	13
halves in heavy syrup	1 cup	188	0	tr	0.1	0.6	3	3
halves in heavy syrup	1 half	68	0	tr	tr	0.2	1	1
halves in light syrup	1 half	45	0	tr	tr	0.1	1	1
halves juice pack	1 cup	123	14	tr	tr	0.5	–	4
halves water pack	1 half	22	0	tr	tr	tr	1	1

FOOD	PORTION	CALS	VIT A	THIA	RIBO	NIACIN	FOLIC	VIT C
pear	1	98	33	tr	0.1	0.2	12	7
sliced w/ skin	1 cup	97	33	tr	0.1	0.2	12	7
Chiquita								
Pear	1 med (5.8 oz)	100	0	—	—	—	—	6
Del Monte								
Fruit Cup Diced In Heavy Syrup	1 pkg (4 oz)	80	0	—	—	—	—	12
Fruit Cup Diced Extra Light Syrup	1 pkg (4 oz)	50	0	—	—	—	—	12
Fruit To Go Peachy Peaches	1 pkg (4 oz)	70	200	—	—	—	—	60
Halves Fruit Naturals	½ cup (4.4 oz)	60	300	—	—	—	—	5
Halves In Extra Light Syrup	½ cup (4.4 oz)	60	0	—	—	—	—	2
Halves In Heavy Syrup	½ cup (4.5 oz)	100	0	—	—	—	—	2
Orchard Select Sliced Bartlett	½ cup (4.4 oz)	80	300	—	—	—	—	48
Sliced In Extra Light Syrup	½ cup (4.5 oz)	60	0	—	—	—	—	2
PEAR JUICE								
nectar	1 cup	149	1	tr	tr	0.3	—	3
PEAS								
green cooked	½ cup	63	534	0.2	0.1	1.2	47	8
green raw	½ cup	58	461	0.2	0.1	1.5	47	29
pea & potato curry	1 serv (7 oz)	284	550	0.1	0.1	2	—	12
pea curry	1 serv (4.4 oz)	438	2600	0.2	0.1	2.5	—	14
snap peas cooked	1 pkg (10 oz)	132	421	0.1	0.1	1.4	—	56
snap peas cooked	½ cup	34	104	0.1	0.1	0.4	—	38
snap peas raw	½ cup	30	105	0.1	0.1	0.4	—	43
split cooked	1 cup	231	14	0.4	0.1	1.7	127	1
Birds Eye								
Butter Peas	½ cup	110	0	—	—	—	—	1
Crowder	½ cup	120	0	—	—	—	—	1
Field Peas w/ Snaps	⅔ cup	130	0	—	—	—	—	2
Green	½ cup	70	500	—	—	—	—	15

FOOD	PORTION	CALS	VIT A	THIA	RIBO	NIACIN	FOLIC	VIT C
Purple Hull Peas	½ cup	110	0	–	–	–	–	1
Sugar Snap	½ cup	40	500	–	–	–	–	15
Tiny Tender	¾ cup	40	1500	–	–	–	–	5
Del Monte								
Sweet	½ cup (4.4 oz)	60	300	–	–	–	–	9
Sweet Very Young Small	½ cup (4.4 oz)	60	300	–	–	–	–	9
Fresh Like								
Garden	3.5 oz	85	698	0.3	0.1	2.1	–	20
La Choy								
Snow Pea Pods	½ pkg (3 oz)	35	200	–	–	–	–	15
S&W								
Petite	½ cup (4.4 oz)	70	500	–	–	–	–	9
Small	½ cup (4.4 oz)	70	500	–	–	–	–	9
TastyBite								
Agra Peas & Greens	½ pkg (5 oz)	260	0	–	–	–	–	0
Tree Of Life								
Peas	⅓ cup (3.1 oz)	70	300	–	–	–	–	9
Veg-All								
Tender Sweet	½ cup	60	300	–	–	–	–	9
PECANS								
halves dried	1 cup	721	138	0.9	0.1	1	42	2
PECTIN								
Sure Jell								
For Lower Sugar Recipes	1 tsp (2.8 g)	20	0	–	–	–	–	0
Fruit Pectin	1 tsp (3.6 g)	20	0	–	–	–	–	0
PEPEAO								
dried	½ cup	36	0	–	tr	0.4	–	tr
raw sliced	1 cup	25	0	0.1	0.2	0.1	–	1
PEPPER								
cayenne	1 tsp	6	749	tr	tr	0.2	–	1
red	1 tsp	6	749	tr	tr	0.2	–	1
PEPPERS								
ancho	1 (0.6 oz)	48	3474	tr	0.4	1.1	12	0
banana fresh	1 cup (4.4 oz)	33	422	0.1	0.1	1.5	36	27
banana fresh	1 (4 in) (1.2 oz)	9	112	tr	tr	0.4	10	27

FOOD	PORTION	CALS	VIT A	THIA	RIBO	NIACIN	FOLIC	VIT C
chili green	1 cup (5.5 oz)	29	175	tr	tr	0.9	75	0
chili green hot chopped	½ cup	17	415	tr	tr	0.5	—	46
chili green hot fresh	1	18	346	tr	tr	0.4	11	109
chili red fresh chopped	½ cup	30	8063	0.1	0.1	0.7	18	182
chili red hot	1 (2.6 oz)	18	8681	tr	tr	0.6	—	50
green	1 tbsp	1	25	tr	tr	tr	1	8
green chopped cooked	½ cup	19	403	tr	tr	0.3	11	51
green cooked	1 (2.6 oz)	20	432	tr	tr	0.3	11	54
green fresh	1 (2.6 oz)	20	468	tr	tr	0.4	16	95
green fresh chopped	½ cup	13	316	tr	tr	0.3	11	45
habanero chile	1 tsp	9	85	tr	0.1	0.2	7	27
hungarian fresh	1 (0.9 oz)	8	38	tr	tr	0.3	14	0
jalapeno chopped	½ cup	17	1156	tr	tr	0.3	—	9
jalapeno fresh	1 (0.5 oz)	4	30	tr	tr	0.2	7	6
jalapeno fresh sliced	1 cup (3.2 oz)	27	194	0.1	0.1	1	42	6
pasilla	1 (7 g)	24	2503	tr	0.2	0.5	12	0
red	1 tbsp	1	309	tr	tr	tr	1	8
red chopped cooked	½ cup	19	2745	tr	tr	0.3	11	125
red cooked	1 (2.6 oz)	20	2745	tr	tr	0.3	11	125
red fresh	1 (2.6 oz)	20	4218	tr	tr	0.4	16	141
red fresh chopped	½ cup	13	2850	tr	tr	0.3	11	95
serrano fresh	1 (6 g)	2	57	0	0	0.1	1	3
serrano fresh chopped	1 cup (3.7 oz)	34	984	0.1	0.1	1.6	24	3
yellow fresh	10 strips	14	124	tr	tr	0.5	14	95
yellow fresh	1 (6.5 oz)	50	442	0.1	tr	1.7	48	341
Birds Eye								
Diced Green	¾ cup	20	100	—	—	—	—	18
Chiquita								
Pepper	1 med (5.2 oz)	30	400	—	—	—	—	114

FOOD	PORTION	CALS	VIT A	THIA	RIBO	NIACIN	FOLIC	VIT C
Vlasic								
Jalapeno Sliced	1 oz	10	500	–	–	–	–	4
PERCH								
red raw	3.5 oz	114	tr	0.1	0.1	2.5	–	1
PERSIMMONS								
dried japanese	1	93	190	–	tr	0.1	–	0
fresh japanese	1	118	3640	0.1	tr	0.2	13	13
PHEASANT								
breast w/o skin raw	½ breast (6.4 oz)	243	268	0.1	0.2	15.7	–	11
w/ skin raw	½ pheasant (14 oz)	723	706	0.3	0.6	25.7	–	21
w/o skin raw	½ pheasant (12.4 oz)	470	181	0.3	0.5	32.8	–	21
PHYLLO DOUGH								
phyllo dough	1 oz	85	0	0.2	0.1	1.2	5	0
sheet	1	57	0	0.1	0.1	0.8	3	0
Ekizian								
Sheets	½ lb	865	520	1.5	1.1	11.1	61	0
PICKLES								
dill	1 (2.3 oz)	12	214	tr	tr	tr	1	1
dill sliced	1 slice	1	20	tr	tr	tr	0	tr
gerkins	1 oz	6	0	tr	tr	–	–	tr
kosher dill	1 (2.3 oz)	12	214	tr	tr	tr	1	1
polish dill	1 (2.3 oz)	12	214	tr	tr	tr	1	1
quick sour	1 (1.2 oz)	4	51	0	tr	0	–	tr
quick sour sliced	1 slice	1	10	tr	tr	tr	–	tr
sweet	1 (1.2 oz)	41	44	tr	tr	tr	0	tr
sweet gherkin	1 sm (½ oz)	20	10	tr	tr	tr	–	1
sweet sliced	1 slice	7	8	tr	tr	tr	0	tr
PIE								
apple	⅙ of 9 in pie (5.4 oz)	411	90	0.2	0.2	1.9	7	3
banana cream	⅙ of 9 in pie (5.2 oz)	398	386	0.2	0.3	1.6	17	2

FOOD	PORTION	CALS	VIT A	THIA	RIBO	NIACIN	FOLIC	VIT C
blueberry	⅙ of 9 in pie (5.2 oz)	360	61	0.2	0.2	1.8	7	1
butterscotch	⅙ of 9 in pie (4.5 oz)	355	383	0.2	0.3	1.3	14	1
cherry	⅙ of 9 in pie (6.3 oz)	486	737	0.3	0.2	2.3	12	2
coconut creme	⅙ of 9 in pie (4.7 oz)	396	379	0.2	0.3	1.3	14	1
custard	⅙ of 9 in pie (4.5 oz)	262	281	0.1	0.3	0.8	13	1
lemon meringue	⅙ of 9 in pie (4.5 oz)	362	204	0.2	0.2	1.2	11	4
mince	⅙ of 9 in pie (5.8 oz)	477	36	0.2	0.2	2.0	9	10
pecan	⅙ of 8 in pie (4 oz)	452	198	0.1	0.1	0.3	7	1
vanilla cream	⅙ of 9 in pie (4.4 oz)	350	385	0.2	0.3	1.2	14	1
Mrs. Smith's								
Apple	1 slice (4.3 oz)	350	400	–	–	–	–	0
Blueberry	1 slice (4.6 oz)	330	300	–	–	–	–	0
Cappuccino	1 slice (4.2 oz)	300	0	–	–	–	–	0
Cherry	1 slice (4.3 oz)	320	750	–	–	–	–	0
Cherry Crumb	1 slice (4.2 oz)	320	750	–	–	–	–	0
Chocolate Cream	1 slice (4.6 oz)	340	0	–	–	–	–	0
Chocolate Mint Cream	1 slice (4.3 oz)	360	0	–	–	–	–	0
Coconut Custard	1 slice (4.4 oz)	260	300	–	–	–	–	0
Cookies 'N Cream	1 slice (4.3 oz)	360	0	–	–	–	–	0
Dutch Apple	1 slice (4.4 oz)	330	100	–	–	–	–	0

FOOD	PORTION	CALS	VIT A	THIA	RIBO	NIACIN	FOLIC	VIT C
French Silk	1 slice (4.4 oz)	560	300	—	—	—	—	0
Key West Lime	1 slice (4.3 oz)	430	200	—	—	—	—	6
Lemon Cream	1 slice (5 oz)	440	0	—	—	—	—	4
Lemonade	1 slice (4.3 oz)	340	0	—	—	—	—	5
Mince	1 slice (4.6 oz)	380	300	—	—	—	—	0
Mixed Berry	1 slice (4.2 oz)	300	300	—	—	—	—	0
Peach	1 slice (4.6 oz)	320	400	—	—	—	—	0
Peach Lattice	1 slice (4.2 oz)	290	400	—	—	—	—	0
Peanut Butter Silk	1 slice (4.6 oz)	600	200	—	—	—	—	0
Pecan	1 slice (4.8 oz)	560	500	—	—	—	—	0
Pumpkin Custard	1 slice (4.6 oz)	270	5000	—	—	—	—	0
Raspberry	1 slice (4.6 oz)	330	300	—	—	—	—	0
S'Mores Cream	1 slice (4.3 oz)	360	0	—	—	—	—	0
Strawberry Banana	1 slice (4.3 oz)	330	0	—	—	—	—	0
Sweet Potato Custard	1 slice (4.6 oz)	340	3500	—	—	—	—	0
Sara Lee								
Homestyle Peach	⅙ pie (4.6 oz)	320	200	—	—	—	—	21
Homestyle Pumpkin	⅙ pie (4.6 oz)	260	750	—	—	—	—	0

PIE CRUST

FOOD	PORTION	CALS	VIT A	THIA	RIBO	NIACIN	FOLIC	VIT C
as prep	9 in crust (5.6 oz)	801	0	0.5	0.3	3.8	—	0
as prep	⅛ of 9 in pie (0.7 oz)	100	0	0.1	tr	0.5	—	0

FOOD	PORTION	CALS	VIT A	THIA	RIBO	NIACIN	FOLIC	VIT C
chocolate cookie crumb	9 in crust (7.7 oz)	1130	1876	0.3	0.5	4.8	1	tr
chocolate cookie crumb	⅛ of 9 in pie (1 oz)	139	231	tr	0.1	0.6	1	0
graham cracker	9 in crust (8.4 oz)	1181	1876	0.2	0.4	5.1	17	tr
graham cracker	⅛ of 9 in pie (1 oz)	148	238	tr	0.1	0.6	2	0
puff pastry baked	1 shell (1.4 oz)	223	0	0.1	0.1	1.5	4	0
vanilla wafer cracker crumbs	9 in crust (6.1 oz)	937	1950	0.3	0.4	3.7	11	tr
vanilla wafer cracker crumbs	⅛ of 9 in pie (0.8 oz)	119	248	tr	0.1	0.5	1	0

PIE FILLING

FOOD	PORTION	CALS	VIT A	THIA	RIBO	NIACIN	FOLIC	VIT C
pumpkin pie mix	1 cup	282	22405	tr	0.3	1.0	–	10
Comstock								
Red Ruby Cherry	⅓ cup (3.1 oz)	90	100	–	–	–	–	0

PIEROGI

FOOD	PORTION	CALS	VIT A	THIA	RIBO	NIACIN	FOLIC	VIT C
pierogi	¾ cup (4.4 oz)	307	246	0.3	0.2	1.9	8	1
Health Is Wealth								
Potato & Cheddar	2 (2.8 oz)	140	0	–	–	–	–	1
Potato & Onion	2 (2.8 oz)	140	0	–	–	–	–	1
Mrs. T's								
Jalapeno & Cheddar	3 (4.2 oz)	190	100	–	–	–	–	9
Potato & American Cheese	3 (4.2 oz)	220	100	–	–	–	–	6
Potato & Cheddar	3 (4.2 oz)	190	100	–	–	–	–	6
Potato & Onion	3 (4.2 oz)	180	0	–	–	–	–	9
Potato & Roasted Garlic	3 (4.2 oz)	190	200	–	–	–	–	9
Rogies Cheddar & Bacon	7 (3 oz)	140	100	–	–	–	–	4
Rogies Jalapeno & Cheddar	7 (3 oz)	120	0	–	–	–	–	5
Rogies Potato & Cheddar	7 (3 oz)	130	100	–	–	–	–	5

FOOD	PORTION	CALS	VIT A	THIA	RIBO	NIACIN	FOLIC	VIT C
PIG'S EARS AND FEET								
ear simmered	1	184	0	tr	0.1	0.6	0	0
feet pickled	1 lb	921	0	tr	0.2	1.7	18	0
feet pickled	1 oz	58	0	0	tr	0.1	1	0
feet simmered	3 oz	165	0	tr	0.1	0.4	1	0
PIGEON PEAS								
dried cooked	½ cup	102	2	0.1	0.1	0.7	93	0
PIKE								
northern cooked	½ fillet (5.4 oz)	176	125	0.1	0.1	–	–	6
PIMIENTOS								
canned	1 tbsp	3	319	tr	tr	0.1	1	10
canned	1 slice	0	27	0	tr	tr	0	1
PINE NUTS								
pinyon dried	1 oz	161	8	0.4	0.1	1.2	–	1
PINEAPPLE								
chunks in heavy syrup	1 cup	199	37	0.2	0.1	0.7	12	19
chunks juice pack	1 cup	150	95	0.2	tr	0.7	–	24
chunks sweetened	½ cup	104	37	0.1	tr	0.4	–	10
crushed in heavy syrup	1 cup	199	37	0.2	0.1	0.7	12	19
diced	1 cup	77	35	0.1	0.1	0.7	16	24
slice	1 slice	42	19	0.1	tr	0.4	9	13
slices in heavy syrup	1 slice	45	8	0.1	tr	0.2	3	4
slices in light syrup	1 slice	30	9	0.1	tr	0.2	3	4
slices juice pack	1 slice	35	22	0.1	tr	0.2	–	6
slices water pack	1 slice	19	9	0.1	tr	0.2	3	5
tidbits in heavy syrup	1 cup	199	37	0.2	0.1	0.7	12	19
tidbits in juice	1 cup	150	95	0.2	tr	0.7	–	24
tidbits in water	1 cup	79	37	0.2	0.1	0.7	12	19

FOOD	PORTION	CALS	VIT A	THIA	RIBO	NIACIN	FOLIC	VIT C
Del Monte								
Chunks In Heavy Syrup	½ cup (4.3 oz)	90	0	—	—	—	—	12
Chunks In Its Own Juice	½ cup (4.3 oz)	70	0	—	—	—	—	12
Crushed In Heavy Syrup	½ cup (4.3 oz)	90	0	—	—	—	—	12
Crushed In Its Own Juice	½ cup (4.3 oz)	70	0	—	—	—	—	12
Fruit Cup Tidbits	1 pkg (4 oz)	50	0	—	—	—	—	12
Sliced In Heavy Syrup	2 slices (4.1 oz)	90	0	—	—	—	—	12
Sliced In Its Own Juice	½ cup (4 oz)	60	0	—	—	—	—	12
Spears In Its Own Juice	½ cup (4.3 oz)	70	0	—	—	—	—	12
Tidbits In Its Own Juice	½ cup (4.3 oz)	70	0	—	—	—	—	12
Wedges In Its Own Juice	½ cup (4.3 oz)	70	0	—	—	—	—	12
Sunfresh								
In Extra Light Syrup	½ cup (4.6 oz)	80	0	—	—	—	—	42
PINEAPPLE JUICE								
canned	1 cup	139	12	0.1	0.1	0.6	58	27
frzn as prep	1 cup	129	25	0.2	0.1	0.5	—	30
Del Monte								
Juice	6 fl oz	80	0	—	—	—	—	60
PINK BEANS								
dried cooked	1 cup	252	0	0.4	0.1	1	284	0
PINTO BEANS								
cooked	1 cup	235	3	0.3	0.2	0.7	294	4
Eden								
Organic Spicy	½ cup (4.6 oz)	125	200	0.1	0.1	0.8	—	0

FOOD	PORTION	CALS	VIT A	THIA	RIBO	NIACIN	FOLIC	VIT C
PITANGA								
fresh	1 cup	57	2595	0.1	0.1	0.5	–	46
fresh	1	2	105	tr	tr	tr	–	2
PIZZA								
cheese	12 in pie	1121	3051	1.4	1.3	19.8	470	10
cheese pie	⅛ of 12 in	140	382	0.2	0.2	2.5	59	1
cheese deep dish individual	1 (5.5 oz)	460	400	–	–	–	–	1
cheese meat & vegetables	⅛ of 12 in pie	184	524	0.2	0.2	2	27	2
cheese meat & vegetables	12 in pie	1472	4184	1.7	1.4	15.6	215	13
pepperoni	12 in pie	1445	2250	1.1	1.9	24.3	421	13
pepperoni	⅛ of 12 in pie	181	282	0.1	0.2	3.1	53	2
Banquet								
Pepperoni	1 pie (6.75 oz)	490	0	–	–	–	–	0
Pizza Snack Cheese	6 pieces (7.5 oz)	200	100	–	–	–	–	5
Pizza Snack Pepperoni	6 pieces (7.5 oz)	230	100	–	–	–	–	1
Pizza Snack Pepperoni & Sausage	6 pieces (7.5 oz)	210	100	–	–	–	–	5
Health Is Wealth								
Pizza Munchees	6 (3 oz)	190	200	–	–	–	–	2
Healthy Choice								
French Bread Cheese	1 piece (6 oz)	340	100	–	–	–	–	0
French Bread Pepperoni	1 piece (6 oz)	340	300	–	–	–	–	0
French Bread Sausage	1 piece (6 oz)	320	200	–	–	–	–	0
French Bread Supreme	1 piece (6.35 oz)	330	200	–	–	–	–	0
French Bread Vegetable	1 piece (6 oz)	280	200	–	–	–	–	0

FOOD	PORTION	CALS	VIT A	THIA	RIBO	NIACIN	FOLIC	VIT C
Kid Cuisine								
Backpacking Pizza Snack	6 pieces	230	100	–	–	–	–	1
Big League Hamburger	1 meal (8.3 oz)	400	400	–	–	–	–	1
Fire Chief Cheese	1 pie (5.2 oz)	340	500	–	–	–	–	0
Pirate Pizza w/ Cheese	1 meal (8 oz)	430	100	–	–	–	–	0
Poolside Pepperoni	1 (5.2 oz)	380	500	–	–	–	–	0
Lean Cuisine								
Everyday Favorites French Bread Cheese	1 pkg (6 oz)	320	300	–	–	–	–	4
Everyday Favorites French Bread Deluxe	1 pkg (6.1 oz)	290	200	–	–	–	–	6
Everyday Favorites French Bread Pepperoni	1 pkg (5.25 oz)	300	200	–	–	–	–	1
Everyday Favorites French Bread Sun Dried Tomatoes	1 serv (6 oz)	340	200	–	–	–	–	1
Marie Callender's								
French Bread Cheese	1 (7.2 oz)	530	300	–	–	–	–	0
French Bread Pepperoni	1 (7.5 oz)	570	500	–	–	–	–	0
French Bread Supreme	1 (7.5 oz)	510	400	–	–	–	–	0

PIZZA DOUGH

FOOD	PORTION	CALS	VIT A	THIA	RIBO	NIACIN	FOLIC	VIT C
crust	1 slice (1.7 oz)	130	0	0.2	0.1	1.6	40	0
Boboli								
Thin Crust	⅓ crust (2 oz)	160	0	0.2	0.1	1.2	40	0

FOOD	PORTION	CALS	VIT A	THIA	RIBO	NIACIN	FOLIC	VIT C
PIZZA SAUCE								
Muir Glen								
Organic	¼ cup (2.2 oz)	40	100	–	–	–	–	1
PLANTAINS								
fresh uncooked	1 (6.3 oz)	218	2017	0.1	0.1	1.2	39	33
ripe fried	2.8 oz	214	80	0.1	tr	0.6	–	10
sliced cooked	½ cup	89	700	tr	tr	0.6	20	8
PLUMS								
plum	1	36	213	tr	0.1	0.3	1	6
purple in heavy syrup	3	119	344	tr	0.1	0.4	3	1
purple in heavy syrup	1 cup	320	668	tr	0.1	0.8	7	1
purple in light syrup	1 cup	158	666	tr	0.1	0.7	6	1
purple in light syrup	3	83	352	tr	0.1	0.4	3	1
purple juice pack	3	55	958	tr	0.1	0.4	–	3
purple water pack	3	39	868	tr	tr	0.4	3	3
sliced	1 cup	91	533	0.1	0.1	0.8	4	16
Chiquita								
Purple	2 med (4.6 oz)	80	300	–	–	–	–	12
Eden								
Umeboshi Paste	1 tsp	5	0	–	–	–	–	0
Umeboshi Plums	1	5	0	–	–	–	–	0
POI								
poi	½ cup	134	24	0.2	tr	1.3	–	5
POKEBERRY SHOOTS								
cooked	½ cup	16	7134	0.1	0.2	0.9	–	67
fresh	½ cup	18	6960	0.1	0.3	1	–	109
POPCORN								
air-popped	1 cup (0.3 oz)	31	16	tr	tr	0.2	2	0
caramel coated	1 cup (1.2 oz)	152	18	tr	tr	0.8	–	0
caramel coated w/ peanuts	⅔ cup (1 oz)	114	18	tr	tr	0.6	–	0
cheese	1 cup (0.4 oz)	58	27	tr	tr	0.2	–	tr
oil popped	1 cup (0.4 oz)	55	17	tr	tr	0.2	2	0

FOOD	PORTION	CALS	VIT A	THIA	RIBO	NIACIN	FOLIC	VIT C
Cracker Jack								
Original	½ cup (1 oz)	120	0	–	–	–	–	0
Husman's								
Cheese Corn	2¼ cups (1 oz)	160	0	–	–	–	–	0
POPOVER								
home recipe as prep w/ 2% milk	1 (1.4 oz)	87	117	0.1	0.1	0.7	7	tr
home recipe as prep w/ whole milk	1 (1.4 oz)	90	97	0.1	0.1	0.7	7	tr
PORK								
boston blade roast lean & fat cooked	3 oz	229	6	0.5	0.3	3.5	4	1
boston blade steak lean & fat cooked	3 oz	220	8	0.6	0.4	3.5	3	1
center loin roast lean bone in cooked	3 oz	169	6	0.8	0.2	4.6	3	1
center loin chop lean bone in cooked	3 oz	172	6	0.7	0.2	4.1	3	1
center rib chop lean & fat bone in cooked	3 oz	213	6	0.5	0.2	4.2	2	tr
center rib roast lean & fat bone in cooked	3 oz	217	5	0.6	0.3	5.2	3	tr
chicharrones pork cracklings fried	1 cup	844	20	tr	0.2	4.9	–	0
fresh ham rump lean roasted	3 oz	175	8	0.7	0.3	4.2	3	tr
fresh ham rump lean & fat roasted	3 oz	214	8	0.6	0.3	4	3	tr
fresh ham shank lean roasted	3 oz	183	7	0.5	0.3	4.2	5	tr

FOOD	PORTION	CALS	VIT A	THIA	RIBO	NIACIN	FOLIC	VIT C
fresh ham shank lean & fat roasted	3 oz	246	8	0.5	0.3	3.8	4	tr
fresh ham whole lean roasted	3 oz	179	8	0.5	0.3	4.2	10	tr
fresh ham whole lean roasted diced	1 cup	285	12	0.9	0.5	6.7	16	tr
fresh ham whole lean & fat roasted	3 oz	232	9	0.5	0.3	3.9	9	tr
fresh ham whole lean & fat roasted diced	1 cup	369	14	0.9	0.4	6.2	14	tr
ground cooked	3 oz	252	7	0.6	0.2	3.6	5	1
loin chop lean bone in braised	3 oz	191	6	0.5	0.2	3.3	3	1
loin chop lean bone in broiled	3 oz	199	6	0.6	0.3	3.9	3	1
loin roast lean bone in roasted	3 oz	210	7	0.5	0.3	4	4	tr
loin whole lean & fat braised	3 oz	203	6	0.5	0.2	3.8	3	1
loin whole lean & fat broiled	3 oz	206	6	0.8	0.3	4.3	4	1
loin whole lean & fat roasted	3 oz	211	8	0.8	0.3	4.7	5	1
lungs braised	3 oz	84	0	0.1	0.3	1.2	2	7
pancreas cooked	3 oz	186	0	0.1	0.6	2.7	4	5
ribs country style lean & fat braised	3 oz	252	7	0.4	0.2	3.3	3	1
shoulder arm picnic lean & fat roasted	3 oz	269	7	0.4	0.3	3.3	3	tr
shoulder whole lean & fat roasted	3 oz	248	7	0.5	0.3	3.4	4	tr
shoulder whole lean & fat roasted diced	1 cup	394	11	0.8	0.4	5.4	7	tr
shoulder whole lean roasted	3 oz	196	6	0.5	0.3	3.6	4	1

FOOD	PORTION	CALS	VIT A	THIA	RIBO	NIACIN	FOLIC	VIT C
shoulder whole lean roasted diced	1 cup	311	9	0.9	0.5	5.8	7	1
sirloin chop lean & fat bone in braised	3 oz	208	6	0.6	0.2	3.2	3	1
sirloin roast lean & fat bone in cooked	3 oz	222	7	0.6	0.3	4.5	5	tr
spareribs braised	3 oz	338	9	0.4	0.3	4.7	3	0
spleen braised	3 oz	127	0	0.1	0.2	5	3	10
tail simmered	3 oz	336	0	0.1	0.1	1	3	0
tenderloin lean roasted	3 oz	139	6	0.8	0.3	4	5	tr
top loin chop boneless lean & fat cooked	3 oz	198	6	0.5	0.2	3.9	3	tr
top loin roast boneless lean & fat cooked	3 oz	192	7	0.5	0.3	4.4	7	tr
Freirich								
Porkette	4 oz	220	0	—	—	—	—	0

PORK DISHES
Smithfield

FOOD	PORTION	CALS	VIT A	THIA	RIBO	NIACIN	FOLIC	VIT C
Pulled Pork w/ Barbecue Sauce	2 oz	90	0	—	—	—	—	2
Tyson								
Lemon Pepper Pork Roast	1 serv (3 oz)	110	0	—	—	—	—	1

POT PIE

FOOD	PORTION	CALS	VIT A	THIA	RIBO	NIACIN	FOLIC	VIT C
beef	⅓ of 9 in pie (7.4 oz)	515	4220	0.3	0.3	4.8	—	6
chicken	⅓ of 9 in pie (8.1 oz)	545	7220	0.3	0.3	4.9	—	5
Banquet								
Beef	1 (7 oz)	400	750	—	—	—	—	0
Cheesy Potato & Broccoli w/ Ham	1 (7 oz)	410	0	—	—	—	—	0
Chicken	1 (7 oz)	380	1000	—	—	—	—	1
Chicken & Broccoli	1 (7 oz)	350	1000	—	—	—	—	0

FOOD	PORTION	CALS	VIT A	THIA	RIBO	NIACIN	FOLIC	VIT C
Family Size Hearty Chicken	1 cup	460	750	–	–	–	–	0
Macaroni & Cheese	1 pkg (6.5 oz)	210	0	–	–	–	–	0
Turkey	1 (7 oz)	370	750	–	–	–	–	0
Vegetable Cheese	1 (7 oz)	340	1250	–	–	–	–	0
Healthy Choice								
Colonial Chicken	1 (9.5 oz)	310	1500	–	–	–	–	4
Lean Cuisine								
Everyday Favorites Chicken Pie	1 pkg (9.5 oz)	300	2250	–	–	–	–	15
Everyday Favorites Vegetable Eggroll	1 pkg (9 oz)	300	2250	–	–	–	–	9
Marie Callender's								
Beef	1 (9.5 oz)	680	1000	–	–	–	–	0
Chicken	1 (9.5 oz)	680	1000	–	–	–	–	0
Chicken & Broccoli	1 (9.5 oz)	670	2000	–	–	–	–	0
Chicken Au Gratin	1 (9.5 oz)	690	1000	–	–	–	–	0
Turkey	1 (9.5 oz)	680	2250	–	–	–	–	0
Morton								
Macaroni & Cheese	1 (6.5 oz)	210	0	–	–	–	–	0
Vegetable w/ Beef	1 (7 oz)	340	500	–	–	–	–	0
Vegetable w/ Chicken	1 (7 oz)	320	500	–	–	–	–	0
Vegetable w/ Turkey	1 (7 oz)	310	500	–	–	–	–	0
Swanson								
Beef	1 (7 oz)	376	1471	–	–	–	–	1
Chicken	1 (7 oz)	416	1968	–	–	–	–	2
Turkey	1 (7 oz)	440	998	–	–	–	–	2
POTATO								
au gratin as prep	½ cup	160	322	0.1	0.1	1.2	10	12
au gratin w/ cheese	½ cup	178	392	0.1	0.2	1.1	–	12
baked skin only	1 skin (2 oz)	115	0	0.1	0.1	1.8	–	8
baked topped w/ cheese sauce	1	475	834	0.2	0.2	3.4	28	26

FOOD	PORTION	CALS	VIT A	THIA	RIBO	NIACIN	FOLIC	VIT C
baked topped w/ cheese sauce & bacon	1	451	627	0.3	0.2	4	28	29
baked topped w/ cheese sauce & broccoli	1	402	1695	0.3	0.3	3.6	61	49
baked topped w/ cheese sauce & chili	1	481	768	0.3	0.3	4.2	50	32
baked topped w/ sour cream & chives	1	394	1346	0.3	0.2	3.7	32	34
baked w/ skin	1 (6.5 oz)	220	0	0.2	0.1	3.3	22	26
baked w/o skin	1 (5 oz)	145	0	0.2	tr	2.2	14	20
boiled	½ cup	68	0	0.1	tr	1.1	8	10
curry	1 serv (6 oz)	292	1000	0.1	tr	1.8	–	14
french fries	1 reg	235	22	0.1	0	1.7	25	4
french fries	1 lg	355	33	0.2	0	2.6	38	6
hash brown	½ cup (2.5 oz)	151	18	0.1	tr	1.1	8	6
instant mashed flakes as prep w/ whole milk & butter	½ cup	118	189	0.1	0.1	0.7	8	10
instant mashed granules not prep	½ cup	372	9	0.5	0.3	4.8	40	37
mashed	½ cup	111	177	0.1	tr	1.1	0	6
mustard potato salad	3.5 oz	120	500	0.2	0.1	2	–	12
o'brien	1 cup	157	934	0.1	0.1	2	16	32
potato pancakes	1 (1.3 oz)	101	53	0.1	0.1	0.8	9	8
potato puffs as prep	1	16	1	tr	tr	0.2	1	1
potato salad	½ cup	179	261	0.1	0.1	1.1	8	13
scalloped	½ cup	105	165	0.1	0.1	1.3	10	13
Birds Eye								
Baby Gourmet	7 (4 oz)	100	0	–	–	–	–	0
Whole	3	50	0	–	–	–	–	2
Del Monte								
New Sliced	⅔ cup (5.4 oz)	60	0	–	–	–	–	9
New Whole	2 med (5.5 oz)	60	0	–	–	–	–	9

FOOD	PORTION	CALS	VIT A	THIA	RIBO	NIACIN	FOLIC	VIT C
Healthy Choice								
Cheddar Broccoli Potatoes	1 meal (10.5 oz)	330	300	–	–	–	–	27
Lean Cuisine								
Everyday Favorites Deluxe Cheddar Potato	1 pkg (10.4 oz)	250	300	–	–	–	–	18
Everyday Favorites Roasted Potatoes w/ Broccoli	1 pkg (10.25 oz)	260	750	–	–	–	–	12
Oh Boy!								
Stuffed With Cheddar Cheese	1 (5 oz)	130	100	–	–	–	–	1
S&W								
Whole Small	2 (5.5 oz)	60	0	–	–	–	–	9
TastyBite								
Bombay Potatoes	½ pkg (5 oz)	190	0	–	–	–	–	0
Mumbai Pav Bhaji	½ pkg (5 oz)	229	50	–	–	–	–	1
Simla Potatoes	½ pkg (5 oz)	180	0	–	–	–	–	0
Tree Of Life								
Organic French Fries	20 pieces (3 oz)	110	0	–	–	–	–	0

PRETZELS

FOOD	PORTION	CALS	VIT A	THIA	RIBO	NIACIN	FOLIC	VIT C
dutch twist	4 (2.1 oz)	229	0	0.3	0.4	3.1	–	0
pretzels	1 oz	108	0	0.1	0.2	1.5	–	0
rods	4 (2 oz)	229	0	0.3	0.4	3.1	–	0
sticks	10	10	0	tr	tr	0.1	–	0
sticks	120 (2 oz)	229	0	0.3	0.4	3.1	–	0
twist	1 (½ oz)	65	0	0.1	tr	0.7	–	0
twists	10 (2.1 oz)	229	0	0.3	0.4	3.1	–	0
Rold Gold								
Sharp Cheddar	22 (1 oz)	110	0	–	–	–	–	0
Snyder's Of Hanover								
Snaps	24 (1 oz)	120	0	–	–	–	–	0

PRUNE JUICE

FOOD	PORTION	CALS	VIT A	THIA	RIBO	NIACIN	FOLIC	VIT C
canned	1 cup	181	9	tr	0.2	2	1	11

FOOD	PORTION	CALS	VIT A	THIA	RIBO	NIACIN	FOLIC	VIT C
PRUNES								
canned in heavy syrup	5	90	686	tr	0.1	0.7	–	2
dried	10	201	1669	0.1	0.1	1.6	3	3
PUDDING								
banana as prep w/ 2% milk	½ cup (4.9 oz)	142	251	tr	0.2	0.1	5	1
banana as prep w/ whole milk	½ cup (4.9 oz)	157	155	tr	0.2	0.1	5	1
blancmange	1 serv (4.7 oz)	154	350	tr	0.2	1.1	–	tr
bread pudding	½ cup (4.4 oz)	212	304	0.1	0.3	0.8	16	1
bread w/ raisins	½ cup	180	125	0.1	0.2	0.4	13	1
chocolate	½ cup (5.5 oz)	221	193	tr	0.2	0.2	7	1
chocolate	1 pkg (5 oz)	189	51	tr	0.2	0.5	4	3
chocolate as prep w/ whole milk	½ cup (5 oz)	158	157	tr	0.2	0.1	–	1
coconut cream	½ cup (4.9 oz)	148	251	tr	0.2	0.1	–	1
corn	⅔ cup	181	411	0.7	0.2	1.6	42	5
instant banana as prep w/ 2% milk	½ cup (5.2 oz)	152	250	–	0.2	0.1	6	1
instant banana as prep w/ whole milk	½ cup (5.2 oz)	167	154	–	0.2	0.1	6	1
instant chocolate	½ cup (5.2 oz)	149	254	0.1	0.2	0.1	6	1
instant chocolate as prep w/ whole milk	½ cup (5.2 oz)	164	157	tr	0.2	0.1	6	1
instant lemon	½ cup (5.2 oz)	155	250	tr	0.2	0.1	6	1
instant vanilla	½ cup (5 oz)	147	242	tr	0.2	0.1	6	1
lemon	½ cup (5.1 oz)	163	117	–	–	–	–	0

FOOD	PORTION	CALS	VIT A	THIA	RIBO	NIACIN	FOLIC	VIT C
queen of puddings	1 serv (4.4 oz)	266	625	0.1	0.2	1.8	—	1
rice pudding	1 serv (3 oz)	110	255	tr	0.1	0.9	—	1
rice w/ raisins	½ cup	246	161	0.1	0.3	0.7	21	1
tapioca	½ cup (5.3 oz)	189	314	0.1	0.3	0.1	14	1
vanilla	½ cup (4.3 oz)	130	153	tr	0.2	0.1	5	1
vanilla	1 pkg (4 oz)	146	23	tr	0.2	0.3	0	0
vanilla as prep w/ 2% milk	½ cup (4.9 oz)	141	251	tr	0.2	0.1	—	1
vanilla as prep w/ whole milk	½ cup (4.9 oz)	155	155	tr	0.2	0.1	—	1
yorkshire	1 serv (3 oz)	177	270	0.1	0.2	0.4	3	0
Jell-O								
Fat Free Chocolate Fudge & Caramel	1 serv (4 oz)	100	100	—	—	—	—	0
Fat Free Tapioca	1 serv (4 oz)	100	100	—	—	—	—	0
Vanilla as prep w/ 2% milk	½ cup (5.1 oz)	150	200	—	—	—	—	0
Uncle Ben's								
Rice Pudding Cinnamon & Raisins as prep	½ cup (1.5 oz)	160	0	0.1	—	—	32	0

PUDDING POPS

FOOD	PORTION	CALS	VIT A	THIA	RIBO	NIACIN	FOLIC	VIT C
chocolate	1 (1.6 oz)	72	52	tr	0.1	0.1	1	tr
vanilla	1 (1.6 oz)	75	81	tr	0.1	tr	2	tr

PUFFERFISH

FOOD	PORTION	CALS	VIT A	THIA	RIBO	NIACIN	FOLIC	VIT C
raw	3 oz	72	0	tr	0.2	3.4	—	0

PUMMELO

FOOD	PORTION	CALS	VIT A	THIA	RIBO	NIACIN	FOLIC	VIT C
fresh	1	228	0	0.2	0.2	1.3	—	372
sections	1 cup	71	0	0.1	0.1	0.4	—	116

PUMPKIN

FOOD	PORTION	CALS	VIT A	THIA	RIBO	NIACIN	FOLIC	VIT C
cooked mashed	½ cup	24	1320	tr	0.1	0.5	—	6
flowers cooked	½ cup	10	1162	tr	tr	0.2	—	3
leaves cooked	½ cup	7	866	tr	tr	0.3	—	tr

FOOD	PORTION	CALS	VIT A	THIA	RIBO	NIACIN	FOLIC	VIT C
PURSLANE								
cooked	1 cup	21	2130	tr	0.1	0.5	–	12
fresh	1 cup	7	568	tr	tr	0.2	–	9
QUAIL								
breast w/o skin raw	1 (2 oz)	69	21	0.1	0.1	4.6	–	3
w/ skin raw	1 quail (3.8 oz)	210	265	0.3	0.3	8.2	8	7
QUICHE								
cheese	1 slice (3 oz)	283	910	0.1	0.2	3.2	–	tr
lorraine	⅛ of 8 in pie	600	1640	0.1	0.3	tr	–	tr
mushroom	1 slice (3 oz)	256	745	0.1	0.2	3.2	–	tr
QUINCE								
fresh	1	53	37	tr	tr	0.2	–	14
QUINOA								
quinoa not prep	1 cup (6 oz)	636	0	0.3	0.7	5	83	0
RADICCHIO								
raw shredded	½ cup	5	5	tr	tr	0.1	12	2
RADISHES								
chinese dried	½ cup	157	0	0.2	0.4	2	–	0
chinese raw	1 (12 oz)	62	0	0.1	0.1	0.7	–	74
chinese raw sliced	½ cup	8	0	tr	tr	0.1	–	10
chinese sliced cooked	½ cup	13	0	0	tr	0.1	–	11
daikon dried	½ cup	157	0	0.2	0.4	2	–	0
daikon raw	1 (12 oz)	62	0	0.1	0.1	0.7	–	74
daikon raw sliced	½ cup	8	0	tr	tr	tr	–	10
daikon sliced cooked	½ cup	13	0	0	tr	0.1	–	11
moo namul saengche korean salad	1 serv (3.7 oz)	34	81	0	tr	0.2	15	13
red raw	10	7	3	tr	tr	0.1	12	10
red sliced	½ cup	10	4	tr	tr	0.2	16	13
white icicle raw	1 (½ oz)	2	0	tr	tr	0.1	2	5

FOOD	PORTION	CALS	VIT A	THIA	RIBO	NIACIN	FOLIC	VIT C
white icicle raw sliced	½ cup	7	0	tr	tr	0.2	7	15
Eden								
Daikon Dried Shredded	2 tbsp	45	0	0	0	0	0	0
Daikon Pickled	2 slices	5	200	0	0	0	0	0

RAISINS

FOOD	PORTION	CALS	VIT A	THIA	RIBO	NIACIN	FOLIC	VIT C
chocolate coated	10 (0.4 oz)	39	4	tr	tr	tr	—	0
chocolate coated	1 cup (6.7 oz)	741	71	0.2	0.3	0.8	—	tr
golden seedless	1 cup	437	64	tr	0.3	1.7	5	5
seedless	1 cup	434	11	0.2	0.1	1.2	5	5
sultanas	1 oz	88	20	tr	tr	0.2	—	0
Mariana								
Fruitn Yogurt Milk Chocolate Covered Raisins	32 pieces (1 oz)	130	0	—	—	—	—	0
Tree Of Life								
Organic	¼ cup (1.4 oz)	130	0	—	—	—	—	9

RASPBERRIES

FOOD	PORTION	CALS	VIT A	THIA	RIBO	NIACIN	FOLIC	VIT C
canned in heavy syrup	½ cup	117	43	tr	tr	0.6	13	11
fresh	1 cup	61	160	tr	0.1	1.1	—	31
fresh	1 pint	154	406	0.1	0.3	2.8	—	78
frozen sweetened	1 cup	256	149	tr	0.1	0.6	65	41
frozen sweetened	1 pkg (10 oz)	291	169	0.1	0.1	0.7	74	47
Tree Of Life								
Organic	⅔ cup (5 oz)	50	0	—	—	—	—	18

RASPBERRY JUICE

Fresh Samantha

FOOD	PORTION	CALS	VIT A	THIA	RIBO	NIACIN	FOLIC	VIT C
Raspberry Dream	1 cup (8 oz)	120	200	0.1	0.1	0.8	40	48

RED BEANS

Bean Cuisine

FOOD	PORTION	CALS	VIT A	THIA	RIBO	NIACIN	FOLIC	VIT C
Pasta & Beans Barcelona Red With Radiatore	1 serv	210	1000	—	—	—	—	42

FOOD	PORTION	CALS	VIT A	THIA	RIBO	NIACIN	FOLIC	VIT C
RELISH								
cranberry orange	½ cup	246	97	tr	tr	0.1	–	25
hamburger	1 tbsp	19	40	tr	tr	0.1	–	tr
hot dog	1 tbsp	14	25	tr	tr	0.1	–	tr
sweet	1 tbsp	19	23	0	tr	tr	–	tr
RENNIN								
tablet	1 (0.9 g)	1	0	0	0	0	–	0
RHUBARB								
fresh	½ cup	13	61	tr	tr	0.2	4	5
frzn as prep w/ sugar	½ cup	139	83	tr	tr	0.2	6	4
RICE								
brown long grain cooked	1 cup (6.8 oz)	216	0	0.2	tr	3	8	0
brown medium grain cooked	1 cup (6.8 oz)	218	0	0.2	tr	2.6	8	0
glutinous cooked	1 cup (6.1 oz)	169	0	tr	tr	0.5	2	0
nasi goreng indonesian rice & vegetables	1 cup (4.9 oz)	130	2250	–	–	–	–	5
paella	1 serv (7 oz)	308	0	0.1	0.1	5.2	–	10
pilaf	½ cup	84	726	0.1	0.1	1.1	24	15
risotto	6.6 oz	426	730	0.3	tr	4.2	–	tr
spanish	¾ cup	363	763	0.3	0.2	3.2	14	26
white long grain cooked	1 cup (5.5 oz)	205	0	0.3	tr	2.3	92	0
white long grain instant cooked	1 cup (5.8 oz)	162	0	0.1	0.1	1.5	68	0
white medium grain cooked	1 cup (6.5 oz)	242	0	0.3	tr	3.4	108	0
white short grain cooked	1 cup (6.5 oz)	242	0	0.3	tr	2.8	110	0
Lipton								
Oriental Stir Fry as prep	1 cup	270	750	0.2	0	2	80	2

FOOD	PORTION	CALS	VIT A	THIA	RIBO	NIACIN	FOLIC	VIT C
Rice & Sauce Alfredo Broccoli as prep	1 cup	320	500	0.4	0.2	3	100	6
Rice & Sauce Beef as prep	1 cup	270	200	0.4	0.1	3	80	0
Rice & Sauce Cajun Style as prep	1 cup	270	500	0.4	0.2	3	80	4
Rice & Sauce Cajun Style w/ Beans as prep	1 cup	310	500	0.2	0.1	2	100	1
Rice & Sauce Cheddar Broccoli as prep	1 cup	280	400	0.4	0.1	3	100	5
Rice & Sauce Chicken & Parmesan Risotto as prep	1 cup	270	200	0.4	0.1	3	100	0
Rice & Sauce Chicken Broccoli as prep	1 cup	280	500	0.4	0.1	3	100	6
Rice & Sauce Chicken Flavor as prep	1 cup	280	300	0.4	0.1	3	60	0
Rice & Sauce Creamy Chicken as prep	1 cup	290	750	0.4	0.1	3	80	0
Rice & Sauce Herb & Butter as prep	1 cup	280	300	0.4	0.1	3	80	0
Rice & Sauce Medley as prep	1 cup	270	500	0.4	0.1	3	80	0
Rice & Sauce Mushroom as prep	1 cup	270	0	0.4	0.1	3	80	0
Rice & Sauce Mushroom & Herb as prep	1 cup	290	300	0.6	0.1	4	80	1
Rice & Sauce Oriental as prep	1 cup	280	750	0.2	0.1	2	60	2
Rice & Sauce Pilaf as prep	1 cup	260	400	0.4	0.1	3	80	0

FOOD	PORTION	CALS	VIT A	THIA	RIBO	NIACIN	FOLIC	VIT C
Rice & Sauce Scampi Style as prep	1 cup	270	200	0.4	0.1	2	80	0
Rice & Sauce Spanish as prep	1 cup	270	500	0.5	0.1	3	80	5
Rice & Sauce Teriyaki as prep	1 cup	270	300	0.4	0.1	3	80	0
Roasted Chicken as prep	1 cup	260	500	0.2	0	2	80	0
Salsa Style as prep	1 cup	220	400	0.2	0	2	60	4
Southwestern Chicken Flavor as prep	1 cup	260	750	0.2	0	2	80	2
Minute								
Boil-In-Bag White as prep	1 cup (5.7 oz)	190	0	0.2	0	1.6	80	0
Instant White as prep	1 cup (5.7 oz)	160	0	0.2	0	1.2	60	0
Long Grain & Wild Seasoned w/ Herbs as prep	1 cup (7.8 oz)	230	0	0.2	tr	2	80	0
Success								
Broccoli & Cheese	½ cup	130	200	0.1	—	0.8	32	1
Classic Chicken	½ cup	90	200	0.1	0	0.8	32	2
Long Grain & Wild	½ cup	120	200	0.1	—	1.2	32	4
Pilaf	½ cup	120	300	0.2	0.2	8	40	0
Spanish	½ cup	120	400	0.1	—	1.2	32	2

ROLL

FOOD	PORTION	CALS	VIT A	THIA	RIBO	NIACIN	FOLIC	VIT C
brioche sweet roll	1 (3.5 oz)	410	950	0.4	0.3	2.2	—	tr
cinnamon raisin	1 (2¾ in)	223	129	0.2	0.2	1.4	14	1
crescent	1 (1 oz)	98	0	0.1	0.1	0.9	—	0
hard	1 (3½ in)	167	0	0.3	0.2	2.4	8	0
hot cross bun	1	202	220	0.1	0.1	1.8	—	0
kaiser	1 (3½ in)	167	0	0.3	0.2	2.4	8	0
submarine	1 (4.7 oz)	155	0	0.2	0.1	1.7	—	0
wheat	1 (1 oz)	77	0	0.1	0.1	1.2	—	0
whole wheat	1 (1 oz)	75	0	0.1	tr	1	8	0
Bread Du Jour								
Cracked Wheat	1 (1.2 oz)	100	0	0.2	0.1	1.2	16	0
Italian	1 (1.2 oz)	90	0	0.2	0.1	1.2	16	0

FOOD	PORTION	CALS	VIT A	THIA	RIBO	NIACIN	FOLIC	VIT C
Sourdough	1 (1.2 oz)	90	0	0.1	0.1	1.6	24	0
Freihofer's								
Brown 'N Serve	1 (1 oz)	80	0	0.1	0.1	0.8	24	0
Pepperidge Farm								
Dinner Rolls Finger Poppy	1 (0.9 oz)	80	0	0.1	0.1	1.2	24	0
Parker House	1 (0.9 oz)	80	0	0.1	0.1	1.2	24	0
Stroehmann								
Hamburger	1 (1.4 oz)	100	0	0.2	0.1	1.2	40	0
Hamburger Potato	1 (1.9 oz)	140	100	0.2	0.2	1.6	60	0
Hot Dog	1 (1.4 oz)	100	0	0.2	0.1	1.2	40	0
Hot Dog Potato	1 (1.9 oz)	140	100	0.2	0.2	1.6	60	0
Wonder								
Brown & Serve	1 (1 oz)	80	0	0.1	tr	1.6	24	0
Brown & Serve Sourdough	1 (1 oz)	70	0	0.1	0.1	0.8	24	0
Brown & Serve Wheat	1 (1 oz)	80	0	0.1	0.1	0.8	16	0
Bun	1 (3 oz)	220	0	0.4	0.2	3	60	0
Dinner	2 (1.6 oz)	130	0	0.2	0.1	1.6	32	0
Dinner Honey Rich	1 (1.3 oz)	100	0	0.3	0.1	0.8	32	0
Dinner Wheat	2 (1.6 oz)	140	0	0.1	0.1	2	16	0
Hamburger	1 (2.5 oz)	190	0	0.4	0.2	2	60	0
Hamburger	1 (1.5 oz)	110	0	0.2	0.1	1.2	32	0
Hamburger	1 (2 oz)	150	0	0.3	0.1	2	40	0
Hamburger Wheat	1 (1.9 oz)	140	0	0.2	0.1	2	32	0
Potato Bun	1 (1.5 oz)	110	0	0.2	0.1	2	24	0
Steak	1 (2.5 oz)	190	0	0.3	0.2	2	60	0

ROSE APPLE

FOOD	PORTION	CALS	VIT A	THIA	RIBO	NIACIN	FOLIC	VIT C
fresh	3.5 oz	32	tr	tr	tr	0.8	–	22

ROSELLE

FOOD	PORTION	CALS	VIT A	THIA	RIBO	NIACIN	FOLIC	VIT C
fresh	1 cup	28	163	tr	tr	0.2	–	7

ROSEMARY

FOOD	PORTION	CALS	VIT A	THIA	RIBO	NIACIN	FOLIC	VIT C
dried	1 tsp	4	38	tr	–	tr	–	1

RUTABAGA

FOOD	PORTION	CALS	VIT A	THIA	RIBO	NIACIN	FOLIC	VIT C
cooked mashed	½ cup	41	0	0.1	tr	0.8	19	26

FOOD	PORTION	CALS	VIT A	THIA	RIBO	NIACIN	FOLIC	VIT C
SAGE								
ground	1 tsp	2	41	tr	tr	tr	—	tr
SALAD								
chef w/o dressing	1½ cups	386	1197	0.4	0.4	3.2	56	15
tossed w/o dressing	¾ cup	16	1182	0	0	0.6	39	24\
tossed w/o dressing	1½ cups	32	2352	0	0.1	1.2	77	48
tossed w/o dressing w/ cheese & egg	1½ cups	102	822	0.1	0.2	1	85	10
tossed w/o dressing w/ chicken	1½ cups	105	935	0.1	0.1	5.9	67	17
tossed w/o dressing w/ pasta & seafood	1½ cups (14.6 oz)	380	6245	0.3	0.2	3.6	100	38
tossed w/o dressing w/ shrimp	1½ cups	107	791	0.1	0.2	1.2	87	9
waldorf	½ cup	79	125	tr	tr	0.1	6	2
Dole								
Salad-In-A-Minute Spinach	3.5 oz	180	1000	0.1	0.1	<0.4	<8	9
SALAD DRESSING								
blue cheese	1 tbsp	77	32	0	0	0	—	tr
russian	1 tbsp	76	106	tr	tr	0.1	—	1
SALMON								
pink w/ bone	3 oz	118	47	tr	0.2	5.6	13	0
pink w/ bone	1 can (15.9 oz)	631	250	0.1	0.8	29.7	70	0
salmon cake	1 (3 oz)	241	446	0.1	0.2	5.8	7	tr
Bumble Bee								
Keta	½ cup (3.5 oz)	160	0	0.1	0.2	6	—	0
Red	½ cup (3.5 oz)	180	100	tr	0.2	7	—	0
SALSIFY								
fresh sliced cooked	½ cup	46	0	tr	0.1	0.3	—	3

FOOD	PORTION	CALS	VIT A	THIA	RIBO	NIACIN	FOLIC	VIT C
SALT/SEASONED SALT								
Eden								
Atlantic Sea Salt	¼ tsp	0	0	0	0	0	0	0
Brittany Sea Salt	¼ tsp	0	0	0	0	0	0	0
SANDWICHES								
chicken fillet plain	1	515	100	0.3	0.2	6.8	28	9
chicken fillet w/ cheese lettuce mayonnaise & tomato	1	632	620	0.4	0.5	9.1	46	3
croque monsieur	1 (12.4 oz)	765	2240	0.7	0.8	4.5	41	9
fish fillet w/ tartar sauce	1	431	110	0.3	0.2	3.4	44	3
fish fillet w/ tartar sauce & cheese	1	524	432	0.5	0.4	4.2	32	3
fried egg w/ cheese	1	340	668	0.3	0.6	2.1	36	2
fried egg w/ cheese & ham	1	348	561	0.4	0.6	4.2	43	3
ham w/ cheese	1	353	319	0.3	0.5	2.7	71	3
roast beef submarine sandwich w/ tomato lettuce & mayonnaise	1	411	412	0.4	0.4	6	45	6
roast beef w/ cheese	1	402	193	0.4	0.5	5.9	41	0
roast beef plain	1	346	210	0.4	0.3	5.9	40	2
steak w/ tomato lettuce salt & mayonnaise	1	459	367	0.4	0.4	7.3	89	6
tuna salad submarine sandwich w/ lettuce & oil	1	584	188	0.5	0.4	11.3	58	4
SAPODILLA								
fresh	1	140	102	—	tr	0.3	—	25

FOOD	PORTION	CALS	VIT A	THIA	RIBO	NIACIN	FOLIC	VIT C
SAPOTES								
fresh	1	301	923	tr	tr	4	–	45
SARDINES								
pacific in tomato sauce w/ bone	1	68	139	tr	0.1	1.6	9	tr
SAUCE								
fish sauce chinese	1 tbsp	9	90	0	tr	0.4	–	0
fish sauce vietnamese nuoc mam	1 tbsp	6	0	0	tr	0.4	9	0
hoisin	1 tbsp	35	0	0	tr	0.2	4	0
oyster	1 tbsp	8	4	0	tr	0.2	2	0
teriyaki	1 tbsp	15	0	tr	tr	0.2	4	0
SAUERKRAUT								
canned	½ cup	22	21	tr	tr	0.2	–	17
Eden								
Organic	½ cup	25	0	0.1	tr	1.6	0	12
SAUSAGE								
chipolata	3.5 oz	342	tr	0.3	0.2	2.8	3	1
chorizo	3.5 oz	499	tr	0.6	0.3	5.6	3	0
pork	1 patty (1 oz)	100	tr	0.2	0	1.2	–	0
SAUSAGE DISHES								
sausage roll	1 (2.3 oz)	311	405	0.1	tr	2.1	–	0
SAUSAGE SUBSTITUTES								
nonmeat sausage	1 patty (38 g)	97	243	0.9	0.2	4.3	10	0
nonmeat sausage	1 link (25 g)	64	160	0.6	0.1	2.8	7	0
Yves								
Veggie Breakfast Patties	1 (2 oz)	70	0	0.5	0.2	4	–	0
SCONE								
cheese	1 (3.5 oz)	364	850	0.2	0.2	3.2	–	tr
plain	1 (3.5 oz)	362	700	0.2	tr	2.6	–	tr
SEA CUCUMBER								
dried	1 oz	74	37	tr	tr	0.4	–	0

FOOD	PORTION	CALS	VIT A	THIA	RIBO	NIACIN	FOLIC	VIT C
SEA URCHIN								
canned	1 oz	39	0	0	tr	–	–	0
fresh	1 oz	36	0	tr	0.3	0.1	–	3
roe paste	1 tbsp	19	24	0	tr	0.1	–	0
SEAWEED								
agar dried	1 oz	87	0	tr	0.1	0.1	–	0
agar fresh	1 oz	tr	0	tr	tr	tr	–	0
hijiki dried	1 tbsp	9	16	0	tr	0.2	–	0
laver fresh	1 oz	10	1483	tr	0.1	0.4	–	11
nori fresh	1 oz	10	1483	tr	0.1	0.4	–	11
nori sheet dried	1 (8 x 8 in)	5	30	tr	tr	0.2	–	0
wakame fresh	1 oz	13	103	tr	0.1	0.5	–	1
SEMOLINA								
dry	1 cup (5.9 oz)	601	0	1.4	1	10	129	0
SESAME								
sesame butter	1 tbsp	95	8	tr	tr	1.1	–	0
Eden								
Organic Seaweed Gomasio	1 serv (1.5 oz)	10	0	0	0	0	0	0
Organic Gomasio	½ tsp	10	0	0	0	0	0	0
Organic Gomasio Garlic	½ tsp	10	0	0	0	0	0	0
Maranatha								
Roasted Tahini	2 tbsp	210	0	–	–	–	–	0
SESBANIA								
flowers cooked	1 cup	23	0	0.1	tr	0.3	–	39
SHARK								
fin dried	1 oz	32	0	tr	tr	tr	–	0
SHELLIE BEANS								
canned	½ cup	37	278	tr	0.1	0.3	–	4
SHERBET								
orange	½ cup (4 fl oz)	132	73	tr	0.1	0.1	4	4
orange	1 bar (2.75 fl oz)	91	50	tr	tr	0.1	3	3

FOOD	PORTION	CALS	VIT A	THIA	RIBO	NIACIN	FOLIC	VIT C
SHRIMP								
chinese shrimp paste	1 tbsp	15	0	tr	–	–	–	0
jambalaya	¾ cup	188	1256	0.2	0.1	2.9	15	19
SNACKS								
cheese puffs	1 oz	157	75	0.1	0.1	0.9	34	0
oriental mix	1 oz	155	15	0.1	tr	3	25	tr
pork skins	1 oz	154	37	tr	0.1	0.4	–	tr
pork skins barbecue	1 oz	152	427	tr	0.1	1	–	tr
trail mix	1 cup (5.3 oz)	693	27	0.7	0.3	7.1	107	2
trail mix tropical	1 oz	115	14	0.1	tr	0.4	12	2
trail mix w/ chocolate chips	1 cup (5.1 oz)	707	64	0.6	0.3	6.4	95	2
Big Dipper								
Bagel Chips Lowfat Barbeque	12 (1 oz)	110	0	0.2	0.1	0	40	0
Bagel Chips Lowfat Garlic	12 (1 oz)	120	0	0.2	0.1	0	40	0
Bagel Chips Lowfat Original	12 (1 oz)	110	0	0.2	0.1	0	40	0
Chex Mix								
Bold'n Zesty	1 pkg (1.7 oz)	230	0	0.4	tr	5	60	4
Cheddar Cheese	1 pkg (1.7 oz)	220	0	0.4	tr	5	60	4
Hot'n Spicy	1 pkg (1.7 oz)	210	0	0.2	tr	3	60	4
Traditional	1 pkg (1.7 oz)	210	0	0.4	tr	5	60	4
Dakota Gourmet								
Toasted Corn Heart Smart	1 pkg (1.75 oz)	177	338	0.3	0.1	3.5	72	2
Trail Mix Heart Smart	1 pkg (1.75 oz)	172	24	0.1	0.1	0.6	45	1
Pita Puffs								
Barbeque	35 (1 oz)	120	0	0.1	0.2	0	16	0
Lowfat Garlic	35 (1 oz)	110	0	0.2	0.1	0	40	0

FOOD	PORTION	CALS	VIT A	THIA	RIBO	NIACIN	FOLIC	VIT C
Lowfat Original	35 (1 oz)	110	0	0.2	0.1	0	32	0
Lowfat Salsa	35 (1 oz)	110	0	0.2	0.1	0	40	0
Pizza	35 (1 oz)	120	0	0.1	0.2	0	16	0
Ranch	35 (1 oz)	120	0	0.1	0.2	0	24	0
Pumpkorn								
Caramel	⅓ cup	150	100	–	–	–	16	0
Chili	⅓ cup	150	400	–	–	–	16	0
Curry	⅓ cup	150	100	–	–	–	16	0
Maple Vanilla	⅓ cup	150	100	–	–	–	16	0
Mesquite	⅓ cup	150	100	–	–	–	16	0
Original	⅓ cup	150	100	–	–	–	16	0

SNAIL

FOOD	PORTION	CALS	VIT A	THIA	RIBO	NIACIN	FOLIC	VIT C
escargot cooked	5	25	10	0	0	0.3	0	0

SNAKE

FOOD	PORTION	CALS	VIT A	THIA	RIBO	NIACIN	FOLIC	VIT C
fresh	3 oz	78	15	0.1	0.1	0.8	–	3

SODA

FOOD	PORTION	CALS	VIT A	THIA	RIBO	NIACIN	FOLIC	VIT C
club	12 oz	0	0	0	0	0	0	0
cola	12 oz	151	0	0	0	0	0	0
cream	12 oz	191	0	0	0	0	0	0
diet cola	12 oz	2	0	0	0	0	0	0
diet cola w/ equal	12 oz	2	0	tr	0.1	0	0	0
diet cola w/ saccharin	12 oz	2	0	0	0	0	0	0
ginger ale	12 oz can	124	0	0	0	0	0	0
grape	12 oz	161	0	0	0	–	0	0
lemon lime	12 oz	149	0	0	0	0	0	0
orange	12 oz	177	0	0	0	0	0	0
pepper type	12 oz	151	0	0	0	0	0	0
quinine	12 oz	125	0	0	0	0	0	0
root beer	12 oz	152	0	0	0	0	0	0
tonic water	12 oz	125	0	0	0	0	0	0
Lucozade								
Soda	7 oz	136	0	0	0	0	–	0
Yoo-Hoo								
Original	9 fl oz	150	500	tr	0.2	2.0	8	6

SOLE

FOOD	PORTION	CALS	VIT A	THIA	RIBO	NIACIN	FOLIC	VIT C
battered & fried	3.2 oz	211	35	0.1	0.1	1.9	51	0
breaded & fried	3.2 oz	211	35	0.1	0.1	1.9	51	0

FOOD	PORTION	CALS	VIT A	THIA	RIBO	NIACIN	FOLIC	VIT C
SORGHUM								
sorghum	1 cup (6.7 oz)	651	0	0.5	0.3	11.2	—	0
SOUFFLE								
spinach	1 cup	218	3461	0.1	0.3	0.5	62	3
SOUP								
asparagus cream of as prep w/ milk	1 cup	161	599	0.1	0.3	0.9	—	4
asparagus cream of as prep w/ water	1 cup	87	445	0.1	0.1	0.8	—	3
beef broth ready-to-serve	1 cup	16	0	tr	0.1	1.9	—	0
beef broth ready-to-serve	1 can (14 oz)	27	0	tr	0.1	3.1	—	0
beef stew soup	1 cup (8.8 oz)	221	6626	0.2	0.2	3.6	25	14
black bean turtle soup	1 cup	218	10	0.3	0.3	1.5	146	6
brunswick stew soup	1 cup (8.5 oz)	232	433	0.1	0.2	6.6	21	14
celery cream of as prep w/ milk	1 cup	165	461	0.1	0.2	0.4	9	1
celery cream of as prep w/ water	1 cup	90	306	tr	tr	0.3	2	tr
celery cream of not prep	1 can (10¾ oz)	219	746	0.1	0.1	0.8	6	1
cheese as prep w/ milk	1 cup	230	1243	0.1	0.3	0.5	—	1
cheese as prep w/ water	1 cup	155	1088	tr	0.1	0.4	—	0
cheese not prep	1 can (11 oz)	377	2643	tr	0.3	1	—	0
chicken broth as prep w/ water	1 cup	21	40	tr	tr	0.2	—	tr
chicken cream of as prep w/ milk	1 cup	191	715	0.1	0.3	0.9	8	1
chicken cream of as prep w/ water	1 cup	116	560	tr	0.1	0.8	2	tr
chicken gumbo as prep w/water	1 cup	56	136	tr	0.1	0.7	—	5

FOOD	PORTION	CALS	VIT A	THIA	RIBO	NIACIN	FOLIC	VIT C
chicken noodle as prep w/ water	1 cup	53	63	0.1	0.1	0.9	1	tr
clam chowder manhattan as prep w/ water	1 cup	77	963	tr	tr	0.8	10	4
clam chowder new england as prep w/ water	1 cup	95	8	tr	tr	1	4	2
clam chowder new england as prep w/ milk	1 cup	163	164	0.1	0.2	1	10	4
corn & cheese chowder	¾ cup	215	636	0.1	0.3	1	12	7
gazpacho ready-to-serve	1 cup	57	200	tr	tr	0.9	–	3
greek lemon	¾ cup	63	39	0.1	0.1	0.3	8	4
hot & sour	1 serv (14 oz)	173	124	0.3	0.2	2.2	9	1
minestrone as prep w/water	1 cup	83	2337	0.1	tr	0.9	16	1
mushroom cream of as prep w/ milk	1 cup	203	154	0.1	0.3	0.9	–	2
mushroom cream of as prep w/ water	1 cup	129	0	tr	0.1	0.7	–	1
onion soup gratinee	1 serv	492	1145	0.3	0.4	4.3	57	11
oxtail	5 oz	64	0	tr	tr	1.7	–	0
oyster stew as prep w/ milk	1 cup	134	225	0.1	0.2	0.3	–	4
pasta e fagioli	1 cup (8.8 oz)	194	1878	0.2	0.1	1.6	49	12
pepperpot as prep w/ water	1 cup	103	856	0.1	tr	1.2	tr	1
potato cream of as prep w/ milk	1 cup	148	443	0.1	0.2	0.6	9	1
potato cream of as prep w/ water	1 cup	73	288	tr	tr	0.5	3	0
ratatouille	1 cup (7.5 oz)	266	815	0.1	0.1	1.1	34	41
scotch broth as prep w/ water	1 cup	80	2180	tr	tr	1.2	–	1

FOOD	PORTION	CALS	VIT A	THIA	RIBO	NIACIN	FOLIC	VIT C
split pea w/ ham as prep w/ water	1 cup	189	444	0.1	0.1	1.5	3	1
tomato as prep w/ milk	1 cup	160	849	0.1	0.2	1.5	21	68
tomato as prep w/ water	1 cup	102	832	0.1	tr	0.8	7	5
vichyssoise	1 cup	148	443	0.1	0.2	0.6	9	1
vietnamese pho beef noodle	1 serv (7.8 oz)	480	309	0.2	0.2	2.4	33	50
Cup-a-Soup								
Chicken Vegetable as prep	1 serv (6 oz)	50	0	0.1	tr	0.4	16	0
Chicken Broth w/ Pasta Fat Free as prep	1 serv (6 oz)	45	0	0.1	0	0.8	16	0
Chicken Noodle as prep	1 serv (6 oz)	50	0	0.1	0.1	1.2	16	0
Hearty Chicken Noodle as prep	1 serv (6 oz)	60	0	0.1	0.1	1.2	16	0
Ring Noodle as prep	1 serv (6 oz)	50	0	0.1	tr	0.8	16	0
Spring Vegetable as prep	1 serv (6 oz)	45	0	0.1	tr	0.8	16	0
Lipton								
Chicken Noodle w/ White Chicken Meat as prep	1 cup	80	0	0.2	0.1	1.6	24	0
Extra Noodle w/ Chicken Broth as prep	1 cup	90	0	0.4	0.1	1.6	32	0
Giggle Noodle w/ Chicken Broth as prep	1 cup	70	0	0.2	0.1	1.2	16	0
Ring-O-Noodle w/ Chicken Broth as prep	1 cup	70	0	0.2	0.1	1.2	24	0
Soup Secrets Chicken 'N Onion as prep	1 cup	120	0	0.1	0.1	1.2	24	1

FOOD	PORTION	CALS	VIT A	THIA	RIBO	NIACIN	FOLIC	VIT C
Soup Secrets Chicken w/ Pasta & Beans as prep	1 cup	110	500	0.2	0.1	1.6	32	1
Soup Secrets Country Chicken w/ Pasta & Herbs as prep	1 cup	100	0	0.2	0.1	1.2	32	0
Soup Secrets Honestyle Lentil w/ Bow Tie Pasta as prep	1 cup	130	500	tr	—	—	32	0
Soup Secrets Minestrone as prep	1 cup	110	500	0.1	0.1	0.8	49	4
Spiral Pasta w/ Chicken Broth as prep	1 cup	60	0	0.2	0.1	1.2	24	0

SOUR CREAM

FOOD	PORTION	CALS	VIT A	THIA	RIBO	NIACIN	FOLIC	VIT C
sour cream	1 cup (8 oz)	493	1817	0.1	0.3	0.2	25	2
sour cream	1 tbsp (0.4 oz)	26	95	tr	tr	tr	1	tr

SOUR CREAM SUBSTITUTES

FOOD	PORTION	CALS	VIT A	THIA	RIBO	NIACIN	FOLIC	VIT C
nondairy	1 oz	59	0	0	0	0	0	0
nondairy	1 cup	479	0	0	0	0	0	0

SOURSOP

FOOD	PORTION	CALS	VIT A	THIA	RIBO	NIACIN	FOLIC	VIT C
fresh	1	416	15	0.4	0.3	5.6	—	129

SOY

FOOD	PORTION	CALS	VIT A	THIA	RIBO	NIACIN	FOLIC	VIT C
soy milk	1 cup	79	77	0.4	0.2	0.4	4	0
soya cheese	1.4 oz	128	0	0.1	0.3	1.6	—	0

SOY SAUCE

FOOD	PORTION	CALS	VIT A	THIA	RIBO	NIACIN	FOLIC	VIT C
shoyu	1 tbsp	9	0	tr	tr	0.6	3	0
soy sauce	1 tbsp	7	0	tr	tr	0.5	2	0
tamari	1 tbsp	11	0	tr	tr	0.7	3	0
Eden								
Shoyu	1 tbsp	15	0	0	0.1	0	0	0

FOOD	PORTION	CALS	VIT A	THIA	RIBO	NIACIN	FOLIC	VIT C
SOYBEANS								
dried cooked	1 cup	298	15	0.3	0.5	0.7	93	3
dry roasted	½ cup	387	20	0.4	0.6	0.9	176	4
roasted & toasted	1 cup	490	216	0.1	0.2	1.9	244	2
sprouts raw	½ cup	43	4	0.1	tr	0.4	60	5
sprouts stir fried	1 cup	125	17	0.4	0.2	1.1	—	12
Dakota Gourmet								
Soy Nuts	1 oz	129	6	0.1	0.2	0.8	55	1
Eden								
Organic Black	½ cup (4.6 oz)	120	500	0.1	0.1	0.4	24	0
SPAGHETTI SAUCE								
bolognese	5 oz	195	2260	0.1	0.2	4.6	—	7
marinara sauce	1 cup	171	2403	0.1	0.1	4	—	32
spaghetti sauce	1 cup	272	3055	0.1	0.1	3.7	—	28
Di Giorno								
Alfredo	¼ cup (2.2 oz)	180	400	0	0.1	0	0	0
Basil Pesto	¼ cup (2.2 oz)	320	500	0	0.1	0	8	0
Four Cheese	¼ cup (2.2 oz)	160	500	0	0.1	0	0	0
Garlic Pesto	¼ cup (2.1 oz)	340	200	0	0.1	0	0	0
Light Alfredo Sauce	¼ cup (2.4 oz)	140	750	0	0.1	0	0	0
Marinara	½ cup (4.5 oz)	70	500	0.1	0.1	1.6	0	0
Plum Tomato Cream Sauce	½ cup (4.4 oz)	160	750	0.1	0.1	1.2	0	1
Plum Tomato & Mushroom	½ cup (4.4 oz)	60	500	0.1	tr	2	0	0
Roasted Red Bell Pepper Cream Sauce	¼ cup (2.3 oz)	140	1000	0	0.1	0	0	0
Eden								
Organic Lightly Seasoned	½ cup (4.4 oz)	80	2000	tr	1.6	0	0	2

FOOD	PORTION	CALS	VIT A	THIA	RIBO	NIACIN	FOLIC	VIT C
SPANISH FOOD								
burrito w/ apple	1 sm (2.6 oz)	231	405	0.2	0.2	1.9	4	tr
burrito w/ beans	2 (7.6 oz)	448	332	0.6	0.6	4	118	2
burrito w/ beans & cheese	2 (6.5 oz)	377	1250	0.2	0.7	3.6	81	2
burrito w/ beans & chili peppers	2 (7.2 oz)	413	205	0.5	0.7	4.4	118	1
burrito w/ beans & meat	2 (8.1 oz)	508	636	0.5	0.8	5.4	73	2
burrito w/ beans cheese & beef	2 (7.1 oz)	331	799	0.3	0.7	3.9	61	5
burrito w/ beans cheese & chili peppers	2 (11.8 oz)	663	1596	0.6	1.2	7.7	146	7
burrito w/ beef	2 (7.7 oz)	523	277	0.2	0.9	6.5	39	1
burrito w/ beef & chili peppers	2 (7.1 oz)	426	463	0.4	0.8	5.1	37	2
burrito w/ beef cheese & chili peppers	2 (10.7 oz)	634	972	0.6	1.2	8.3	58	4
burrito w/ cherry	1 sm (2.6 oz)	231	405	0.2	0.2	1.9	4	tr
chimichanga w/ beef	1 (6.1 oz)	425	147	0.5	0.6	5.8	31	5
chimichanga w/ beef & cheese	1 (6.4 oz)	443	540	0.4	0.9	4.7	34	3
chimichanga w/ beef & red chili peppers	1 (6.7 oz)	424	262	0.3	0.7	5.3	34	tr
chimichanga w/ beef cheese & red chili peppers	1 (6.3 oz)	364	702	0.2	1	3.5	33	2
enchilada w/ cheese	1 (5.7 oz)	320	1160	0	0.4	1.9	34	tr
enchilada w/ cheese & beef	1 (6.7 oz)	324	1135	0.1	0.4	2.5	192	1
enchirito w/ cheese beef & beans	1 (6.8 oz)	344	1015	0.2	0.7	3	254	5

FOOD	PORTION	CALS	VIT A	THIA	RIBO	NIACIN	FOLIC	VIT C
frijoles w/ cheese	1 cup (5.9 oz)	226	457	0.1	0.3	1.5	111	2
nachos w/ cheese	6 to 8 (4 oz)	345	559	0.2	0.4	1.5	10	1
nachos w/ cheese & jalapeno peppers	6 to 8 (7.2 oz)	607	4061	0.1	0.5	2.8	19	tr
nachos w/ cheese beans ground beef & peppers	6 to 8 (8.9 oz)	568	3401	0.2	0.7	3.4	39	5
nachos w/ cinnamon & sugar	6 to 8 (3.8 oz)	592	108	0.2	0.4	3.9	7	8
taco	1 sm (6 oz)	370	855	0.2	0.5	3.2	23	2
taco salad	1½ cups	279	589	0.1	0.4	2.5	40	4
taco salad w/ chili con carne	1½ cups	288	1573	0.2	0.5	2.5	64	3
tostada w/ beans & cheese	1 (5.1 oz)	223	622	0.1	0.3	1.3	75	1
tostada w/ beans beef & cheese	1 (7.9 oz)	334	1275	0	0.5	2.6	97	4
tostada w/ beef & cheese	1 (5.7 oz)	315	713	0.1	0.6	3.1	15	3
tostada w/ guacamole	2 (9.2 oz)	360	1752	0.1	0.6	2	110	4
Quaker								
Masa Harina De Maiz	2 tortillas	137	0	0.4	0.3	3.5	17	0
Masa Trigo	2 tortillas	149	0	0.4	0.2	3.1	29	0

SPINACH

FOOD	PORTION	CALS	VIT A	THIA	RIBO	NIACIN	FOLIC	VIT C
cooked	½ cup	21	7371	0.1	0.2	0.4	131	9
malabar cooked	1 cup (1.5 oz)	10	510	0.1	0.1	0.4	50	1
raw chopped	½ cup	6	1880	tr	0.1	0.2	54	8
Fresh Like								
Cut Leaf	3.5 oz	21	8194	0.1	0.1	0.4	–	26

SPROUTS

FOOD	PORTION	CALS	VIT A	THIA	RIBO	NIACIN	FOLIC	VIT C
kidney bean cooked	1 lb	152	8	1.6	1.2	13.7	–	162
lentil sprouts	½ cup	40	17	0.1	tr	0.4	38	6
mung bean canned	½ cup	8	14	tr	tr	0.1	6	tr

FOOD	PORTION	CALS	VIT A	THIA	RIBO	NIACIN	FOLIC	VIT C
mung bean cooked	½ cup	13	8	tr	0.1	0.5	–	7
pea	½ cup	77	100	0.1	0.1	1.9	87	6
radish	½ cup	8	74	tr	tr	0.5	18	6

SQUASH

FOOD	PORTION	CALS	VIT A	THIA	RIBO	NIACIN	FOLIC	VIT C
acorn cooked mashed	½ cup	41	315	0.1	tr	0.6	14	8
acorn cubed baked	½ cup	57	437	0.2	tr	0.9	19	11
butternut cooked mashed	½ cup	47	4007	0.1	tr	0.6	–	4
butternut baked	½ cup	41	7141	0.1	tr	1	20	15
crookneck raw sliced	½ cup	12	220	tr	tr	0.3	15	5
crookneck sliced cooked	½ cup	18	259	tr	tr	0.5	18	5
hubbard baked	½ cup	51	6156	0.1	tr	0.6	17	10
hubbard cooked mashed	½ cup	35	4726	0.1	tr	0.4	12	8
scallop sliced cooked	½ cup	14	77	tr	tr	0.4	19	10
spaghetti cooked	½ cup	23	86	tr	tr	0.6	6	3

STARFRUIT

FOOD	PORTION	CALS	VIT A	THIA	RIBO	NIACIN	FOLIC	VIT C
fresh	1	42	626	tr	tr	0.5	–	27

STRAWBERRIES

FOOD	PORTION	CALS	VIT A	THIA	RIBO	NIACIN	FOLIC	VIT C
strawberries	1 cup	45	41	tr	0.1	0.3	26	85
strawberries	1 pint	97	87	0.1	0.1	0.7	57	182
sweetened sliced	1 cup	245	61	tr	0.1	1	38	106

STUFFING/DRESSING

FOOD	PORTION	CALS	VIT A	THIA	RIBO	NIACIN	FOLIC	VIT C
bread	½ cup	195	349	0.2	0.2	1.8	19	2
cornbread	½ cup	179	353	0.1	0.1	1.2	8	1
sausage	½ cup	292	78	0.2	0.1	1.1	3	2
Stove Top								
Chicken as prep w/ margarine	½ cup (3.6 oz)	170	300	0.1	0.1	0.8	16	0
Cornbread as prep w/ margarine	½ cup (3.6 oz)	170	300	0.1	tr	0.8	16	0

FOOD	PORTION	CALS	VIT A	THIA	RIBO	NIACIN	FOLIC	VIT C
Flexible Serve Chicken as prep w/ margarine	½ cup (3.3 oz)	170	300	0.1	0.1	0.8	16	0
Flexible Serve Cornbread as prep w/ margarine	½ cup (3.3 oz)	160	300	0.1	tr	0.8	16	0
Flexible Serve Homestyle Herb as prep w/ margarine	½ cup (3.3 oz)	170	300	0.1	0.1	0.8	16	0
For Beef as prep w/ margarine	½ cup (3.7 oz)	180	500	0.1	0.1	0.8	16	0
For Pork as prep w/ margarine	½ cup (3.6 oz)	170	400	0.1	0.2	0.8	24	0
For Turkey as prep w/ margarine	½ cup (3.6 oz)	170	300	0.1	0.1	0.8	16	0
Long Grain & Wild Rice as prep w/ margarine	½ cup (3.7 oz)	180	300	0.1	0.1	0.8	16	0
Lower Sodium Chicken as prep w/ margarine	½ cup (3.6 oz)	180	300	0.1	0.1	0.8	16	0
Microwave Chicken as prep w/ margarine	½ cup (3.5 oz)	160	200	0.1	0.1	0.8	16	0
Microwave Homestyle Cornbread as prep w/ margarine	½ cup (3 oz)	160	200	0.1	tr	0.8	16	0
Mushroom & Onion as prep w/ margarine	½ cup (3.6 oz)	180	300	0.1	0.1	0.8	16	0
San Francisco Style as prep w/ margarine	½ cup (3.6 oz)	170	500	0.1	0.1	1.2	24	0
Savory Herb as prep w/ margarine	½ cup (3.6 oz)	170	300	0.1	0.1	0.8	16	0

FOOD	PORTION	CALS	VIT A	THIA	RIBO	NIACIN	FOLIC	VIT C
Traditional Sage as prep w/ margarine	½ cup (3.6 oz)	180	500	0.1	0.1	0.8	16	0
SUGAR								
brown packed	1 cup (7.7 oz)	828	0	tr	0.1	0.2	1	0
maple	1 piece (1 oz)	100	0	tr	tr	tr	0	0
powdered	1 tbsp (0.3 oz)	31	0	0	0	0	0	0
white	1 cup (7 oz)	773	0	tr	0	0	0	0
white	1 tsp (4 g)	15	0	0	tr	0	0	0
SUGAR-APPLE								
fresh	1	146	9	0.2	0.2	1.4	–	66
SUNCHOKE								
fresh raw sliced	½ cup	57	15	0.2	tr	1	–	3
SUNFLOWER								
Dakota Gourmet								
Lightly Salted Kernels	1 pkg (1 oz)	168	12	0.6	0.1	1.1	0	0
SunGold								
SunButter	2 tbsp	200	0	0.8	–	0.8	–	0
SUSHI								
california roll	1 piece (0.8 oz)	28	39	tr	tr	0.1	5	1
sashimi	1 serv (6 oz)	198	1035	0.3	0.5	9.4	8	4
tuna roll	1 piece (0.7 oz)	23	255	tr	tr	0.6	1	tr
vegetable roll	1 piece (1.2 oz)	27	371	tr	tr	0.1	16	3
vinegared ginger	⅓ cup (1.6 oz)	48	0	tr	tr	0.3	5	2
wasabi	2 tsp (0.3 oz)	5	0	0	0	0	0	0
yellowtail roll	1 piece (0.6 oz)	25	57	tr	tr	0.3	3	1

FOOD	PORTION	CALS	VIT A	THIA	RIBO	NIACIN	FOLIC	VIT C
SWAMP CABBAGE								
chopped cooked	½ cup	10	2548	tr	0.1	0.2	–	8
SWEET POTATO								
baked w/ skin	1 (3½ oz)	118	24877	0.1	0.1	0.7	26	28
candied	3½ oz	144	4399	tr	tr	0.4	12	7
canned in syrup	½ cup	106	7014	tr	tr	0.3	–	11
leaves cooked	½ cup	11	293	tr	0.1	0.3	–	1
mashed	½ cup	172	27968	0.1	0.2	1.1	18	28
SWEETBREADS								
beef braised	3 oz	230	0	0.2	0.4	3.4	–	17
SWISS CHARD								
cooked	½ cup	18	2762	tr	0.1	0.3	–	16
SWORDFISH								
cooked	3 oz	132	117	tr	0.1	10	–	1
SYRUP								
corn	2 tbsp	122	0	0	0	0	0	0
malt	1 tbsp (0.8 oz)	76	0	–	0.1	1.9	3	0
Eden								
Organic Barley Malt	1 tbsp	60	0	0	0	0	0	0
TAMARIND								
fresh	1	5	1	tr	tr	tr	–	tr
fresh cut up	1 cup	287	36	0.5	0.2	2.3	–	4
TANGERINE								
in light syrup	½ cup	76	1058	0.1	0.1	0.6	–	25
juice pack	½ cup	46	1056	0.1	tr	–	–	43
sections	1 cup	86	1794	0.2	tr	0.3	40	60
tangerine	1	37	773	0.1	tr	0.1	17	26
TANGERINE JUICE								
fresh	1 cup	106	1037	0.1	tr	0.2	–	77
frzn sweetened as prep	1 cup	110	1382	0.1	tr	0.2	11	58
Fresh Samantha								
Fresh Juice	1 cup (8 oz)	110	1000	0.2	tr	0	8	66

FOOD	PORTION	CALS	VIT A	THIA	RIBO	NIACIN	FOLIC	VIT C
TAPIOCA								
pearl dry	½ cup (2.7 oz)	272	0	tr	0	0	3	0
TARO								
chips	10 (0.8 oz)	115	0	tr	tr	0.1	–	1
leaves cooked	½ cup	18	3136	0.1	0.3	0.9	–	26
TEA/HERBAL TEA								
brewed tea	6 oz	2	0	0	tr	0	9	0
chamomile brewed	1 cup	2	47	tr	tr	0	1	0
instant unsweetened as prep w/ water	8 oz	2	0	0	tr	0.1	1	0
Eden								
Organic Genmaicha Tea	1 cup	0	0	0	0	0	0	0
Organic Kukicha Tea	1 cup	0	0	0	0	0	0	0
Silk								
Chai	1 cup	140	300	–	0.4	–	–	0
TEMPEH								
tempeh	½ cup	165	569	0.1	0.1	3.8	43	0
TOFU								
firm	¼ block (3 oz)	118	134	0.1	0.1	0.3	24	tr
firm	½ cup	183	209	0.2	0.1	0.5	37	tr
fresh fried	1 piece (0.5 oz)	35	0	tr	tr	tr	4	0
koyadofu dried frozen	1 piece (½ oz)	82	88	0.1	0.1	0.2	16	tr
okara	½ cup	47	0	tr	tr	0.1	–	0
regular	¼ block (4 oz)	88	99	0.1	0.1	0.2	17	tr
regular	½ cup	94	105	0.1	0.1	0.2	19	tr
TOMATILLO								
fresh	1 (1.2 oz)	11	39	tr	tr	0.6	2	4
fresh chopped	½ cup	21	75	tr	tr	1.2	4	8

FOOD	PORTION	CALS	VIT A	THIA	RIBO	NIACIN	FOLIC	VIT C
TOMATO								
cooked	½ cup	32	892	0.1	0.1	0.9	16	27
green	1	30	789	0.1	tr	0.6	–	29
paste	½ cup	110	3234	0.2	0.2	4.2	–	55
puree	1 cup	102	3402	0.2	0.1	4.3	–	88
red	1 (4.5 oz)	26	766	0.1	0.1	0.8	18	24
red chopped	1 cup	35	2039	0.1	0.1	1.1	17	32
sauce	½ cup	37	1195	0.1	0.1	1.4	–	16
sauce w/ mushrooms	½ cup	42	1165	0.1	0.1	1.5	–	15
sauce w/ onion	½ cup	52	1038	0.1	0.2	1.5	–	16
stewed	1 cup	80	673	0.1	0.1	1.1	11	18
sun dried	1 piece	5	17	tr	tr	0.2	1	1
sun dried in oil	1 piece (3 g)	6	39	tr	tr	0.2	1	3
w/ green chiles	½ cup	18	468	tr	tr	0.8	–	8
wedges in tomato juice	½ cup	34	757	0.1	tr	0.9	–	19
Eden								
Organic Diced	½ cup	30	1000	0.1	tr	1.2	0	18
Organic Diced w/ Green Chilies	½ cup	30	1000	0.1	tr	1.2	0	9
TOMATO JUICE								
clam & tomato	1 can (5½ oz)	77	357	0.1	0.1	0.3	–	7
tomato juice	½ cup	21	678	0.1	tr	0.8	24	22
TONGUE								
pork braised	3 oz	230	0	0.3	0.4	4.5	3	1
TORTILLA								
flour w/o salt	1–8 in diam (1.2 oz)	114	0	0.2	0.1	1.3	4	0
TREE FERN								
chopped cooked	½ cup	28	142	0	0.2	2.5	–	21
TRITICALE								
dry	1 cup (6.7 oz)	645	0	0.8	0.3	2.7	140	0

FOOD	PORTION	CALS	VIT A	THIA	RIBO	NIACIN	FOLIC	VIT C
TROUT								
baked	3 oz	162	54	0.4	0.4	–	13	tr
rainbow cooked	3 oz	129	63	0.1	0.2	–	–	3
TUNA								
light in water	3 oz	99	47	tr	0.1	11.3	3	0
light in water	1 can (5.8 oz)	192	92	0.1	0.1	21.9	6	0
TUNA DISHES								
tuna salad	1 cup	383	199	0.1	–	–	15	5
Tuna Helper								
AuGratin 50% Less Fat Recipe as prep	1 cup	240	400	0.3	0.3	5	60	0
AuGratin as prep	1 cup	300	400	0.3	0.3	5	60	0
Cheesy Broccoli 50% Less Fat Recipe as prep	1 cup	240	300	0.3	0.3	5	60	0
Cheesy Broccoli as prep	1 cup	290	300	0.3	0.3	5	60	0
Cheesy Pasta 50% Less Fat Recipe as prep	1 cup	230	400	0.3	0.3	5	60	0
Cheesy Pasta as prep	1 cup	280	400	0.3	0.3	5	60	0
Creamy Broccoli 50% Less Fat Recipe as prep	1 cup	240	400	0.3	0.3	5	60	0
Creamy Broccoli as prep	1 cup	310	400	0.3	0.3	5	60	0
Creamy Pasta 50% Less Fat Recipe as prep	1 cup	230	500	0.3	0.3	5	40	0
Creamy Pasta as prep	1 cup	300	500	0.3	0.3	5	40	0
Fettuccine Alfredo 50% Less Fat Recipe as prep	1 cup	240	400	0.3	0.3	5	60	0

FOOD	PORTION	CALS	VIT A	THIA	RIBO	NIACIN	FOLIC	VIT C
Fettuccine Alfredo as prep	1 cup	310	400	0.3	0.3	5	60	0
Garden Cheddar 50% Less Fat Recipe as prep	1 cup	240	750	0.4	0.3	5	80	0
Garden Cheddar as prep	1 cup	290	750	0.4	0.3	5	80	0
Pasta Salad Low Fat Recipe as prep	⅔ cup	230	100	0.2	0.1	4	40	0
Pasta Salad as prep	⅔ cup	380	100	0.2	0.1	4	40	0
Tetrazzini 50% Less Fat Recipe as prep	1 cup	230	400	0.4	0.3	7	100	0
Tetrazzini as prep	1 cup	300	400	0.4	0.3	7	100	0
Tuna Melt Reduced Fat Recipe as prep	1 cup	240	400	0.3	0.3	5	80	0
Tuna Melt as prep	1 cup	300	400	0.3	0.3	5	80	0
Tuna Pot Pie as prep	1 cup	440	1250	0.2	0.3	5	60	0
Tuna Romanoff 50% Less Fat Recipe as prep	1 cup	240	200	0.3	0.3	6	60	0
Tuna Romanoff as prep	1 cup	280	200	0.3	0.3	6	60	0

TURKEY

FOOD	PORTION	CALS	VIT A	THIA	RIBO	NIACIN	FOLIC	VIT C
back w/ skin roasted	½ back (9 oz)	637	0	0.1	0.6	9	21	0
breast	1 slice (0.75 oz)	23	0	tr	tr	1.7	—	0
breast w/ skin roasted	4 oz	212	0	0.1	0.1	7.1	7	0
ground cooked	3 oz	188	0	tr	0.1	4	5	0
leg w/ skin roasted	1 (1.2 lbs)	1133	0	0.3	1.3	19.4	49	0
neck simmered	1 (5.3 oz)	274	0	0.1	0.3	2.6	12	0
poultry salad sandwich spread	1 tbsp	109	18	tr	tr	0.2	1	0

FOOD	PORTION	CALS	VIT A	THIA	RIBO	NIACIN	FOLIC	VIT C
prebasted breast w/ skin roasted	½ breast (1.9 lbs)	1087	0	0.5	1.1	78.3	—	0
skin roasted	1 oz	141	0	tr	tr	0.9	1	0
turkey loaf breast meat	2 slices (1.5 oz)	47	0	tr	tr	3.5	—	0
w/ broth	½ can (2.5 oz)	116	0	tr	0.1	4.7	—	1
w/o skin roasted	1 cup (5 oz)	238	0	0.1	0.3	7.6	10	0
wing w/ skin roasted	1 (6.5 oz)	426	0	0.1	0.2	10.7	10	0

TURKEY SUBSTITUTES
Yves

FOOD	PORTION	CALS	VIT A	THIA	RIBO	NIACIN	FOLIC	VIT C
Veggie Turkey Deli Slices	1 serv (2.2 oz)	85	0	0.3	—	—	—	1

TURNIPS

FOOD	PORTION	CALS	VIT A	THIA	RIBO	NIACIN	FOLIC	VIT C
canned greens	½ cup	17	4196	tr	0.1	0.4	48	18
cooked mashed	½ cup (4.2 oz)	47	674	0.1	tr	0.9	19	23

VEAL DISHES

FOOD	PORTION	CALS	VIT A	THIA	RIBO	NIACIN	FOLIC	VIT C
parmigiana	4.2 oz	279	1204	0.1	0.3	4.2	11	15

VEGETABLE JUICE

FOOD	PORTION	CALS	VIT A	THIA	RIBO	NIACIN	FOLIC	VIT C
vegetable juice cocktail	½ cup	22	1416	0.1	tr	0.9	—	34

VEGETABLES MIXED

FOOD	PORTION	CALS	VIT A	THIA	RIBO	NIACIN	FOLIC	VIT C
buddha's delight	1 serv (16 oz)	174	1790	0.2	0.3	5.3	161	64
curry	1 serv (7.7 oz)	398	7845	0.2	0.1	2.2	—	26
gyoza potstickers vegetable	8 (4.9 oz)	210	500	—	—	—	—	0
mixed vegetables	½ cup	39	9551	tr	tr	0.5	19	4
pakoras	1 (2 oz)	108	390	0.1	tr	1	—	3
peas & carrots cooked	½ cup	38	6209	0.1	0.1	0.9	21	7
peas & onions cooked	½ cup	40	313	0.1	0.1	0.9	—	6
ratatouille	1 serv (3.5 oz)	96	0	tr	tr	1.2	36	50

FOOD	PORTION	CALS	VIT A	THIA	RIBO	NIACIN	FOLIC	VIT C
samosa	2 (4 oz)	519	170	0.1	tr	1.3	—	4
succotash	½ cup	102	187	tr	0.1	0.8	59	9
Fresh Like								
California Blend	3.5 oz	31	6797	0.1	0.1	0.6	—	40
Midwestern Blend	3.5 oz	42	5388	0.1	0.1	0.6	—	32
Mixed	3.5 oz	69	5199	0.1	0.1	1.1	—	10
Oriental Blend	3.5 oz	26	1362	0.1	0.1	0.5	—	55
Winter Blend	3.5 oz	26	1362	0.1	0.1	0.5	—	55

VINEGAR

FOOD	PORTION	CALS	VIT A	THIA	RIBO	NIACIN	FOLIC	VIT C
cider	1 tbsp	tr	0	0	0	0	0	0
Eden								
Organic Brown Rice	1 tbsp	2	0	0	0	0	0	0

WAFFLES

FOOD	PORTION	CALS	VIT A	THIA	RIBO	NIACIN	FOLIC	VIT C
buttermilk	1 4 in sq (1.2 oz)	88	448	0.2	0.2	1.6	17	0
plain	1 (7 in diam)	218	140	0.2	0.2	1.5	—	tr
Eggo								
Apple Cinnamon	2 (2.7 oz)	220	1000	0.3	0.3	4	40	0
Banana Bread	2 (2.7 oz)	200	1000	0.3	0.3	4	40	0
Blueberry	2 (2.7 oz)	220	1000	0.3	0.3	4	40	0
Buttermilk	2 (2.7 oz)	220	1000	0.3	0.3	4	40	0
Golden Oat	2 (2.7 oz)	150	1000	0.3	0.3	4	32	0
Homestyle	2 (2.7 oz)	220	1000	0.3	0.3	4	40	0
Minis Cinnamon Toast	12 (3.2 oz)	290	1500	0.5	0.5	6	40	0
Minis Cinnamon Toast	12 (3.2 oz)	280	1500	0.5	0.5	6	120	0
Minis Homestyle	12 (3.3 oz)	260	1500	0.5	0.5	6	60	0
Nut & Honey	2 (2.7 oz)	240	1000	0.3	0.3	4	40	0
Nutri-Grain	2 (2.7 oz)	190	1000	0.3	0.3	4	40	0
Nutri-Grain Multi-Bran	2 (2.7 oz)	180	1000	0.3	0.3	4	20	0
Nutri-Grain Raisin & Bran	2 (2.9 oz)	210	1000	0.3	0.3	4	20	0
Special K	2 (2 oz)	120	1000	0.3	0.3	4	40	0
Strawberry	2 (2.7 oz)	220	1000	0.3	0.3	4	40	0

FOOD	PORTION	CALS	VIT A	THIA	RIBO	NIACIN	FOLIC	VIT C
Kellogg's								
Homestyle Low Fat	2 (2.7 oz)	180	1000	0.3	0.3	4	60	0
Nutri-Grain Low Fat	2 (2.7 oz)	160	1000	0.3	0.3	4	40	0
Nutri-Grain Low Fat Blueberry	2 (2.7 oz)	160	1000	0.3	0.3	4	40	0
Thomas'								
Buttermilk	1 (1.6 oz)	130	1000	0.3	0.3	4	40	0
WALNUTS								
english dried	1 oz	182	35	0.1	tr	0.3	19	1
english dried chopped	1 cup	770	148	0.5	0.2	1.3	79	4
WATER								
ice cubes	3	0	0	0	0	0	0	0
tap water	8 oz	0	0	0	0	0	0	0
Glaceau								
Vitamin Water Tropical Citrus	1 cup (8 oz)	40	1250	–	–	5	–	60
Reebok								
Fitness Water Berry	1 bottle (24 oz)	30	0	–	–	–	100	0
Fitness Water Natural	1 bottle (24 oz)	0	0	–	–	–	100	0
WATER CHESTNUTS								
chinese sliced canned	½ cup	35	3	tr	tr	0.3	–	1
fresh sliced	½ cup	66	0	0.1	0.1	0.6	–	3
WATERCRESS								
garden fresh	½ cup	8	2325	tr	0.1	0.3	–	17
WATERMELON								
cut up	1 cup	50	585	0.1	tr	0.3	3	15
seeds dried	1 cup	602	0	0.1	tr	1	16	0
wedge ·	1⁄16	152	1762	0.4	0.1	1	10	47
WHEAT								
sprouted	1 cup (3.8 oz)	214	0	0.2	0.2	3.3	41	3

FOOD	PORTION	CALS	VIT A	THIA	RIBO	NIACIN	FOLIC	VIT C
WHEAT GERM								
plain toasted	¼ cup (1 oz)	108	0	0.5	0.2	1.6	100	2
Kretschmer								
Honey Crunch	¼ cup	105	0	0.3	0.2	1.2	82	0
WHEY								
acid dry	1 tbsp (3 g)	10	2	tr	0.1	tr	1	tr
acid fluid	1 cup (8 fl oz)	59	17	0.1	0.3	0.2	5	tr
sweet dry	1 tbsp (8 g)	26	3	tr	0.2	0.1	1	tr
sweet fluid	1 cup (8 fl oz)	66	39	0.1	0.4	0.2	2	tr
whey cheese	1 oz	126	356	tr	0.8	2.3	—	tr
WHIPPED TOPPINGS								
cream pressurized	1 tbsp (3 g)	8	27	tr	tr	tr	—	0
nondairy frzn	1 tbsp	13	34	0	0	0	0	0
nondairy pressurized	1 tbsp (4 g)	11	19	0	0	0	0	0
WHITE BEANS								
canned	1 cup	306	0	0.3	0.1	0.3	171	0
dried regular cooked	1 cup	249	0	0.2	0.1	0.3	145	0
dried small cooked	1 cup	253	0	0.4	0.1	0.5	245	0
WILD RICE								
cooked	1 cup (5.7 oz)	166	0	0.1	0.1	2.1	43	0
WINE								
port	3.5 oz	156	0	0	tr	tr	—	0
red	3½ oz	74	0	tr	tr	0.1	2	0
white	3½ oz	70	0	tr	tr	0.1	tr	0
WINGED BEANS								
dried cooked	1 cup	252	0	0.5	0.2	1.4	18	0
YAM								
mountain yam hawaii cooked	½ cup	59	0	0.1	tr	0.1	—	0
yam cubed cooked	½ cup	79	0	0.1	tr	0.4	11	8
YAMBEAN								
cooked	¾ cup	38	19	tr	tr	0.2	8	14

FOOD	PORTION	CALS	VIT A	THIA	RIBO	NIACIN	FOLIC	VIT C
YARDLONG BEANS								
dried cooked	1 cup	202	27	0.4	0.1	0.9	249	1
YAUTIA (TANNIER)								
fresh sliced	1 cup (4.7 oz)	132	15	0.1	0.1	0.9	23	16
YEAST								
brewer's dry	1 tbsp	25	tr	1.3	0.3	3	—	tr
YELLOW BEANS								
canned	½ cup	13	237	tr	tr	0.1	22	3
dried cooked	1 cup	254	4	0.3	0.2	1.3	143	3
fresh cooked	½ cup	22	50	tr	0.1	0.4	21	6
fresh raw	½ cup	17	59	tr	0.1	0.4	20	9
YELLOWTAIL								
baked	3 oz	159	88	0.1	tr	7.4	3	2
YOGURT								
coffee lowfat	8 oz	194	123	0.1	0.5	0.2	24	2
fruit lowfat	8 oz	225	111	0.1	0.4	0.2	19	1
fruit lowfat	4 oz	113	56	tr	0.2	0.1	10	1
plain	8 oz	139	279	0.1	0.3	0.2	17	1
plain lowfat	8 oz	144	150	0.1	0.5	0.3	25	2
plain no fat	8 oz	127	16	0.1	0.5	0.3	28	2
vanilla lowfat	8 oz	194	123	0.1	0.5	0.2	24	2
Colombo								
99% Fat Free Peach	4 oz	110	500	—	0.2	—	—	6
99% Fat Free Strawberry	4 oz	110	500	—	0.2	—	—	0
YOGURT FROZEN								
vanilla soft serve	½ cup (4 fl oz)	114	152	tr	0.2	0.2	4	1
ZUCCHINI								
baby raw	1 (0.5 oz)	3	78	tr	tr	0.1	3	6
canned italian style	½ cup	33	615	tr	tr	0.6	—	3
raw sliced	½ cup	9	221	tr	tr	0.3	14	6
sliced cooked	½ cup	14	216	tr	tr	0.4	15	4

PART TWO

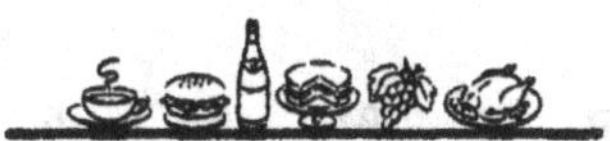

Minerals in Food

FOOD	PORTION	CALS	CALCI	IRON	POTAS	SOD	ZINC
ABALONE							
fresh fried	3 oz	161	32	3	—	502	1
raw	3 oz	89	27	3	—	255	1
ADZUKI BEANS							
dried cooked	1 cup	294	63	5	1224	18	4
ALFALFA							
sprouts	1 cup	40	10	tr	26	2	tr
sprouts	1 tbsp	1	1	tr	2	0	tr
ALLSPICE							
ground	1 tsp	5	13	tr	20	1	tr
ALMONDS							
almond butter honey & cinnamon	1 tbsp	96	43	1	120	2	tr
almond butter w/ salt	1 tbsp	101	43	1	121	75	tr
almond butter w/o salt	1 tbsp	101	43	1	121	2	tr
almond paste	1 oz	127	65	1	184	3	1
dried	1 oz	167	75	1	208	3	1
dry roasted	1 oz	167	80	1	219	3	1
dry roasted salted	1 oz	167	80	1	219	260	1
dry roasted w/ salt	24 nuts (1 oz)	170	80	1	210	100	1
oil roasted	1 oz	174	55	2	197	3	tr
oil roasted salted	1 oz	174	55	2	197	3	tr
toasted	1 oz	167	80	1	220	3	1
AMARANTH							
uncooked	1 cup (6.8 oz)	729	298	15	714	41	6
ANCHOVY							
canned in oil	5	42	46	1	109	734	tr
canned in oil	1 can (1.6 oz)	95	104	2	245	1651	1
fresh raw	3 oz	62	125	3	325	88	1

FOOD	PORTION	CALS	CALCI	IRON	POTAS	SOD	ZINC
ANISE							
seed	1 tsp	7	14	1	30	tr	tr
ANTELOPE							
roasted	3 oz	127	4	4	316	46	1
APPLE							
baked	1 (5.3 oz)	126	10	tr	159	1	tr
baked no sugar	1 (5.9 oz)	82	14	tr	161	6	tr
cooked w/ sugar dried	½ cup	116	4	tr	137	27	tr
cooked w/o sugar dried	½ cup	172	4	tr	134	26	tr
rings dried	10	155	9	1	288	56	tr
sliced sweetened canned	1 cup	136	4	tr	138	7	tr
w/o skin sliced	1 cup	62	4	tr	124	0	tr
w/o skin sliced & cooked	1 cup	91	8	tr	150	1	tr
w/o skin sliced & microwaved	1 cup	96	8	tr	159	1	tr
APPLE JUICE							
frozen as prep	1 cup	111	14	1	301	17	tr
frozen not prep	6 oz	349	43	2	945	54	tr
juice	1 cup	116	16	1	296	7	tr
APPLESAUCE							
sweetened	½ cup	97	5	tr	78	4	tr
unsweetened	½ cup	53	4	tr	91	2	tr
Eden							
Organic	½ cup	50	0	0	107	15	0
Organic Sweet Cinnamon	½ cup	50	0	0	150	0	0
APRICOT JUICE							
nectar	1 cup	141	17	1	286	9	tr
APRICOTS							
fresh	3	51	15	1	313	1	tr
frozen sweetened	½ cup	119	12	1	277	5	tr
halves dried	10	83	16	2	482	3	tr

FOOD	PORTION	CALS	CALCI	IRON	POTAS	SOD	ZINC
halves heavy syrup pack w/ skin	1 cup (9.1 oz)	214	22	1	361	10	tr
halves water pack w/ skin	1 cup (8.5 oz)	65	19	1	465	7	tr
halves water pack w/o skin	1 cup (8 oz)	51	19	1	350	25	tr
heavy syrup w/ skin	3 halves	70	7	tr	119	3	tr
juice pack w/ skin	3 halves	40	10	tr	139	3	tr
light syrup w/ skin	3 halves	54	10	tr	117	3	tr
puree from heavy syrup pack w/ skin	¾ cup (9.1 oz)	214	22	1	361	10	tr
puree from light pack w/ skin	¾ cup (8.9 oz)	160	28	1	349	10	tr
puree from water pack w/ skin	¾ cup (8.5 oz)	65	19	1	465	7	tr
puree juice pack w/ skin	1 cup (8.7 oz)	119	30	1	409	9	tr
water pack w/ skin	3 halves	22	7	tr	161	2	tr
water pack w/o skin	4 halves	20	8	tr	139	10	tr

ARROWROOT

FOOD	PORTION	CALS	CALCI	IRON	POTAS	SOD	ZINC
flour	1 cup (4.5 oz)	457	51	tr	14	3	tr

ARTICHOKE

FOOD	PORTION	CALS	CALCI	IRON	POTAS	SOD	ZINC
boiled	1 med (4 oz)	60	54	2	425	114	1
frozen cooked	1 pkg (9 oz)	108	50	1	634	127	1
hearts cooked	½ cup	42	38	1	297	80	tr

ASIAN FOOD

FOOD	PORTION	CALS	CALCI	IRON	POTAS	SOD	ZINC
buddha's delight w/ cellophane noodles fat choi jai	1 serv (7.6 oz)	211	77	2	986	772	1
chicken teriyaki	¾ cup	399	39	3	511	2190	2
chop suey w/ pork	1 cup	375	36	3	584	1378	3
chow mein pork	1 cup	425	75	5	1050	1673	5
chow mein shrimp	1 cup	221	105	3	701	1658	1
filipino chicken adobo	1 serv (15 oz)	555	56	3	366	468	3
phad thai	1 serv (9.2 oz)	232	111	6	282	426	1
wonton fried	½ cup (1 oz)	111	10	1	33	147	tr

FOOD	PORTION	CALS	CALCI	IRON	POTAS	SOD	ZINC
wonton soup	1 cup	205	32	3	226	322	1
wonton wrappers	1	23	4	tr	7	46	tr
ASPARAGUS							
fresh cooked	4 spears	14	12	tr	96	7	tr
fresh cooked	½ cup	22	18	1	144	10	tr
fresh raw	½ cup	16	14	1	183	2	tr
fresh raw	4 spears	14	12	1	158	1	tr
frozen cooked	4 spears	17	14	tr	131	2	tr
frozen cooked	1 pkg (10 oz)	82	68	2	640	12	2
AVOCADO							
fresh	1	324	22	2	1204	21	1
fresh mashed	1 cup	370	25	2	1378	24	1
guacamole	1 serv (2.2 oz)	105	9	1	378	187	tr
BACON							
breakfast strips cooked	3 strips	156	5	1	—	714	1
pan fried	3 strips	109	2	tr	—	303	1
BACON SUBSTITUTES							
bacon substitute	1 strip	25	2	tr	14	117	tr
BAGEL							
egg	1 (3½ in)	197	9	3	48	359	1
egg toasted	1 (3½ in)	197	9	3	48	358	1
onion	1 (3½ in)	195	53	3	72	379	1
plain	1 (3½ in)	195	53	3	72	379	1
plain toasted	1 (3½ in)	195	53	3	72	379	1
poppy seed	1 (3½ in)	195	53	3	72	379	1
BAKING POWDER							
low sodium	1 tsp	5	217	tr	505	4	tr
BAKING SODA							
baking soda	1 tsp	0	0	0	0	1259	0
BANANA							
banana chips	1 oz	147	5	tr	152	2	tr
fresh	1	105	7	tr	451	1	tr
fresh mashed	1 cup	207	13	1	890	2	tr
powder	1 tbsp	21	1	tr	92	0	tr

FOOD	PORTION	CALS	CALCI	IRON	POTAS	SOD	ZINC
BARLEY							
flour	1 cup (5.2 oz)	511	47	4	457	6	3
malt flour	1 cup (5.7 oz)	585	60	8	363	18	3
pearled cooked	1 cup (5.5 oz)	193	17	2	146	5	1
Quaker							
Medium Pearled	¼ cup	172	11	1	130	0	0
Quick Pearled	¼ cup	172	11	1	130	0	0
Scotch							
Medium Pearled	¼ cup	172	11	1	130	0	0
Quick Pearled	¼ cup	172	11	1	130	0	0
BARRACUDA							
fresh	3 oz	122	11	2	234	57	1
BASIL							
ground	1 tsp	4	30	1	48	tr	tr
BASS							
freshwater raw	3 oz	97	68	1	303	59	1
sea cooked	3 oz	105	11	tr	279	74	tr
sea raw	3 oz	82	9	tr	218	58	tr
BAY LEAF							
crumbled	1 tsp	2	5	tr	3	tr	tr
BEANS							
baked beans plain	½ cup	118	64	tr	376	504	2
baked beans vegetarian	½ cup	118	64	tr	376	504	2
baked beans w/ beef	½ cup	161	60	2	426	632	2
baked beans w/ franks	½ cup	182	61	2	301	551	2
baked beans w/ pork	½ cup	133	66	2	389	522	2
baked beans w/ pork & sweet sauce	½ cup	140	77	2	335	423	2
baked beans w/ pork & tomato sauce	½ cup	123	70	4	378	554	7
refried beans	½ cup	134	59	2	495	534	2

FOOD	PORTION	CALS	CALCI	IRON	POTAS	SOD	ZINC
three bean salad	¼ cup	230	58	3	270	500	tr
Eden							
Organic Baked w/ Sorghum & Mustard	½ cup (4.6 oz)	150	100	4	460	130	2

BEEF

FOOD	PORTION	CALS	CALCI	IRON	POTAS	SOD	ZINC
bottom round lean & fat trim 0 in Select braised	3 oz	171	4	3	259	43	5
bottom round lean & fat trim 0 in Select roasted	3 oz	150	4	3	330	56	4
bottom round lean & fat trim 0 in braised	3 oz	193	4	3	257	43	5
bottom round lean & fat trim ¼ in Choice braised	3 oz	241	5	3	239	42	4
bottom round lean & fat trim ¼ in Choice roasted	3 oz	221	5	2	302	53	4
brisket flat half lean & fat trim 0 in braised	3 oz	183	5	2	246	53	5
brisket flat half lean & fat trim ¼ in braised	3 oz	309	5	2	206	48	4
brisket point half lean & fat trim 0 in braised	3 oz	304	7	2	198	57	5
brisket point half lean & fat trim ¼ in braised	3 oz	343	7	2	188	55	5
brisket whole lean & fat trim 0 in braised	3 oz	247	6	2	220	55	5

FOOD	PORTION	CALS	CALCI	IRON	POTAS	SOD	ZINC
brisket whole lean & fat trim ¼ in braised	3 oz	327	7	2	196	52	4
chuck arm pot roast lean & fat trim 0 in braised	3 oz	238	8	3	224	53	6
chuck arm pot roast lean & fat trim ¼ in braised	3 oz	282	9	3	210	51	6
chuck blade roast lean & fat trim 0 in braised	3 oz	284	11	3	200	56	7
chuck blade roast lean & fat trim ¼ in braised	3 oz	293	11	3	197	55	7
corned beef brisket cooked	3 oz	213	7	2	123	964	4
eye of round lean & fat trim 0 in Choice roasted	3 oz	153	4	2	333	53	4
eye of round lean & fat trim ¼ in Choice roasted	3 oz	205	5	2	305	50	4
flank lean & fat trim 0 in braised	3 oz	224	6	3	287	60	5
flank lean & fat trim 0 in broiled	3 oz	192	6	2	342	69	4
ground extra lean broiled medium	3 oz	217	6	2	266	59	5
ground extra lean broiled well done	3 oz	225	7	2	314	70	5
ground extra lean fried medium	3 oz	216	6	2	265	59	5
ground extra lean fried well done	3 oz	224	7	2	306	69	5
ground extra lean raw	4 oz	265	7	2	321	75	5

FOOD	PORTION	CALS	CALCI	IRON	POTAS	SOD	ZINC
ground lean broiled medium	3 oz	231	9	2	256	65	5
ground lean broiled well done	3 oz	238	10	2	296	76	5
ground regular broiled medium	3 oz	246	9	2	248	70	4
ground regular broiled well done	3 oz	248	10	2	278	79	5
patties broiled medium	3 oz	240	9	2	250	66	5
porterhouse steak lean & fat trim ¼ in Choice broiled	3 oz	260	7	2	299	52	4
porterhouse steak lean only trim ¼ in Prime broiled	3 oz	185	6	3	346	56	5
rib eye small end lean & fat trim 0 in Choice broiled	3 oz	261	11	2	293	54	5
rib large end lean & fat trim 0 in roasted	3 oz	300	8	2	251	55	5
rib large end lean & fat trim ¼ in broiled	3 oz	295	9	2	258	54	4
rib large end lean & fat trim ¼ in roasted	3 oz	310	8	2	245	54	5
rib small end lean & fat trim 0 in broiled	3 oz	252	11	2	293	54	5
rib small end lean & fat trim ¼ in broiled	3 oz	285	11	2	276	53	5
rib small end lean & fat trim ¼ in roasted	3 oz	295	11	2	272	53	4

FOOD	PORTION	CALS	CALCI	IRON	POTAS	SOD	ZINC
rib whole lean & fat trim ¼ in Choice broiled	3 oz	306	10	2	262	53	4
rib whole lean & fat trim ¼ in Choice roasted	3 oz	320	9	2	252	53	4
rib whole lean & fat trim ¼ in Prime roasted	3 oz	348	10	2	254	54	4
shank crosscut lean & fat trim ¼ in Choice simmered	3 oz	224	25	3	344	52	8
short loin top loin lean & fat trim 0 in Choice broiled	1 steak (5.4 oz)	353	13	4	597	104	8
short loin top loin lean & fat trim 0 in Choice broiled	3 oz	193	7	2	327	57	4
short loin top loin lean & fat trim ¼ in Choice braised	3 oz	253	8	2	294	54	4
short loin top loin lean & fat trim ¼ in Choice broiled	1 steak (6.3 oz)	536	16	4	623	114	8
short loin top loin lean & fat trim ¼ in Prime broiled	1 steak (6.3 oz)	582	16	4	623	114	8
short loin top loin lean only trim 0 in Choice broiled	1 steak (5.2 oz)	311	12	4	590	101	8
short loin top loin lean only trim ¼ in Choice broiled	1 steak (5.2 oz)	314	12	4	582	100	8
shortribs lean & fat Choice braised	3 oz	400	10	2	191	43	4

FOOD	PORTION	CALS	CALCI	IRON	POTAS	SOD	ZINC
t-bone steak lean & fat trim ¼ in Choice broiled	3 oz	253	7	2	302	52	4
t-bone steak lean only trim ¼ in Choice broiled	3 oz	182	6	3	346	56	5
tenderloin lean & fat trim ¼ in Choice broiled	3 oz	259	7	3	310	50	4
tenderloin lean & fat trim ¼ in Choice roasted	3 oz	288	8	3	340	55	3
tenderloin lean & fat trim ¼ in Choice broiled	3 oz	208	6	3	338	52	5
tenderloin lean & fat trim ¼ in Prime broiled	3 oz	270	7	3	308	50	4
tenderloin lean only trim ¼ in Choice broiled	3 oz	188	6	3	356	54	5
tip round lean & fat trim 0 in Choice roasted	3 oz	170	5	2	319	54	6
tip round lean & fat trim ¼ in Choice roasted	3 oz	210	5	2	301	53	5
tip round lean & fat trim ¼ in Prime roasted	3 oz	233	5	2	299	53	5
top round lean & fat trim 0 in Choice braised	3 oz	184	3	3	280	38	4
top round lean & fat trim ¼ in Choice braised	3 oz	221	4	3	266	38	4
top round lean & fat trim ¼ in Choice broiled	3 oz	190	6	2	356	51	4

FOOD	PORTION	CALS	CALCI	IRON	POTAS	SOD	ZINC
top round lean & fat trim ¼ in Choice fried	3 oz	235	5	2	399	58	4
top round lean & fat trim ¼ in Prime broiled	3 oz	195	5	2	367	51	5
top sirloin lean & fat trim 0 in Choice broiled	3 oz	194	10	3	328	55	5
top sirloin lean & fat trim ¼ in Choice broiled	3 oz	228	10	3	309	53	5
top sirloin lean & fat trim ¼ in Choice fried	3 oz	277	10	3	336	59	5
Double J							
Filet	3.5 oz	130	12	4	350	54	4
NY Strip	3.5 oz	133	13	4	354	57	4
Rib Eye	3.5 oz	134	12	4	350	55	4
Top Butt	3.5 oz	136	12	4	350	55	4
BEEF DISHES							
bulgoghi korean grilled beef	1 serv (5.2 oz)	256	19	3	367	834	6
greek moussaka	1 serv (8.5 oz)	450	243	2	423	763	4
stroganoff	¾ cup	260	60	2	244	503	2
swiss steak	4.6 oz	214	17	3	435	139	4
BEEFALO							
roasted	3 oz	160	21	3	390	70	5
BEER AND ALE							
alcohol free beer	7 fl oz	50	5	tr	40	3	tr
beer light	12 oz can	100	18	tr	64	10	tr
beer regular	12 oz can	146	18	tr	89	19	tr
pilsener lager beer	7 fl oz	85	4	12	55	4	tr
BEETS							
greens cooked fresh	½ cup	20	82	1	654	173	tr

FOOD	PORTION	CALS	CALCI	IRON	POTAS	SOD	ZINC
greens raw chopped fresh	½ cup	4	23	1	104	38	tr
greens raw fresh	½ cup	4	23	1	104	38	tr
pickled canned	½ cup	75	13	tr	169	301	tr
raw sliced fresh	½ cup (2.4 oz)	29	11	1	221	53	tr
sliced cooked fresh	½ cup (3 oz)	38	14	1	259	65	tr
whole cooked fresh	2 (3.5 oz)	44	16	1	306	77	tr
whole raw	2 (5.7 oz)	70	27	1	530	126	1

BISCUIT

FOOD	PORTION	CALS	CALCI	IRON	POTAS	SOD	ZINC
buttermilk ready-to-eat	1 (2 oz)	212	141	2	73	348	tr
buttermilk refrigerated	1 (1 oz)	98	6	1	45	341	tr
buttermilk mix	1 (2 oz)	191	105	1	107	544	tr
plain ready-to-eat	1 (35 g)	276	90	2	86	584	tr
plain refrigerated	1 (1 oz)	98	6	1	45	341	tr
plain mix	1 (2 oz)	191	105	1	107	544	tr
w/ egg	1 (4.8 oz)	316	154	3	160	654	1
w/ egg & bacon	1 (5.2 oz)	458	189	4	251	999	2
w/ egg & ham	1 (6.7 oz)	442	221	5	319	1382	2
w/ egg & sausage	1 (6.3 oz)	581	155	4	320	1141	2
w/ egg & steak	1 (5.2 oz)	410	138	5	306	888	3
w/ egg cheese & bacon	1 (5.1 oz)	477	164	3	230	1260	2
w/ ham	1 (4 oz)	386	160	3	197	1433	2
w/ sausage	1 (4.4 oz)	485	128	3	198	1071	2
w/ steak	1 (4.9 oz)	455	116	4	234	795	3

BISON

FOOD	PORTION	CALS	CALCI	IRON	POTAS	SOD	ZINC
roasted	3 oz	122	7	3	307	48	3

BLACK BEANS

FOOD	PORTION	CALS	CALCI	IRON	POTAS	SOD	ZINC
dried cooked	1 cup	227	47	4	611	1	2
Eden							
Organic	½ cup (4.6 oz)	100	60	2	280	15	1

BLACKBERRIES

FOOD	PORTION	CALS	CALCI	IRON	POTAS	SOD	ZINC
canned in heavy syrup	½ cup	118	27	1	127	3	tr
fresh	½ cup	37	23	tr	141	0	tr
unsweetened frzn	1 cup	97	44	1	211	2	tr

FOOD	PORTION	CALS	CALCI	IRON	POTAS	SOD	ZINC
BLACKEYE PEAS							
dried cooked	1 cup	198	42	4	476	6	2
w/pork canned	½ cup	199	21	3	427	840	2
Eden							
Organic	½ cup (4.6 oz)	90	30	2	210	25	2
BLUEBERRIES							
canned in heavy syrup	1 cup	225	7	1	102	9	tr
fresh	1 cup	82	9	tr	129	9	tr
unsweetened frzn	1 cup	78	12	tr	83	1	tr
BLUEFIN							
fillet baked	4.1 oz	186	10	1	558	90	1
BLUEFISH							
fresh baked	3 oz	135	8	1	405	65	1
BOYSENBERRIES							
in heavy syrup	1 cup	226	23	1	230	9	tr
unsweetened frzn	1 cup	66	36	1	183	2	tr
BRAINS							
beef pan-fried	3 oz	167	8	2	301	134	1
beef simmered	3 oz	136	8	2	204	102	1
lamb braised	3 oz	124	10	1	175	114	1
lamb fried	3 oz	232	18	2	304	133	2
pork braised	3 oz	117	8	2	–	77	1
veal braised	3 oz	115	13	1	181	133	1
veal fried	3 oz	181	9	1	401	150	2
BRAN							
corn	1 cup (2.7 oz)	170	32	2	33	5	1
oat	½ cup (1.6 oz)	116	27	3	266	2	2
oat cooked	½ cup (3.8 oz)	44	11	1	101	1	1
rice	½ cup (2.1 oz)	187	34	11	786	3	4
wheat	½ cup (2 oz)	63	21	3	343	1	2
Kretschmer							
Toasted Wheat Bran	⅓ cup	57	26	4	399	2	3
Quaker							
Unprocessed	2 tbsp	8	6	1	121	0	1

FOOD	PORTION	CALS	CALCI	IRON	POTAS	SOD	ZINC
BRAZIL NUTS							
dried	1 oz	186	50	1	170	0	1
BREAD							
boston brown canned	1 slice (1.6 oz)	88	31	1	143	284	tr
chapatis as prep w/ fat	1 bread (1.6 oz)	95	10	1	101	180	1
cornbread mix	1 piece (2 oz)	189	44	1	77	467	tr
cornstick	1 (1.3 oz)	101	37	tr	36	195	tr
cracked wheat	1 slice	65	11	1	44	135	tr
egg	1 slice (1.4 oz)	115	37	1	46	197	tr
focaccia onion	1 piece (4.6 oz)	282	20	3	114	536	tr
focaccia rosemary	1 piece (3.5 oz)	251	13	3	68	535	tr
focaccia tomato olive	1 piece (4.7 oz)	270	31	3	122	683	tr
french	1 slice (1 oz)	78	21	1	32	172	tr
irish soda bread	1 slice (2 oz)	174	49	2	160	239	tr
italian	1 slice (1 oz)	81	23	1	33	175	tr
naan	1 bread (3.5 oz)	286	54	3	107	546	1
navajo fry	1 (5 in diam)	296	210	3	67	625	tr
navajo fry	1 (10.5 in diam)	527	373	6	118	1112	1
oatmeal	1 slice	73	18	1	38	162	tr
paratha	1 bread (2.1 oz)	201	10	1	78	268	1
pita	1 reg (2 oz)	165	52	2	72	322	1
pita	1 sm (1 oz)	78	24	1	34	152	tr
pumpernickel	1 slice	80	22	1	661	215	tr
raisin	1 slice	71	17	1	59	101	tr
rye	1 slice	83	23	1	53	211	tr
seven grain	1 slice	65	24	1	53	127	tr
sourdough	1 slice (1 oz)	78	21	1	32	172	tr
vienna	1 slice (1 oz)	78	21	1	32	172	tr
wheat berry	1 slice	65	26	1	50	132	tr
wheat bran	1 slice	89	27	1	82	175	tr
white	1 slice	67	27	1	30	135	tr

FOOD	PORTION	CALS	CALCI	IRON	POTAS	SOD	ZINC
white reduced calorie	1 slice	48	22	1	18	104	tr
white toasted	1 slice	67	27	1	30	136	tr
whole wheat	1 slice	70	20	1	71	149	1
Natural Ovens							
Cracked Wheat	2 slices (2.4 oz)	140	200	2	—	140	5
English Muffin Bread	2 slices (2.4 oz)	140	100	1	—	140	1
Executive Fitness Sunny Millet	2 slices (2.6 oz)	160	200	2	—	70	3
Glorious Cinnamon & Raisin Fat Free	2 slices (2.1 oz)	110	250	1	—	140	3
Honey 'N Flax	2 slices (2.5 oz)	140	120	1	—	140	3
Hunger Filler Bread	2 slices (2.1 oz)	110	300	2	—	140	5
Light Wheat	2 slices (2.2 oz)	84	200	2	—	140	6
Nutty Natural Wheat Bread	2 slices (2.5 oz)	140	300	2	—	140	6
Seven Grain Herb	2 slices (2.5 oz)	140	200	2	—	140	3
Soft Hearth Whole Wheat	2 slices (2 oz)	100	300	2	—	140	5
Soft Sandwich Very Low Fat	2 slices (2.3 oz)	110	200	2	—	140	3
Stay Slim	2 slices (2 oz)	100	240	4	—	140	5

BREADCRUMBS

FOOD	PORTION	CALS	CALCI	IRON	POTAS	SOD	ZINC
dry	1 cup	426	245	7	239	930	1
dry seasonsed	1 cup (4 oz)	441	119	4	324	3180	1
fresh	½ cup	76	31	1	34	153	tr

BREADFRUIT

FOOD	PORTION	CALS	CALCI	IRON	POTAS	SOD	ZINC
fresh	¼ small	99	17	1	470	2	tr

BREADSTICKS

FOOD	PORTION	CALS	CALCI	IRON	POTAS	SOD	ZINC
plain	1 sm	25	2	tr	12	66	tr
plain	1	41	2	tr	12	66	tr

FOOD	PORTION	CALS	CALCI	IRON	POTAS	SOD	ZINC
BREAKFAST DRINKS							
orange drink powder	3 rounded tsp	93	46	tr	40	4	tr
orange drink powder as prep w/water	6 oz	86	46	tr	37	9	tr
Carnation							
Instant Breakfast French Vanilla as prep w/ 2% milk	1 serv	250	500	5	620	220	4
Instant Breakfast French Vanilla as prep w/ fat free milk	1 serv	220	500	5	650	230	4
Instant Breakfast French Vanilla as prep w/ whole milk	1 serv	280	500	5	610	220	4
BROAD BEANS							
canned	1 cup	183	67	3	620	1161	2
dried cooked	1 cup	186	62	3	456	8	2
BROCCOFLOWER							
fresh raw	½ cup (1.8 oz)	16	16	tr	150	12	tr
BROCCOLI							
chinese broccoli (gai lan) cooked	1 cup (3.1 oz)	19	88	tr	230	6	tr
chopped cooked	½ cup	22	36	1	228	20	tr
chopped cooked frozen	½ cup	25	47	1	166	22	tr
raw chopped	½ cup	12	21	tr	143	12	tr
spears cooked frozen	10 oz pkg	69	127	2	451	60	1
spears cooked frozen	½ cup	25	127	1	166	22	tr
BROWNIE							
plain	1 lg (2 oz)	227	16	1	84	175	tr
plain	1 sm (1 oz)	115	8	1	42	88	tr

FOOD	PORTION	CALS	CALCI	IRON	POTAS	SOD	ZINC
plain mix	1 (1.2 oz)	139	6	1	61	83	tr
plain mix low calorie	1 (0.8 oz)	84	3	tr	69	21	tr
BRUSSELS SPROUTS							
fresh cooked	½ cup	30	28	1	247	17	tr
fresh cooked	1 sprout	8	7	tr	67	4	tr
frozen cooked	½ cup	33	19	1	254	18	tr
raw	½ cup	19	18	1	171	11	tr
raw	1 sprout	8	8	tr	74	5	tr
BUCKWHEAT							
groats roasted cooked	1 cup (5.9 oz)	647	12	1	148	7	1
groats roasted uncooked	1 cup (5.7 oz)	567	28	4	525	18	4
BUFFALO							
water buffalo roasted	3 oz	111	13	2	266	48	2
BULGUR							
cooked	1 cup (6.3 oz)	151	18	2	124	9	1
uncooked	1 cup (4.9 oz)	479	49	3	574	24	3
BURBOT (FISH)							
fresh baked	3 oz	98	54	1	440	106	1
BUTTER							
stick	1 stick (4 oz)	813	27	tr	29	937	tr
stick	1 pat (5 g)	36	1	tr	1	41	tr
whipped	4 oz	542	18	tr	20	625	tr
whipped	1 pat (4 g)	27	1	tr	1	31	tr
Crystal							
Salted Stick	1 tbsp (0.5 oz)	102	3	0	4	89	0
Unsalted Stick	1 tbsp (0.5 oz)	102	3	0	4	1	0
BUTTERNUTS							
dried	1 oz	174	15	1	119	0	1
CABBAGE							
chinese pe-tsai raw shredded	1 cup	12	58	tr	181	7	tr

FOOD	PORTION	CALS	CALCI	IRON	POTAS	SOD	ZINC
chinese pe-tsai shredded cooked	1 cup	16	38	tr	268	11	tr
danish raw	1 head (2 lbs)	228	431	5	2231	164	2
danish raw shredded	½ cup (1.2 oz)	9	17	tr	86	6	tr
danish shredded cooked	½ cup (2.6 oz)	17	23	tr	73	6	tr
green raw	1 head (2 lbs)	228	431	5	2231	164	2
green raw shredded	½ cup (1.2 oz)	9	17	tr	86	6	tr
green shredded cooked	½ cup (2.6 oz)	17	23	tr	73	6	tr
napa cooked	1 cup (3.8 oz)	13	32	1	95	12	4
red raw shredded	½ cup	10	18	tr	72	4	tr
red shredded cooked	½ cup	16	28	tr	105	6	tr
stuffed cabbage	1 (6 oz)	373	339	3	335	1007	3

CACTUS

FOOD	PORTION	CALS	CALCI	IRON	POTAS	SOD	ZINC
napoles fresh sliced	½ cup (1.5 oz)	7	70	tr	137	9	tr

CAKE

FOOD	PORTION	CALS	CALCI	IRON	POTAS	SOD	ZINC
angelfood	1 cake (11.9 oz)	876	477	2	318	2548	tr
angelfood home recipe	½12 cake (1.9 oz)	142	3	tr	116	96	tr
angelfood ready-to-eat	½12 cake (1 oz)	73	40	tr	26	212	tr
apple crisp home recipe	1 recipe 6 serv (29.6 oz)	1377	239	6	821	1537	1
apple crisp ready-to-eat	½ cup (5 oz)	230	40	1	137	257	1
baklava	1 oz	126	23	1	62	78	tr
boston cream pie frzn	⅙ cake (3.2 oz)	232	21	tr	36	132	tr
carrot w/ cream cheese icing	½12 cake (3.9 oz)	484	27	1	124	273	1
cheesecake	⅙ cake (2.8 oz)	256	50	1	72	165	tr

FOOD	PORTION	CALS	CALCI	IRON	POTAS	SOD	ZINC
cheesecake home recipe	½ cake (4.5 oz)	456	74	2	131	362	1
cheesecake w/ cherry topping	½ cake (5 oz)	359	54	2	116	254	1
chocolate w/o frosting home recipe	½ cake (3.3 oz)	340	57	2	133	299	1
chocolate w/o frosting home recipe	2 layers (39.9 oz)	4067	679	18	1596	3581	8
coffeecake cheese	⅛ cake (2.7 oz)	258	45	tr	—	257	tr
coffeecake creme-filled chocolate frosting home recipe	⅛ cake (3.2 oz)	298	35	tr	—	290	tr
coffeecake crumb topped cheese	⅛ cake (2.7 oz)	258	45	tr	—	257	tr
coffeecake crumb topped cinnamon	⅑ cake (2.2 oz)	263	34	1	77	221	1
coffeecake crumb topped cinnamon home recipe	½ cake (2.1 oz)	240	67	1	144	233	tr
coffeecake fruit	⅛ cake (1.8 oz)	156	23	1	45	192	tr
cream puff shell home recipe	1 (2.3 oz)	239	24	1	64	368	tr
cream puff w/ custard filling	1 (4.6 oz)	336	86	2	149	444	1
crumpet	1 (2.3 oz)	131	79	1	61	535	tr
eclair home recipe	1 (3 oz)	262	63	1	117	337	1
fruitcake	1 piece (1.5 oz)	139	14	1	66	116	tr
gingerbread	⅑ cake (2.6 oz)	264	52	2	325	242	tr
pineapple upside down	⅑ cake (4 oz)	367	137	2	129	367	tr
pound	⅒ cake (1 oz)	117	11	tr	36	119	tr

FOOD	PORTION	CALS	CALCI	IRON	POTAS	SOD	ZINC
pound fat free	1 cake (12 oz)	961	146	7	373	1158	1
shortcake home recipe	1 (2.3 oz)	225	133	2	69	329	tr
sour cream pound	1/10 cake (1 oz)	117	19	tr	32	120	tr
sponge	1/12 cake (1.3 oz)	110	26	1	38	93	tr
sponge home recipe	1/12 cake (2.2 oz)	140	20	1	66	107	tr
strudel apple	1 piece (2½ oz)	195	11	tr	—	191	tr
tiramisu	1 cake (4.4 lbs)	5732	1602	14.7	2953	1107	11
toaster pastry apple	1 (1¾ oz)	204	14	2	58	218	tr
toaster pastry blueberry	1 (1¾ oz)	204	14	2	58	218	tr
toaster pastry brown sugar cinnamon	1 (1¾ oz)	206	17	2	57	212	tr
toaster pastry cherry	1 (1¾ oz)	204	14	2	58	218	tr
toaster pastry strawberry	1 (1¾ oz)	204	14	2	58	218	tr
white w/ coconut frosting home recipe	1/12 cake (3.9 oz)	399	101	1	111	318	tr
white w/o frosting home recipe	1/12 cake (2.6 oz)	264	96	1	70	242	tr
yellow w/ chocolate frosting	1/8 cake (2.2 oz)	242	24	1	114	216	tr
yellow w/o frosting home recipe	1/12 cake (2.4 oz)	245	99	1	62	233	tr
yellow w/o frosting home recipe	2 layers (28.7 oz)	2947	1192	13	740	2803	4

Kellogg's

FOOD	PORTION	CALS	CALCI	IRON	POTAS	SOD	ZINC
Pop-Tarts Frosted Chocolate Vanilla Creme	1 (1.8 oz)	200	0	2	60	220	tr
Pop-Tarts Frosted Chocolate Fudge	1 (1.8 oz)	200	0	2	80	220	tr

FOOD	PORTION	CALS	CALCI	IRON	POTAS	SOD	ZINC
CAKE ICING							
chocolate as prep w/ butter home recipe	1 recipe (21.1 oz)	2409	104	5	544	1144	2
chocolate as prep w/ butter home recipe	½ recipe (1.8 oz)	200	9	tr	45	95	tr
chocolate as prep w/ margarine home recipe	1 recipe (21.1 oz)	2411	106	5	557	1235	2
chocolate as prep w/ margarine home recipe	½ recipe (1.8 oz)	200	9	tr	46	103	tr
chocolate ready-to-use	½ pkg (1.3 oz)	151	3	1	74	70	tr
chocolate ready-to-use	1 pkg (16 oz)	1834	37	7	905	845	1
coconut ready-to-use	½ pkg (1.3 oz)	157	5	tr	71	74	tr
coconut ready-to-use	1 pkg (16 oz)	1903	62	3	858	899	2
cream cheese ready-to-use	½ pkg (1.3 oz)	157	1	tr	13	90	0
cream cheese ready-to-use	1 pkg (16 oz)	1906	15	1	163	1094	0
glaze home recipe	1 recipe (11.5 oz)	1173	73	tr	97	307	tr
glaze home recipe	½ recipe (1 oz)	97	6	tr	8	25	tr
seven minute home recipe	1 recipe (13.6 oz)	1231	9	tr	246	859	tr
seven minute home recipe	½ recipe (1.1 oz)	102	1	tr	20	55	tr
sour cream ready-to-use	½ pkg (1.3 oz)	157	1	tr	74	78	0
sour cream ready-to-use	1 pkg (16 oz)	1904	11	tr	896	943	tr
vanilla as prep w/ butter home recipe	½ recipe (1.7 oz)	165	11	tr	14	31	tr

FOOD	PORTION	CALS	CALCI	IRON	POTAS	SOD	ZINC
vanilla as prep w/ butter home recipe	1 recipe (20.1 oz)	1972	128	tr	168	366	1
vanilla as prep w/ margarine home recipe	½ recipe (1.7 oz)	195	6	tr	9	98	tr
vanilla as prep w/ margarine home recipe	1 recipe (20.1 oz)	2326	75	tr	103	1175	tr
vanilla ready-to-use	½ pkg (1.3 oz)	159	1	tr	14	34	0
vanilla ready-to-use	1 pkg (16 oz)	1936	14	1	169	418	0

CAKE MIX

FOOD	PORTION	CALS	CALCI	IRON	POTAS	SOD	ZINC
angelfood	10 in cake (20.9 oz)	1535	503	1	808	3036	1
angelfood	½ cake (1.8 oz)	129	42	tr	68	255	tr
carrot w/o frosting	2 layers (29.6 oz)	2886	927	11	1011	3001	3
carrot w/o frosting	½ cake (2.5 oz)	239	77	1	64	249	tr
cheesecake no-bake	⅛ cake (3.5 oz)	271	170	tr	209	377	tr
chocolate pudding type w/o frosting	2 layers (32.4 oz)	3234	765	17	1926	4815	7
chocolate pudding type w/o frosting	½ cake (2.7 oz)	270	64	1	161	402	tr
chocolate w/o frosting	2 layers (26.8 oz)	2393	843	25	1851	4464	5
chocolate w/o frosting	½ cake (2.3 oz)	198	70	2	153	370	tr
chocolate w/o frosting low sodium	⅒ cake (1.3 oz)	116	11	1	82	130	tr
coffeecake crumb topped cinnamon	⅛ cake (2 oz)	178	76	1	63	236	tr

FOOD	PORTION	CALS	CALCI	IRON	POTAS	SOD	ZINC
devil's food w/o frosting	½ cake (2.3 oz)	198	70	2	153	370	tr
fudge w/o frosting	½ cake (2.3 oz)	198	70	2	153	370	tr
german chocolate pudding type w/ coconut nut frosting	½ cake (3.9 oz)	404	54	1	151	369	tr
lemon w/o frosting no sugar low sodium	⅒ cake (1.3 oz)	118	8	1	50	83	tr
marble pudding type w/o frosting	½ cake (2.6 oz)	253	40	1	68	242	tr
marble pudding type w/o frosting	2 layers (30.6 oz)	3021	475	11	816	2884	4
white pudding type w/o frosting	2 layers (29 oz)	2915	417	7	508	3654	1
white pudding type w/o frosting	½ cake (2.4 oz)	244	35	1	42	305	tr
white w/o frosting	2 layer cake (26 oz)	2265	1016	7	700	3593	3
white w/o frosting	½ cake (2.2 oz)	190	85	1	59	301	tr
white w/o frosting no sugar low sodium	⅒ cake (1.3 oz)	118	8	1	50	83	tr
yellow pudding-type w/o frosting	2 layers (31 oz)	3084	681	10	509	3800	3
yellow pudding-type w/o frosting	½ cake (2.6 oz)	257	57	1	42	317	tr
yellow w/o frosting	2 layers (26.5 oz)	2415	761	9	552	3580	3
yellow w/o frosting	½ cake (2.2 oz)	202	64	1	46	299	tr

FOOD	PORTION	CALS	CALCI	IRON	POTAS	SOD	ZINC
CANADIAN BACON							
grilled	1 pkg (6 oz)	257	14	1	—	2149	2
CANADIAN BACON SUBSTITUTES							
Yves							
Canadian Veggie Bacon	1 serv (2 oz)	80	20	5	170	480	4
CANDY							
butterscotch	1 piece (6 g)	24	0	0	0	3	0
butterscotch	1 oz	112	1	tr	1	12	tr
caramels	1 piece (8 g)	31	11	tr	17	20	tr
caramels	1 pkg (2.5 oz)	271	98	tr	152	174	tr
crisped rice bar almond	1 bar (1 oz)	130	21	2	65	66	2
crisped rice bar chocolate chip	1 bar (1 oz)	115	6	2	48	79	tr
fondant chocolate coated	1 lg (1.2 oz)	128	6	1	59	9	tr
fondant chocolate coated	1 sm (0.4 oz)	40	2	tr	18	3	tr
fudge brown sugar w/ nuts	1 piece (0.5 oz)	56	16	tr	52	14	tr
fudge chocolate marshmallow	1 piece (0.7 oz)	84	9	tr	28	21	tr
fudge chocolate marshmallow w/ nuts	1 piece (0.8 oz)	96	11	tr	37	21	tr
fudge chocolate w/ nuts	1 piece (0.7 oz)	81	9	tr	30	11	tr
fudge peanut butter	1 piece (0.6 oz)	59	7	tr	21	12	tr
fudge vanilla w/ nuts	1 piece (0.5 oz)	62	7	tr	17	9	tr
gumdrops	10 sm (0.4 oz)	135	1	tr	2	15	0
gumdrops	10 lg (3.8 oz)	420	3	tr	5	48	tr
hard candy	1 oz	106	1	tr	1	11	0
jelly beans	10 lg (1 oz)	104	1	tr	11	7	0
jelly beans	10 sm (0.4 oz)	40	0	tr	4	3	tr
lollipop	1 (6 g)	22	0	tr	0	2	0

FOOD	PORTION	CALS	CALCI	IRON	POTAS	SOD	ZINC
milk chocolate	1 bar (1.55 oz)	226	84	1	169	36	1
milk chocolate crisp	1 bar (1.45 oz)	203	70	tr	141	59	tr
milk chocolate w/ almonds	1 bar (1.45 oz)	215	92	1	182	30	1
peanut brittle	1 oz	128	8	tr	59	128	tr
praline	1 piece (1.4 oz)	177	12	tr	82	24	1
sweet chocolate	1 oz	143	7	1	82	5	tr
sweet chocolate	1 bar (1.45 oz)	201	10	1	119	7	1
taffy	1 piece (0.5 oz)	56	0	tr	1	13	0
toffee	1 piece (0.4 oz)	65	4	tr	6	22	tr
truffles	1 piece (0.4 oz)	59	19	tr	37	8	tr
Body Smarts							
Chocolate Peanut Crunch	2 bars (1.8 oz)	210	200	5	—	70	4
CANTALOUPE							
fresh cubed	1 cup	57	17	tr	494	14	tr
fresh half	½	94	28	1	825	23	tr
CARAWAY							
seed	1 tsp	7	14	tr	28	tr	tr
CARDAMOM							
ground	1 tsp	6	8	tr	22	tr	tr
CARIBOU							
roasted	3 oz	142	19	5	264	51	4
CAROB							
carob mix as prep w/ whole milk	9 oz	195	291	1	370	132	1
flour	1 tbsp	14	28	tr	66	3	tr
flour	1 cup	185	359	3	852	36	1
CARP							
fresh	3 oz	108	15	1	283	42	1

FOOD	PORTION	CALS	CALCI	IRON	POTAS	SOD	ZINC
fresh cooked	3 oz	138	44	1	363	54	2
fresh cooked	1 fillet (6 oz)	276	89	3	726	107	3

CARROT JUICE
FOOD	PORTION	CALS	CALCI	IRON	POTAS	SOD	ZINC
canned	6 oz	73	44	1	538	54	tr

CARROTS
FOOD	PORTION	CALS	CALCI	IRON	POTAS	SOD	ZINC
raw	1 (2.5 oz)	31	19	tr	233	25	tr
raw shredded	½ cup	24	15	tr	178	19	tr
slices canned	½ cup	17	19	tr	131	176	tr
slices low sodium canned	½ cup	17	19	tr	131	31	tr
slices cooked fresh	½ cup	35	24	tr	177	52	tr
slices cooked frozen	½ cup	26	21	tr	115	43	tr

CASHEWS
FOOD	PORTION	CALS	CALCI	IRON	POTAS	SOD	ZINC
cashew butter w/o salt	1 tbsp	94	7	1	87	2	1
dry roasted salted	1 oz	163	13	2	160	213	2
dry roasted w/ salt	18 nuts (1 oz)	160	13	2	160	180	1
oil roasted	1 oz	163	12	1	151	5	1
oil roasted salted	1 oz	163	12	1	151	209	1

CATFISH
FOOD	PORTION	CALS	CALCI	IRON	POTAS	SOD	ZINC
channel breaded & fried	3 oz	194	37	1	289	238	1
channel raw	3 oz	99	34	1	296	54	1

CAULIFLOWER
FOOD	PORTION	CALS	CALCI	IRON	POTAS	SOD	ZINC
flowerets raw	3 (2 oz)	14	12	tr	170	17	tr
fresh cooked	½ cup (2.2 oz)	14	10	tr	88	9	tr
fresh flowerets cooked	3 (2 oz)	12	9	tr	76	8	tr
fresh green cooked	1½ cup (3.2 oz)	29	29	1	250	21	1
frozen cooked	½ cup	17	15	tr	125	16	tr
green raw	1 head 7 in diam (18 oz)	158	169	4	1533	118	3

FOOD	PORTION	CALS	CALCI	IRON	POTAS	SOD	ZINC
green raw	1 cup (2.2 oz)	20	21	tr	192	15	tr
green raw floweret	1 (0.9 oz)	8	8	tr	75	6	tr
raw	½ cup (1.8 oz)	13	11	tr	151	15	tr
CELERY							
diced cooked	½ cup	13	32	tr	213	68	tr
fresh	1 stalk (1.3 oz)	6	16	tr	115	35	tr
raw diced	½ cup	10	24	tr	172	52	tr
seed	1 tsp	8	35	1	28	3	tr
CEREAL							
corn flakes low sodium	1 cup (0.9 oz)	100	11	1	18	3	tr
corn grits white regular & quick as prep w/ water & salt	¾ cup (6.4 oz)	109	0	tr	40	406	tr
corn grits white regular or quick as prep	¾ cup (6.4 oz)	109	0	1	40	0	tr
corn grits yellow regular & quick as prep w/ water & salt	¾ cup (6.4 oz)	109	0	1	40	406	tr
corn grits yellow regular & quick not prep	1 cup (5.5 oz)	579	3	6	214	2	1
crispy rice	1 cup (1 oz)	111	5	1	27	206	tr
crispy rice low sodium	1 cup (0.9 oz)	105	17	1	20	3	tr
farina as prep w/ water	¾ cup (6.1 oz)	88	4	1	23	0	tr
farina not prep	1 tbsp (0.4 oz)	40	2	tr	10	0	tr
granola	½ cup (2.1 oz)	285	45	3	328	15	2
oatmeal instant w/ cinnamon & spice as prep w/ water	1 pkg (5.6 oz)	177	172	7	105	280	1
oatmeal instant w/ raisins & spice as prep w/ water	1 cup (5.5 oz)	161	166	7	150	226	1

FOOD	PORTION	CALS	CALCI	IRON	POTAS	SOD	ZINC
oatmeal instant w/ bran & raisins as prep w/ water	1 pkg (6.8 oz)	158	174	8	236	248	1
oatmeal istant as prep w/ water	1 cup (8.2 oz)	138	215	8	131	377	1
oatmeal regular & quick as prep w/ water	¾ cup (6.1 oz)	149	14	1	98	2	1
oatmeal regular & quick not prep	⅓ cup (0.9 oz)	104	14	1	95	1	1
puffed rice	1 cup (0.5 oz)	56	1	4	16	0	tr
puffed wheat	1 cup (0.4 oz)	44	3	4	42	0	tr
shredded mini wheats	1 cup (1.1 oz)	107	11	1	108	3	1
shredded wheat rectangular	1 biscuit (0.8 oz)	85	10	1	77	0	1
shredded wheat round	2 biscuits (1.3 oz)	136	15	1	124	1	1
whole wheat hot natural as prep w/ water	¾ cup (6.4 oz)	113	13	1	129	0	1

Alpen

FOOD	PORTION	CALS	CALCI	IRON	POTAS	SOD	ZINC
Corn Flakes	1 serv (1 oz)	110	13	1	22	2	tr

Aunt Jemima

FOOD	PORTION	CALS	CALCI	IRON	POTAS	SOD	ZINC
Enriched White Hominy Grits Regular	3 tbsp	101	1	1	39	1	0

Cap'n Crunch

FOOD	PORTION	CALS	CALCI	IRON	POTAS	SOD	ZINC
Original	¾ cup	113	6	5	36	241	2

General Mills

FOOD	PORTION	CALS	CALCI	IRON	POTAS	SOD	ZINC
Basic 4	1 cup (1.9 oz)	200	250	5	150	320	4
Boo Berry	1 cup (1 oz)	120	20	5	15	210	4
Cheerios	1 cup (1 oz)	110	100	8	95	280	4
Cheerios Apple Cinnamon	¾ cup (1 oz)	120	100	5	60	120	4
Cheerios Frosted	1 cup (1 oz)	120	100	5	55	210	4
Cheerios Honey Nut	1 cup (1 oz)	120	100	5	90	270	4
Cheerios Multi Grain	1 cup (1 oz)	110	100	18	85	200	15
Cheerios Team	1 cup (1 oz)	120	100	5	70	210	4

FOOD	PORTION	CALS	CALCI	IRON	POTAS	SOD	ZINC
Chex Corn	1 cup (1 oz)	110	100	9	25	280	4
Chex Morning Mix Cinnamon	1 pkg (1.1 oz)	130	100	5	75	180	2
Chex Morning Mix Fruit & Nut	1 pkg (1.1 oz)	180	100	5	75	190	2
Chex Morning Mix Honey Nut	1 pkg (1.1 oz)	130	100	5	80	190	2
Chex Multi-Bran	1 cup (2 oz)	200	100	16	220	380	4
Chex Rice	1¼ cup (1.1 oz)	120	100	9	35	290	4
Cinnamon Grahams	¾ cup (1 oz)	120	100	5	—	240	4
Cinnamon Toast Crunch	¾ cup (1 oz)	130	100	5	45	210	4
Cocoa Puffs	1 cup (1 oz)	120	100	5	50	170	4
Cookie Crisp	1 cup (1 oz)	120	100	5	25	180	4
Count Chocula	1 cup (1 oz)	120	20	5	—	180	4
Country Corn Flakes	1 cup (1 oz)	120	250	8	30	270	4
Fiber One	½ cup (1 oz)	60	100	5	230	130	4
Franken Berry	1 cup (1 oz)	120	20	5	15	210	4
French Toast Crunch	¾ cup (1 oz)	120	60	5	—	180	4
Golden Grahams	¾ cup (1 oz)	120	350	5	50	270	4
Harmony	1¼ cups (1.9 oz)	200	600	9	90	350	8
Honey Nut Clusters	1 cup (1.9 oz)	210	20	5	135	270	4
Kaboom	1¼ cup (1 oz)	120	100	8	65	290	4
Kix	1⅓ cup (1 oz)	120	150	8	35	270	4
Kix Berry Berry	¾ cup (1 oz)	120	40	5	25	180	4
Lucky Charms	1 cup (1 oz)	120	100	5	60	210	4
Nature Valley Low Fat Fruit Granola	⅔ cup (1.9 oz)	210	20	1	150	210	1
Newquick	¾ cup (1 oz)	120	100	5	65	190	4
Oatmeal Crisp Almond	1 cup (1.9 oz)	220	20	5	180	240	4
Oatmeal Crisp Apple Cinnamon	1 cup (1.9 oz)	210	20	5	170	250	4
Oatmeal Crisp Raisin	1 cup (1.9 oz)	210	20	5	200	220	4

FOOD	PORTION	CALS	CALCI	IRON	POTAS	SOD	ZINC
Raisin Nut Bran	¾ cup (1.9 oz)	200	20	5	230	250	4
Reese's Puffs	¾ cup	130	100	5	45	170	4
Sunrise Organic	¾ cup (1 oz)	110	0	5	50	190	4
Total Brown Sugar & Oat	¾ cup (1 oz)	110	1000	18	80	200	15
Total Corn Flakes	1⅓ cup (1 oz)	110	1000	18	30	210	15
Total Raisin Bran	1 cup (1.9 oz)	170	1000	18	350	240	15
Total Whole Grain	¾ cup (1 oz)	110	1000	18	90	190	15
Trix	1 cup (1 oz)	120	100	5	15	190	4
Wheat Hearts	¼ cup (1.3 oz)	130	0	11	130	0	1
Wheaties	1 cup (1 oz)	110	20	8	105	220	8
Wheaties Raisin Bran	1 cup (1.9 oz)	180	20	8	230	250	8
Grainfield's							
Brown Rice	1 serv (1 oz)	110	14	1	81	4	tr
Raisin Bran	1 serv (1 oz)	90	16	1	130	4	tr
Wheat Flakes	1 serv (1 oz)	100	28	tr	99	2	tr
Grist Mill							
Granola Low Fat w/ Raisins	⅔ cup (1.9 oz)	220	0	2	40	100	4
Oat & Honey Natural	½ cup (1.9 oz)	270	60	1	—	10	1
Oat Honey & Raisin Natural	½ cup (1.9 oz)	260	40	1	—	10	1
Healthy Choice							
Almond Crunch With Raisins	1 cup (2 oz)	210	20	6	200	230	2
Golden Multi-Grain Flakes	¾ cup (1.1 oz)	110	0	6	100	180	2
Toasted Brown Sugar Squares	1 cup (2 oz)	190	0	6	210	5	2
Kellogg's							
All-Bran	½ cup (1.1 oz)	80	150	5	390	65	4
All-Bran Bran Buds	⅓ cup (1 oz)	80	0	5	290	210	4
All-Bran Extra Fiber	½ cup (0.9 oz)	50	100	5	270	120	4
Apple Jacks	1 cup (1.2 oz)	120	0	5	35	150	4
Cocoa Krispies	¾ cup (1.1 oz)	120	0	2	65	220	2
Complete Oat Bran Flakes	¾ cup (1 oz)	110	0	8	120	270	4

FOOD	PORTION	CALS	CALCI	IRON	POTAS	SOD	ZINC
Complete Wheat Bran Flakes	¾ cup (1 oz)	90	0	8	170	220	4
Cracklin' Oat Bran	¾ cup (1.7 oz)	190	20	2	220	170	2
Crispix	1 cup (1 oz)	110	0	8	35	210	2
Granola Low Fat	½ cup (1.7 oz)	190	20	2	120	120	4
Just Right Crunchy Nuggets	1 cup (2 oz)	210	0	16	120	320	1
Just Right Fruit & Nut	1 cup (2.1 oz)	220	0	16	170	280	9
Low Fat With Raisins	⅔ cup (2.1 oz)	220	20	2	170	150	4
Mini-Wheat Frosted	1 cup (1.8 oz)	180	0	15	170	5	2
Mini-Wheat Strawberry Squares	¾ cup (1.8 oz)	170	20	16	170	15	2
Mini-Wheats Apple Cinnamon Squares	¾ cup (1.9 oz)	180	20	16	170	20	2
Mini-Wheats Blueberry Squares	¾ cup (1.9 oz)	180	0	16	180	20	2
Mini-Wheats Frosted Bite Size	24 pieces (2.1 oz)	200	0	17	200	5	2
Mini-Wheats Raisin Squares	¾ cup (1.9 oz)	180	0	16	250	5	2
Mueslix Apple & Almond Crunch	¾ cups (1.9 oz)	200	40	5	200	260	3
Mueslix Raisin & Almond	⅔ cup (1.9 oz)	200	20	5	240	160	4
Nutri-Grain Almond Raisin	1¼ cup (1.7 oz)	180	150	1	190	170	4
Nutri-Grain Golden Wheat	¾ cup (1 oz)	100	0	1	110	210	4
Product 19	1 cup (1 oz)	100	0	18	50	210	15
Raisin Bran	1 cup (2.1 oz)	200	40	5	360	370	4
Rice Krispies	1¼ cup (1.2 oz)	120	0	2	40	350	1
Rice Krispies Razzle Dazzle	¾ cup (1 oz)	110	0	2	25	170	1

FOOD	PORTION	CALS	CALCI	IRON	POTAS	SOD	ZINC
Smacks	¾ cup (1 oz)	100	0	2	40	50	tr
Smart Start	1 cup (1.8 oz)	180	0	18	100	310	15
Special K	1 cup (1.1 oz)	110	0	9	60	220	1
Morning Traditions							
Banana Nut Crunch	1 cup (2 oz)	250	0	2	170	240	2
Blueberry Morning	1¼ cup (1.9 oz)	220	20	2	95	250	1
Cranberry Almond Crunch	1 cup (1.9 oz)	220	0	2	100	200	2
Great Grains Crunchy Pecan	⅔ cup (1.9 oz)	220	0	3	150	190	1
Great Grains Raisins Dates & Pecans	⅔ cup (1.9 oz)	210	0	4	120	160	1
Mueslix							
Crispy Blend	⅔ cup (1.9 oz)	200	20	5	200	190	4
Nabisco							
100% Bran	⅓ cup (1 oz)	80	20	8	270	120	4
Frosted Shredded Wheat Bite Size	1 cup (1.8 oz)	190	0	2	170	10	2
Honey Nut Shredded Wheat Bite Size	1 cup (1.8 oz)	200	0	2	200	40	2
Original Shredded Wheat	2 biscuits (1.6 oz)	160	20	1	200	0	1
Original Shredded Wheat 'N Bran	1¼ cup (2.1 oz)	200	20	3	250	0	2
Original Shredded Wheat Spoon Size	1 cup (1.7 oz)	170	20	1	200	0	1
Post							
Alpha-Bits	1 cup (1 oz)	130	0	3	60	210	2
Alpha-Bits Marshmallow	1 cup (1 oz)	120	0	3	30	160	2
Bran Flakes	¾ cup (1 oz)	100	0	8	190	220	2
Cocoa Pebbles	¾ cup (1 oz)	120	0	2	40	160	2
Fruit & Fibre Dates Raisins & Walnuts	1 cup (1.9 oz)	210	20	6	250	250	2

FOOD	PORTION	CALS	CALCI	IRON	POTAS	SOD	ZINC
Fruit & Fibre Peaches Raisins & Almonds	1 cup (1.9 oz)	210	20	5	260	260	2
Fruity Pebbles	¾ cup (1 oz)	110	0	2	30	160	2
Golden Crisp	¾ cup (1 oz)	110	0	2	35	40	2
Grape-Nuts	¾ cup (1 oz)	100	0	8	80	140	1
Grape-Nuts Flakes	¾ cup (1 oz)	100	0	8	80	140	1
Honey Bunches Of Oats	¾ cup (1 oz)	120	0	3	50	190	tr
Honey Bunches Of Oats With Almonds	¾ cup (1.1 oz)	130	0	3	65	180	tr
Honeycomb	1⅓ cups (1 oz)	110	0	3	35	220	2
Post Toasties	1 cup (1 oz)	100	0	tr	30	270	0
Raisin Bran	1 cup (2 oz)	190	20	11	340	300	2
Selects Blueberry Morning	¾ cup (1.3 oz)	140	0	1	60	150	tr
Waffle Crisp	1 cup (1 oz)	130	0	2	35	120	2
Quaker							
Enriched White Hominy Grits Quick	3 tbsp	101	1	1	39	1	0
Enriched Yellow Hominy Quick Grits	3 tbsp	101	1	1	30	1	0
Instant Grits With Imitation Bacon Bits	1 pkg	101	7	8	62	590	0
Instant Grits With Imitation Ham Bits	1 pkg	99	7	8	56	800	0
Instant Grits With Real Cheddar Cheese	1 pkg	104	14	8	40	497	0
King Vitaman	1½ cup	110	6	8	50	280	tr
Life Cinnamon	⅔ cup	101	89	8	167	182	1
Life Original	⅔ cup	101	93	8	171	186	1
Puffed Rice	1 cup	54	1	tr	18	1	tr
Puffed Wheat	1 cup	50	3	1	53	1	tr
Shredded Wheat	2 biscuits	132	16	1	147	1	1

FOOD	PORTION	CALS	CALCI	IRON	POTAS	SOD	ZINC
Ralston							
Almond Delight	1 cup (1.8 oz)	210	20	2	—	410	2
Bran Flakes	¾ cup (1.1 oz)	110	0	18	—	220	5
Cookie Crisp	1 cup (1 oz)	120	0	5	—	110	2
Crisp Crunch	¾ cup (1.1 oz)	120	0	5	—	240	2
Crisp Rice	1¼ cup	130	0	2	—	330	tr
Fruit Rings	¾ cup (0.9 oz)	100	0	4	—	115	3
Magic Stair	¾ cup (1.1 oz)	120	20	5	—	160	2
Muesli Blueberry	1 cup (1.9 oz)	200	0	5	—	170	2
Muesli Cranberry	¾ cup (1.9 oz)	200	0	5	—	180	2
Muesli Peach	¾ cup (1.9 oz)	200	0	5	—	170	2
Muesli Raspberry	¾ cup (2 oz)	220	0	5	—	170	2
Muesli Strawberry	1 cup (1.9 oz)	210	0	5	—	170	2
Multi Vitamin Whole Grain Flakes	1 cup (1.1 oz)	120	200	18	—	300	15
Nutty Nuggets	½ cup (1.7 oz)	180	0	13	—	220	2
Raisin Bran	¾ cup (1.9 oz)	190	20	23	—	290	5
Tasteeos	1¼ cup (1.1 oz)	130	60	9	—	260	2
Tasteeos Apple Cinnamon	1 cup (1.2 oz)	130	20	5	—	150	2
Tasteeos Honey Nut	1 cup (1.2 oz)	130	40	5	—	250	2
CEREAL BARS							
granola	1 (1 oz)	134	17	1	95	83	tr
Dolly Madison							
Apple	1 (1.3 oz)	120	20	5	—	90	4
Blueberry	1 (1.3 oz)	120	20	5	—	90	4
Raspberry	1 (1.3 oz)	120	20	5	—	100	4
Strawberry	1 (1.3 oz)	120	20	5	—	100	4
General Mills							
Milk 'N Cereal Bars Chex	1 bar (1.6 oz)	160	250	5	105	150	5
Milk 'N Cereal Bars Cinnamon Toast Crunch	1 bar (1.6 oz)	180	250	5	115	160	5
Hostess							
Apple	1 (1.3 oz)	120	20	5	—	90	4
Banana Nut	1 (1.3 oz)	120	20	5	—	80	4

FOOD	PORTION	CALS	CALCI	IRON	POTAS	SOD	ZINC
Blueberry	1 (1.3 oz)	120	20	5	–	90	4
Raspberry	1 (1.3 oz)	120	20	5	–	100	4
Strawberry	1 (1.3 oz)	120	20	5	–	100	4
Kellogg's							
Nutri-Grain Apple Cinnamon	1 (1.3 oz)	140	20	2	75	110	2
Nutri-Grain Peach	1 (1.3 oz)	140	20	2	75	110	2
Nutri-Grain Raspberry	1 (1.3 oz)	140	20	2	70	110	2
Nutri-Grain Strawberry	1 (1.3 oz)	140	20	1	55	110	2
Nutri-Grain							
Blueberry	1 (1.3 oz)	140	20	2	75	110	2
Cherry	1 (1.3 oz)	140	20	2	70	110	2
Fruit-full Squares Apple	1 (1.7 oz)	180	0	2	–	95	2
Fruit-full Squares Banana	1 (1.7 oz)	190	0	2	–	95	2
Fruit-full Squares Cinnamon Raisin	1 (1.7 oz)	180	0	2	–	95	2
Minis Strawberry	1 pkg (1.5 oz)	160	200	2	–	115	2
Mixed Berry	1 (1.3 oz)	140	20	2	80	110	2
SnackWell's							
Country Fruit Medley	1 (1.3 oz)	130	20	4	–	75	4
Fat Free Apple Cinnamon	1 (1.3 oz)	120	20	4	–	115	4
Fat Free Blueberry	1 (1.3 oz)	120	20	5	–	85	4
Fat Free Strawberry	1 (1.3 oz)	120	20	5	–	115	4
Hearty Fruit'n Grain Crisp Autumn Apple	1 (1.3 oz)	130	20	5	–	95	4
Hearty Fruit'n Grain Mixed Berry	1 (1.3 oz)	120	20	5	–	95	4
Hearty Fruit'n Grain Orchard Cherry	1 (1.3 oz)	130	20	4	–	90	4
CHAYOTE							
raw cut up	1 cup	32	25	1	34	198	5

FOOD	PORTION	CALS	CALCI	IRON	POTAS	SOD	ZINC
CHEESE							
american	1 oz	93	163	tr	79	337	1
american cheese food	1 pkg (8 oz)	745	1303	2	633	2700	7
american cheese spread	1 jar (5 oz)	412	798	tr	343	1910	4
american cheese spread	1 oz	82	159	tr	69	381	1
blue	1 oz	100	150	tr	73	396	1
blue crumbled	1 cup (4.7 oz)	477	712	tr	346	1884	4
brick	1 oz	105	191	tr	38	159	1
camembert	1 oz	85	110	tr	53	239	tr
camembert	1 wedge (1⅓ oz)	114	147	tr	71	320	1
cheddar	1 oz	114	204	tr	28	176	1
cheddar low sodium	1 oz	113	200	tr	32	6	1
cheddar shredded	1 cup	455	815	1	111	701	4
colby	1 oz	112	194	tr	36	171	1
colby low sodium	1 oz	113	200	tr	32	6	1
edam	1 oz	101	207	tr	53	274	1
emmentaler	1 oz	115	291	tr	31	129	1
feta	1 oz	75	140	tr	18	316	1
goat hard	1 oz	128	254	1	14	98	tr
goat semisoft	1 oz	103	84	tr	45	146	tr
goat soft	1 oz	76	40	1	7	104	tr
gouda	1 oz	101	198	tr	34	232	1
limburger	1 oz	93	141	tr	36	227	1
monterey	1 oz	106	212	tr	23	152	1
mozzarella	1 lb	1276	2345	1	304	1692	10
mozzarella	1 oz	80	147	tr	19	106	1
mozzarella part skim	1 oz	72	183	tr	24	132	1
muenster	1 oz	104	203	tr	38	178	1
parmesan grated	1 oz	129	390	tr	30	528	1
parmesan grated	1 tbsp (5 g)	23	69	tr	5	93	tr
parmesan hard	1 oz	111	336	tr	26	454	1
pimento	1 oz	106	174	tr	46	405	1
provolone	1 oz	100	214	tr	39	248	1

FOOD	PORTION	CALS	CALCI	IRON	POTAS	SOD	ZINC
quark 20% fat	1 oz	33	24	tr	25	10	tr
quark 40% fat	1 oz	48	27	tr	23	10	tr
quark made w/ skim milk	1 oz	22	26	tr	27	11	tr
queso anego	1 oz	106	193	tr	25	321	1
queso asadero	1 oz	101	188	tr	25	186	1
queso chichuahua	1 oz	106	185	tr	15	175	1
queso manchego	1 oz	107	237	tr	57	341	1
ricotta part skim	½ cup (4.4 oz)	171	337	1	155	155	2
ricotta part skim	1 cup (8.6 oz)	340	669	1	308	307	3
ricotta whole milk	1 cup (8.6 oz)	428	509	1	257	207	3
ricotta whole milk	½ cup (4.4 oz)	216	257	tr	130	104	1
roquefort	1 oz	105	188	tr	26	513	1
swiss	1 oz	107	272	tr	31	74	1
swiss processed	1 oz	95	219	tr	61	388	1
tilsit	1 oz	96	198	tr	18	213	1
Cheez Whiz							
Light	2 tbsp (1.2 oz)	80	150	0	110	540	1
Cracker Barrel							
Baby Swiss	1 oz	110	200	0	15	110	1
Cheddar Extra Sharp	1 oz	120	200	0	30	180	1
Cheddar Marbled Sharp	1 oz	110	200	0	30	180	1
Cheddar New York Aged	1 oz	120	200	0	30	180	1
Cheddar Sharp	1 oz	120	200	0	30	180	1
Cheddar Vermont Sharp	1 oz	110	200	0	30	180	1
Reduced Fat Cheddar Extra Sharp	1 oz	90	200	0	45	240	1
Reduced Fat Cheddar Sharp	1 oz	90	200	0	45	240	1
Reduced Fat Cheddar Vermont Sharp	1 oz	90	200	0	45	240	1

FOOD	PORTION	CALS	CALCI	IRON	POTAS	SOD	ZINC
Whipped Spreadable Cream Cheese & Extra Sharp Cheddar	2 tbsp (0.9 oz)	80	80	0	25	180	tr
Whipped Spreadable Cream Cheese & Sharp Cheddar	2 tbsp (0.9 oz)	80	80	0	20	180	tr
Whipped Spreadable Cream Cheese & Sharp Cheddar w/ Herbs	2 tbsp (0.9 oz)	80	80	0	25	180	tr
Kraft							
Cheddar Extra Sharp	1 oz	120	200	0	30	180	1
Cheddar Medium	1 oz	110	200	0	30	180	1
Cheddar Mild	1 oz	110	200	0	30	180	1
Cheddar Sharp	1 oz	120	200	0	30	180	1
Cheddary Melts Medium Cheddar	1 oz	110	150	0	50	390	1
Cheddary Melts Mild Cheddar	1 oz	110	150	0	50	390	1
Cheddary Melts Shreds Medium Cheddar	¼ cup (1.1 oz)	120	150	0	55	420	1
Cheddary Melts Shreds Mild Cheddar	¼ cup (1.1 oz)	120	150	0	55	420	1
Cheese Food w/ Garlic	1 oz	90	150	0	75	370	1
Cheese Food w/ Jalapeno Peppers	1 oz	90	150	0	80	370	1
Colby	1 oz	110	200	0	15	180	1
Deluxe American	1 oz	100	150	0	25	430	1
Deluxe American White	1 oz	100	150	0	25	430	1
Deluxe Singles American	1 (1 oz)	110	150	0	25	460	1

FOOD	PORTION	CALS	CALCI	IRON	POTAS	SOD	ZINC
Deluxe Singles American	1 (0.7 oz)	70	100	0	15	310	1
Deluxe Singles Pimento	1 (1 oz)	100	150	0	25	430	1
Deluxe Singles Swiss	1 (1 oz)	90	200	0	20	410	1
Deluxe Singles Swiss	1 slice (0.7 oz)	70	150	0	15	310	1
Free Grated	2 tsp (5 g)	15	0	0	10	75	0
Free Shredded Cheddar	¼ cup (0.9 oz)	40	250	0	35	270	2
Free Shredded Mozzarella	¼ cup (1 oz)	45	250	0	30	340	1
Grated Parm Plus! Garlic Herb	2 tsp (5 g)	15	0	0	20	110	0
Grated Parm Plus! Zesty Red Pepper	2 tsp (5 g)	15	20	0	15	110	0
Grated Parmesan	2 tsp (5 g)	20	60	0	10	85	tr
Grated Romano	2 tsp (5 g)	20	60	0	10	70	0
Marbled Cheddar Mild	1 oz	110	200	0	30	180	1
Marbled Cheddar & Monterey Jack	1 oz	110	200	0	20	190	1
Marbled Cheddar & Whole Milk Mozzarella	1 oz	100	200	0	25	190	1
Monterey Jack	1 oz	110	200	0	15	190	1
Monterey Jack w/ Jalapeno Peppers	1 oz	110	200	0	15	190	1
Mozzarella Part Skim Low Moisture	1 oz	80	200	0	20	200	1
Mozzarella String Cheese Low Moisture Part Skim	1 piece (1 oz)	80	150	0	35	240	1
Pizza Shredded Four Cheese	¼ cup (0.9 oz)	90	200	0	20	220	1

FOOD	PORTION	CALS	CALCI	IRON	POTAS	SOD	ZINC
Pizza Shredded Mozzarella & Cheddar	⅓ cup (1.1 oz)	120	200	0	30	220	1
Pizza Shredded Mozzarella & Provolone w/ Smoke Flavor	¼ cup (0.9 oz)	90	150	0	20	200	1
Reduced Fat Cheddar Mild	1 oz	90	200	0	45	240	1
Reduced Fat Cheddar Sharp	1 oz	90	200	0	45	240	1
Reduced Fat Colby	1 oz	80	200	0	50	220	2
Reduced Fat Monterey Jack	1 oz	80	200	0	45	240	2
Shredded Cheddar Medium	¼ cup (0.9 oz)	100	200	0	25	170	1
Shredded Cheddar Sharp	1 oz (0.9 oz)	110	150	0	25	170	1
Shredded Cheddar & Monterey Jack	¼ cup (0.9 oz)	100	200	0	20	170	1
Shredded Colby & Monterey Jack	¼ cup (0.9 oz)	100	150	0	15	170	1
Shredded Hearty Italian	⅓ cup (1.1 oz)	100	200	0	35	230	1
Shredded Italian Style Classic Garlic	⅓ cup (1.1 oz)	100	200	0	45	240	1
Shredded Italian Style Mozzarella & Parmesan	⅓ cup (1.1 oz)	100	200	0	25	240	1
Shredded Lower Fat Cheddar Mild	¼ cup (0.9 oz)	80	200	0	40	220	1
Shredded Lower Fat Cheddar Sharp	¼ cup (0.9 oz)	80	200	0	40	220	1

FOOD	PORTION	CALS	CALCI	IRON	POTAS	SOD	ZINC
Shredded Lower Fat Colby & Monterey Jack	¼ cup (0.9 oz)	80	200	0	40	210	1
Shredded Lower Fat Mozzarella	⅓ cup (1.1 oz)	80	250	0	25	210	1
Shredded Lower Fat Pizza Cheese	⅓ cup (1.1 oz)	90	250	0	40	240	1
Shredded Mexican Style Cheddar & Monterey Jack	⅓ cup (1.1 oz)	120	200	0	25	200	1
Shredded Mexican Style Cheddar & Monterey Jack w/ Jalapeno Peppers	⅓ cup (1.1 oz)	120	200	0	25	200	1
Shredded Mexican Style Four Cheese	⅓ cup (1.1 oz)	120	200	0	25	210	1
Shredded Mexican Style Taco Cheese	⅓ cup (1.1 oz)	120	200	0	25	240	1
Shredded Monterey Jack	¼ cup (0.9 oz)	100	150	0	15	170	1
Shredded Parmesan	2 tsp (5 g)	20	40	0	0	75	0
Shredded Part Skim Mozzarella	¼ cup (1.1 oz)	90	250	0	20	220	1
Shredded Swiss	¼ cup (0.9 oz)	100	250	0	45	25	1
Shredded Whole Milk Mozzarella	¼ cup (1.1 oz)	100	200	0	25	220	1
Shredded Finely Cheddar Mild	¼ cup (1.1 oz)	120	200	0	30	190	1
Shredded Finely Cheddar Sharp	¼ cup (1.1 oz)	120	200	0	30	190	1

FOOD	PORTION	CALS	CALCI	IRON	POTAS	SOD	ZINC
Shredded Finely Colby & Monterey Jack	¼ cup (1 oz)	110	200	0	15	190	1
Shredded Finely Lower Fat Cheddar Mild	⅓ cup (1.1 oz)	100	200	0	50	260	1
Shredded Finely Lower Fat Cheddar Sharp	⅓ cup (1.1 oz)	100	200	0	50	260	1
Shredded Finely Part Skim Mozzarella	¼ cup (1.1 oz)	90	250	0	20	220	1
Shredded Finely Swiss	¼ cup (0.9 oz)	110	250	0	20	45	1
Singles American	1 (1.2 oz)	110	200	0	80	460	1
Singles American	1 (0.7 oz)	60	100	0	45	260	1
Singles American	1 (0.6 oz)	60	150	0	45	260	1
Singles Mild Mexican	1 (0.7 oz)	70	100	0	50	280	1
Singles Monterey	1 slice (0.7 oz)	70	100	0	55	290	1
Singles Pimento	1 (0.7 oz)	60	100	0	50	260	tr
Singles Reduced Fat American	1 (0.7 oz)	50	150	0	60	320	1
Singles Reduced Fat American White	1 (0.7 oz)	50	150	0	60	320	1
Singles Sharp	1 slice (0.7 oz)	70	100	0	25	300	1
Singles Swiss	1 slice (0.7 oz)	70	150	0	55	320	1
Singles Nonfat American	1 (0.7 oz)	30	150	0	60	270	1
Singles Nonfat American White	1 (0.7 oz)	30	150	0	60	270	1
Singles Nonfat Sharp Cheddar	1 (0.7 oz)	35	150	0	65	300	1
Singles Nonfat Swiss	1 slice (0.7 oz)	30	150	0	55	270	1

FOOD	PORTION	CALS	CALCI	IRON	POTAS	SOD	ZINC
Slices Cheddar Mild	1 (1 oz)	110	200	0	30	180	1
Slices Colby	1 (1.6 oz)	180	300	0	25	290	2
Slices Part Skim Mozzarella	1 (1.6 oz)	130	350	0	30	320	2
Slices Part Skim Mozzarella	1 (1.5 oz)	120	350	0	30	310	2
Slices Provolone Smoke Flavor	1 (1.5 oz)	150	300	0	35	370	2
Slices Swiss	1 (1.5 oz)	170	400	0	75	45	2
Slices Swiss	1 (1.3 oz)	150	350	0	25	65	2
Slices Swiss	1 (0.8 oz)	90	200	0	15	40	1
Slices Swiss	1 (1.6 oz)	180	400	0	75	45	2
Slices Swiss Aged	1 (1.5 oz)	170	400	0	30	75	2
Slices Deli-Thin Part Skim Mozzarella	1 (1 oz)	80	200	0	20	200	1
Slices Deli-Thin Swiss	1 (0.8 oz)	90	200	0	15	40	1
Slices Deli-Thin Swiss Aged	1 (0.8 oz)	90	200	0	15	40	1
Slices Reduced Fat Swiss	1 (1.3 oz)	130	400	0	55	90	2
Spread Bacon	2 tbsp (1.1 oz)	90	150	0	20	570	1
Spread Olive & Pimento	2 tbsp (1.1 oz)	70	20	0	50	220	0
Spread Pimento	2 tbsp (1.1 oz)	80	20	0	60	170	0
Spread Pineapple	2 tbsp (1.1 oz)	70	20	0	55	120	0
Spread Pineapple	2 tbsp (1.1 oz)	70	20	0	55	115	0
Spread Roka Brand Blue	2 tbsp (1.1 oz)	90	150	0	15	520	1
Swiss	1 oz	110	250	0	20	50	1
Lactaid							
American	3.5 oz	328	574	1	279	1189	3
Light N'Lively							
Singles American	1 (0.7 oz)	45	150	0	50	280	1

FOOD	PORTION	CALS	CALCI	IRON	POTAS	SOD	ZINC
Old English							
American Sharp	1 slice (1 oz)	100	150	0	20	460	1
Velveeta							
Light	1 oz	60	150	0	90	440	1
Shredded	¼ cup (1.3 oz)	130	200	0	100	500	1
Shredded Mild Mexican w/ Jalapeno Pepper	¼ cup (1.3 oz)	120	200	0	95	520	1
Spread	1 oz	90	150	0	95	420	1
Spread Hot Mexican	1 oz	90	150	0	90	420	1
Spread Mild Mexican	1 oz	90	150	0	90	420	1

CHEESE DISHES

FOOD	PORTION	CALS	CALCI	IRON	POTAS	SOD	ZINC
fondue	½ cup (3.8 oz)	247	514	tr	113	142	2

CHEESE SUBSTITUTES

FOOD	PORTION	CALS	CALCI	IRON	POTAS	SOD	ZINC
Formagg							
American White	1 slice (0.66 oz)	60	200	1	—	260	1
American Yellow	1 slice (0.66 oz)	60	200	1	—	260	1
Cheddar	1 slice (0.66 oz)	60	200	1	—	260	1
Swiss White	1 slice (0.66 oz)	60	200	1	—	260	1
Sargento							
Mozzarella Shredded	¼ cup (1 oz)	80	150	0	—	320	1

CHERRIES

FOOD	PORTION	CALS	CALCI	IRON	POTAS	SOD	ZINC
sour fresh	1 cup	51	16	tr	178	3	tr
sour in heavy syrup	½ cup	232	26	3	238	18	tr
sour in light syrup	½ cup	189	26	3	238	18	tr
sour unsweetened frozen	1 cup	72	20	1	192	1	tr
sour water packed	1 cup	87	26	3	240	17	tr
sweet fresh	10	49	10	tr	152	0	tr
sweet in heavy syrup	½ cup	107	12	tr	187	3	tr
sweet in light syrup	½ cup	85	12	tr	186	3	tr

FOOD	PORTION	CALS	CALCI	IRON	POTAS	SOD	ZINC
sweet juice pack	½ cup	68	17	1	163	3	tr
sweet sweetened frozen	1 cup	232	31	1	514	3	tr
sweet water pack	½ cup	57	13	tr	162	2	tr

CHERVIL

FOOD	PORTION	CALS	CALCI	IRON	POTAS	SOD	ZINC
seed	1 tsp	1	8	tr	28	tr	tr

CHESTNUTS

FOOD	PORTION	CALS	CALCI	IRON	POTAS	SOD	ZINC
chinese cooked	1 oz	44	3	tr	87	1	tr
chinese dried	1 oz	103	8	1	206	2	tr
chinese raw	1 oz	64	5	tr	127	1	tr
chinese roasted	1 oz	68	5	tr	135	1	tr
cooked	1 oz	37	13	tr	203	8	tr
dried peeled	1 oz	105	18	1	281	11	tr
japanese cooked	1 oz	16	3	tr	34	1	tr
japanese dried	1 oz	102	20	1	218	10	1
japanese raw	1 oz	44	9	tr	94	4	tr
raw peeled	1 oz	56	5	tr	137	1	tr
roasted	2 to 3 (1 oz)	70	8	tr	168	1	tr
roasted	1 cup	350	42	1	846	3	1

CHICKEN

FOOD	PORTION	CALS	CALCI	IRON	POTAS	SOD	ZINC
broiler/fryer back w/ skin batter dipped & fried	½ back (2.5 oz)	238	17	1	130	228	1
broiler/fryer back w/ skin floured & fried	1.5 oz	146	10	1	100	40	1
broiler/fryer back w/ skin roasted	1 oz	96	7	tr	67	28	1
broiler/fryer back w/ skin stewed	½ back (2.1 oz)	158	11	1	89	39	1
broiler/fryer back w/o skin fried	½ back (2 oz)	167	15	1	146	58	2
broiler/fryer breast w/ skin batter dipped & fried	½ breast (4.9 oz)	364	28	1	282	385	1
broiler/fryer breast w/ skin batter dipped & fried	2.9 oz	218	17	1	169	231	1

FOOD	PORTION	CALS	CALCI	IRON	POTAS	SOD	ZINC
broiler/fryer breast w/ skin roasted	½ breast (3.4 oz)	193	14	1	240	69	1
broiler/fryer breast w/ skin roasted	2 oz	115	8	1	142	41	1
broiler/fryer breast w/ skin stewed	½ breast (3.9 oz)	202	14	1	195	68	1
broiler/fryer breast w/o skin fried	½ breast (3 oz)	161	14	1	237	68	1
broiler/fryer breast w/o skin roasted	½ breast (3 oz)	142	13	1	220	63	1
broiler/fryer breast w/o skin stewed	2 oz	86	7	1	107	36	1
broiler/fryer drumstick w/ skin batter dipped & fried	1 (2.6 oz)	193	12	1	134	194	2
broiler/fryer drumstick w/ skin floured & fried	1 (1.7 oz)	120	6	1	112	44	1
broiler/fryer drumstick w/ skin roasted	1 (1.8 oz)	112	6	1	119	47	1
broiler/fryer drumstick w/ skin stewed	1 (2 oz)	116	7	1	105	43	2
broiler/fryer drumstick w/o skin fried	1 (1.5 oz)	82	5	1	105	40	1
broiler/fryer drumstick w/o skin roasted	1 (1.5 oz)	76	5	1	108	42	1
broiler/fryer drumstick w/o skin stewed	1 (1.6 oz)	78	5	1	92	37	1
broiler/fryer leg w/ skin batter dipped & fried	1 (5.5 oz)	431	28	2	299	442	3
broiler/fryer leg w/ skin floured & fried	1 (3.9 oz)	285	15	2	261	99	3

FOOD	PORTION	CALS	CALCI	IRON	POTAS	SOD	ZINC
broiler/fryer leg w/ skin roasted	1 (4 oz)	265	14	2	256	99	3
broiler/fryer leg w/ skin stewed	1 (4.4 oz)	275	14	2	220	92	3
broiler/fryer leg w/o skin fried	1 (3.3 oz)	195	12	1	239	90	3
broiler/fryer leg w/o skin roasted	1 (3.3 oz)	182	12	1	230	87	3
broiler/fryer leg w/o skin stewed	1 (3.5 oz)	187	11	1	192	78	3
broiler/fryer neck w/ skin stewed	1 (1.3 oz)	94	10	1	41	20	1
broiler/fryer skin batter dipped & fried	from ½ chicken (6.7 oz)	748	49	3	143	1105	1
broiler/fryer skin roasted	from ½ chicken (2 oz)	254	8	1	76	36	1
broiler/fryer thigh w/ skin batter dipped & fried	1 (3 oz)	238	16	1	165	248	2
broiler/fryer thigh w/ skin floured & fried	1 (2.2 oz)	162	8	1	147	55	2
broiler/fryer thigh w/ skin roasted	1 (2.2 oz)	153	8	1	137	52	1
broiler/fryer thigh w/ skin stewed	1 (2.4 oz)	158	8	1	115	49	2
broiler/fryer thigh w/o skin fried	1 (1.8 oz)	113	7	1	134	49	1
broiler/fryer thigh w/o skin roasted	1 (1.8 oz)	109	6	1	124	46	1
broiler/fryer thigh w/o skin stewed	1 (1.9 oz)	107	6	1	101	41	1
broiler/fryer w/ skin floured & fried	½ chicken (11 oz)	844	52	4	735	264	6
broiler/fryer w/ skin fried	½ chicken (16.4 oz)	1347	97	6	863	1360	8
broiler/fryer w/ skin roasted	½ chicken (10.5 oz)	715	45	4	667	244	6

FOOD	PORTION	CALS	CALCI	IRON	POTAS	SOD	ZINC
broiler/fryer w/ skin stewed	½ chicken (11.7 oz)	730	44	4	556	224	6
broiler/fryer w/o skin roasted	1 cup (5 oz)	266	21	2	340	120	3
broiler/fryer wing w/ skin batter dipped & fried	1 (1.7 oz)	159	10	1	68	157	1
broiler/fryer wing w/ skin floured & fried	1 (1.1 oz)	103	5	tr	57	25	1
broiler/fryer wing w/ skin roasted	1 (1.2 oz)	99	5	tr	62	28	1
broiler/fryer wing w/ skin stewed	1 (1.4 oz)	100	5	tr	56	27	1
capon w/ skin neck & giblets roasted	1 chicken (3.1 lbs)	3211	211	25	3439	704	27
chicken roll light meat	2 oz	90	24	1	129	331	tr
chicken roll light meat	1 pkg (6 oz)	271	73	2	388	992	1
cornish hen w/ skin roasted	1 hen (8 oz)	595	31	2	562	146	3
cornish hen w/o skin & bone roasted	½ hen (2 oz)	72	7	tr	134	34	1
cornish hen w/o skin & bone roasted	1 hen (3.8 oz)	144	14	1	268	67	2
cornish hen w/skin roasted	½ hen (4 oz)	296	15	1	280	73	2
roaster w/ skin roasted	½ chicken (1.1 lbs)	1071	58	6	1014	349	7
stewing w/ skin stewed	½ chicken (9.2 oz)	744	33	4	476	190	5

CHICKEN DISHES

FOOD	PORTION	CALS	CALCI	IRON	POTAS	SOD	ZINC
boneless breaded & fried w/ barbecue sauce	6 pieces (4.6 oz)	330	21	1	319	830	1

FOOD	PORTION	CALS	CALCI	IRON	POTAS	SOD	ZINC
boneless breaded & fried w/ honey	6 pieces (4 oz)	339	17	1	255	537	1
boneless breaded & fried w/ mustard sauce	6 pieces (4.6 oz)	323	25	1	280	791	1
boneless breaded & fried w/ sweet & sour sauce	6 pieces (4.6 oz)	346	20	1	280	791	1
breast & wing breaded & fried	2 pieces (5.7 oz)	494	60	1	566	975	2
chicken & dumplings	¾ cup	256	61	2	163	1283	2
chicken cacciatore	¾ cup	394	45	4	149	671	2
drumstick breaded & fried	2 pieces (5.2 oz)	430	36	2	446	756	3
groundnut stew hkatenkwan	1 serv (15.7 oz)	576	79	3	973	1009	3
jamaican jerk wings	4 wings (9.9 oz)	709	51	3	402	1045	4
sancocho de pollo dominican chicken stew	1 serv	702	72	5	1324	653	4
thigh breaded & fried	2 pieces (5.2 oz)	430	36	2	446	756	3

CHICKEN SUBSTITUTES
Yves

FOOD	PORTION	CALS	CALCI	IRON	POTAS	SOD	ZINC
Veggie Chicken Burgers	1 (3 oz)	120	80	4	300	390	3

CHICKPEAS

FOOD	PORTION	CALS	CALCI	IRON	POTAS	SOD	ZINC
canned	1 cup	285	78	3	413	718	3
dried cooked	1 cup	269	80	5	477	11	3

CHICORY

FOOD	PORTION	CALS	CALCI	IRON	POTAS	SOD	ZINC
witloof head raw	1 (1.9 oz)	9	10	tr	112	1	tr
witloof raw	½ cup (1.6 oz)	8	9	tr	95	1	tr

CHILI

FOOD	PORTION	CALS	CALCI	IRON	POTAS	SOD	ZINC
chile pepper paste	1 tbsp	6	21	1	40	1445	tr
chili w/ beans	1 cup	286	119	9	932	1330	5

FOOD	PORTION	CALS	CALCI	IRON	POTAS	SOD	ZINC
con carne w/ beans	8.9 oz	254	67	5	691	1008	4
dried pasilla	1 tsp	3	1	tr	22	1	tr
powder	1 tsp	8	7	tr	50	26	tr
CHIPS							
barbecue	1 oz	139	14	1	358	213	tr
barbecue	1 bag (7 oz)	971	96	4	2498	1486	2
corn	1 bag (7 oz)	1067	251	3	281	1248	2
corn	1 oz	153	36	tr	40	179	tr
corn barbecue	1 oz	148	37	tr	67	216	tr
corn barbecue	1 bag (7 oz)	1036	259	3	468	1511	2
corn cones	1 oz	145	1	1	23	290	tr
corn onion	1 oz	142	8	1	40	278	tr
potato	1 bag (8 oz)	1217	54	4	2894	1347	2
potato	1 oz	152	7	tr	361	168	tr
potato cheese	1 oz	140	20	1	433	225	tr
potato cheese	1 bag (6 oz)	842	122	3	2597	1348	2
potato sour cream & onion	1 oz	150	20	tr	377	177	tr
potato sour cream & onion	1 bag (7 oz)	1051	143	3	2634	1237	2
potato sticks	½ cup (0.6 oz)	94	3	tr	223	45	tr
potato sticks	1 oz	148	5	1	351	71	tr
potato sticks	1 pkg (1 oz)	148	5	1	351	71	tr
taco	1 oz	136	44	1	61	223	tr
taco	1 bag (8 oz)	1089	352	5	492	1788	3
tortilla	1 oz	142	44	tr	56	150	tr
tortilla	1 bag (7.5 oz)	1067	327	3	419	1124	3
tortilla nacho	1 oz	141	42	tr	61	201	tr
tortilla nacho	1 bag (8 oz)	1131	354	3	491	1606	3
tortilla ranch	1 oz	139	40	tr	69	174	tr
tortilla ranch	1 bag (7 oz)	969	280	3	483	1212	2
CHITTERLINGS							
pork cooked	3 oz	258	23	3	—	33	4
CHIVES							
fresh chopped	1 tbsp	1	3	tr	9	0	tr
fresh chopped	1 tsp	0	1	tr	3	0	tr

FOOD	PORTION	CALS	CALCI	IRON	POTAS	SOD	ZINC
CHOCOLATE							
baking grated unsweetened	1 cup (4.6 oz)	690	98	8	1100	18	5
baking liquid unsweetened	1 oz	134	15	1	331	3	1
baking squares unsweetened	1 square (1 oz)	148	21	2	236	4	1
chips milk chocolate	1 cup (6 oz)	862	321	2	646	138	2
chips semisweet	1 cup (6 oz)	804	54	5	614	19	3
chips semisweet	60 pieces (1 oz)	136	9	1	104	3	tr
powder	2–3 heaping tsp	75	8	1	128	45	tr
powder as prep w/ whole milk	9 oz	226	300	1	498	165	1
CHOCOLATE SYRUP							
chocolate fudge	1 cup (11.9 oz)	1176	340	4	731	442	3
chocolate fudge	1 tbsp (0.7 oz)	73	21	tr	45	27	tr
syrup	1 cup	653	42	6	672	287	2
syrup	2 tbsp	82	5	1	84	36	tr
syrup as prep w/ whole milk	9 oz	232	297	1	455	156	1
CHUTNEY							
mango	1 tbsp	54	4	tr	11	207	tr
tomato	1 tbsp	32	5	tr	62	26	tr
CILANTRO							
fresh	1 tsp (2 g)	tr	1	tr	8	1	0
fresh	1 cup (1.6 oz)	11	31	1	235	25	tr
CINNAMON							
ground	1 tsp	6	28	1	11	1	tr
CISCO							
smoked	3 oz	151	22	tr	249	409	tr
smoked	1 oz	50	7	tr	82	135	tr
CLAMS							
breaded & fried	20 sm	379	119	26	612	684	3
fresh cooked	3 oz	126	78	24	534	95	2

FOOD	PORTION	CALS	CALCI	IRON	POTAS	SOD	ZINC
fresh cooked	20 sm	133	83	25	565	100	2
fresh raw	3 oz	63	39	12	267	47	1
fresh raw	20 sm (6.3 oz)	133	83	25	565	100	2
fresh raw	9 lg (6.3 oz)	133	83	25	565	100	2
meat only canned	1 cup	236	148	45	1005	179	4
meat only canned	3 oz	126	78	24	534	95	2

CLOVES

FOOD	PORTION	CALS	CALCI	IRON	POTAS	SOD	ZINC
ground	1 tsp	7	14	tr	23	5	tr

COCOA

FOOD	PORTION	CALS	CALCI	IRON	POTAS	SOD	ZINC
hot cocoa	1 cup	218	298	1	480	123	1
mix as prep w/ water	7 oz	103	96	tr	203	149	tr
mix w/ equal as prep w/ water	7 oz	48	90	1	405	173	1
powder unsweetened	1 tbsp (5 g)	11	6	1	76	1	tr
powder unsweetened	1 cup (3 oz)	197	110	12	1310	18	6

COCONUT

FOOD	PORTION	CALS	CALCI	IRON	POTAS	SOD	ZINC
coconut water	1 tbsp	3	4	tr	38	16	tr
coconut water	1 cup	46	58	1	600	252	tr
cream canned	1 cup	568	4	2	299	149	2
cream canned	1 tbsp	36	0	tr	19	10	tr
dried sweetened flaked	7 oz pkg	944	28	4	629	509	3
dried sweetened flaked	1 cup	351	10	1	234	189	1
dried sweetened flaked canned	1 cup	341	11	1	249	15	1
dried sweetened shredded	7 oz pkg	997	30	4	670	522	4
dried sweetened shredded	1 cup	466	14	2	313	244	2
dried toasted	1 oz	168	8	1	157	11	1
dried unsweetened	1 oz	187	7	1	154	11	1
fresh	1 piece (1.5 oz)	159	6	1	160	9	1

FOOD	PORTION	CALS	CALCI	IRON	POTAS	SOD	ZINC
fresh shredded	1 cup	283	12	2	285	16	1
milk canned	1 tbsp	30	3	1	33	2	tr
milk canned	1 cup	445	40	7	497	29	1
milk frozen	1 tbsp	30	1	tr	35	2	tr
milk frozen	1 cup	486	11	2	556	29	1

COD

FOOD	PORTION	CALS	CALCI	IRON	POTAS	SOD	ZINC
atlantic canned	1 can (11 oz)	327	66	2	1647	680	2\
atlantic canned	3 oz	89	18	tr	449	185	tr
atlantic dried	3 oz	246	136	2	1239	5973	1
atlantic fresh cooked	1 fillet (6.3 oz)	189	25	1	440	141	1
atlantic fresh cooked	3 oz	89	12	tr	208	66	tr
atlantic fresh raw	3 oz	70	13	tr	351	46	tr
pacific fresh baked	3 oz	95	8	tr	465	82	tr

COFFEE

FOOD	PORTION	CALS	CALCI	IRON	POTAS	SOD	ZINC
cafe au lait	1 cup (8 fl oz)	77	148	tr	249	62	tr
cafe brulot	1 cup (4.8 fl oz)	48	2	tr	64	2	tr
cappuccino	1 cup (8 fl oz)	77	148	tr	249	62	tr
coffee con leche	1 cup (8 fl oz)	77	148	tr	249	62	tr
decaffeinated instant	1 rounded tsp	4	3	tr	63	0	0
decaffeinated instant as prep	6 oz	4	6	tr	63	6	tr
espresso	1 cup (3 fl oz)	2	2	tr	48	2	tr
irish coffee	1 serv (9 fl oz)	107	20	tr	151	25	tr
latte w/ skim milk	13 oz	88	304	tr	470	128	1
latte w/ whole milk	13 oz	152	293	tr	434	122	1
mocha	1 mug (9.6 fl oz)	202	67	1	228	28	tr
regular instant as prep	6 oz	4	6	tr	64	6	tr
regular instant as prep	6 fl oz	4	5	tr	64	5	tr
regular brewed	8 oz	2	1	tr	16	1	tr
regular w/ chicory instant	1 rounded tsp	6	2	tr	61	5	tr

FOOD	PORTION	CALS	CALCI	IRON	POTAS	SOD	ZINC
regular w/ chicory instant as prep	6 oz	6	6	tr	61	10	tr
COFFEE BEVERAGES							
cappuccino mix as prep	7 oz	62	7	tr	119	104	tr
mocha mix as prep	7 oz	51	7	tr	119	36	tr
Silk							
Coffee Soylatte	1 bottle (11 oz)	220	400	1	100	70	1
COFFEE SUBSTITUTES							
powder	1 tsp	9	1	tr	42	2	tr
COFFEE WHITENERS							
liquid nondairy frzn	1 tbsp (0.5 oz)	20	1	tr	29	12	tr
powder nondairy	1 tsp	11	tr	tr	16	4	tr
COLESLAW							
coleslaw w/ dressing	½ cup	42	27	tr	109	14	tr
COLLARDS							
fresh cooked	½ cup	17	15	tr	84	10	1
frzn chopped cooked	½ cup	31	179	1	214	42	tr
raw chopped	½ cup	6	5	tr	30	4	tr
COOKIES							
animal crackers	11 crackers (1 oz)	126	12	1	28	112	tr
animal crackers	1 box (2.4 oz)	299	11	1	57	274	tr
animal crackers	1 (2.5 g)	11	1	tr	2	10	tr
black & white	1 lg (3 oz)	302	32	2	68	72	tr
butter	1 (5 g)	23	1	tr	6	18	tr
chocolate chip	1 (0.4 oz)	48	2	tr	14	32	tr
chocolate chip	1 box (1.9 oz)	233	20	1	82	188	tr
chocolate chip low fat	1 (0.25 oz)	45	2	tr	12	38	tr

FOOD	PORTION	CALS	CALCI	IRON	POTAS	SOB	ZINC
chocolate chip mix	1 (0.56 oz)	79	7	tr	34	47	tr
chocolate chip refrigerated dough baked	1 (0.42 oz)	59	3	tr	24	28	tr
chocolate chip refrigerated dough unbaked	1 oz	126	7	1	51	59	tr
chocolate chip soft-type	1 (0.5 oz)	69	2	tr	14	49	tr
chocolate w/ creme filling	1 (0.35 oz)	47	3	tr	18	36	tr
chocolate w/ creme filling chocolate coated	1 (0.60 oz)	82	6	1	41	55	tr
chocolate w/ extra creme filling	1 (0.46 oz)	65	3	tr	16	64	tr
chocolate wafer	1 (0.2 oz)	26	2	tr	13	35	tr
cream cheese	1 (1.1 oz)	141	12	1	24	53	tr
fig bars	1 (0.56 oz)	56	10	tr	33	56	tr
finikia	1 (1.2 oz)	171	8	1	26	26	tr
fortune	1 (0.28 oz)	30	1	tr	3	22	tr
fudge	1 (0.73 oz)	73	7	1	29	40	tr
gingersnaps	1 (0.24 oz)	29	5	tr	24	48	tr
graham	1 squares (0.24 oz)	30	2	tr	9	42	tr
graham chocolate covered	1 (0.49 oz)	68	8	1	29	41	tr
graham honey	1 (0.24 oz)	30	2	tr	9	42	tr
hermits	1 (1 oz)	117	16	1	76	54	tr
jumbles coconut	1 (1 oz)	121	5	tr	31	19	tr
koulourakia butter cookie twist	1 (0.9 oz)	113	15	1	16	59	tr
ladyfingers	1 (0.38 oz)	40	5	tr	12	16	tr
macaroons	1 (0.8 oz)	97	12	tr	38	59	tr
madeleines	1 (0.8 oz)	86	7	tr	17	34	tr
marshmallow chocolate coated	1 (0.46 oz)	55	6	tr	24	22	tr
marshmallow pie chocolate coated	1 (1.4 oz)	165	18	1	72	66	tr

FOOD	PORTION	CALS	CALCI	IRON	POTAS	SOD	ZINC
molasses	1 (0.5 oz)	65	11	1	52	69	tr
neapolitan tri-color cookie	1 (0.6 oz)	79	12	tr	36	10	tr
oatmeal	1 (0.6 oz)	81	7	tr	26	69	tr
oatmeal mix	1 (0.6 oz)	74	5	tr	30	75	tr
oatmeal refrigerated dough baked	1 (0.4 oz)	56	4	tr	20	39	tr
oatmeal soft-type	1 (0.5 oz)	61	13	tr	20	52	tr
oatmeal raisin	1 (0.6 oz)	81	7	tr	26	69	tr
oatmeal raisin mix	1 (0.6 oz)	74	5	tr	30	75	tr
oatmeal raisin refrigerated dough baked	1 (0.4 oz)	56	4	tr	20	39	tr
oatmeal raisin soft-type	1 (0.5 oz)	61	13	tr	20	52	tr
peanut butter refrigerated dough baked	1 (0.4 oz)	60	13	tr	41	52	tr
peanut butter refrigerated dough unbaked	1 oz	130	29	tr	87	112	tr
peanut butter sandwich	1 (0.5 oz)	67	7	tr	27	52	tr
peanut butter soft-type	1 (0.5 oz)	69	2	tr	16	50	tr
pinenut cookies	1 (1.1 oz)	134	29	1	130	11	1
raisin soft-type	1 (0.5 oz)	60	7	tr	21	51	tr
reginette queen's biscuit	1 (0.8 oz)	86	27	1	32	83	tr
shortbread	1 (0.28 oz)	40	3	tr	8	36	tr
shortbread pecan	1 (0.49 oz)	79	4	tr	10	39	tr
spritz	1 (0.4 oz)	42	4	tr	11	9	tr
sugar	1 (0.52 oz)	72	3	tr	9	53	tr
sugar refrigerated dough	1 (0.42 oz)	58	11	tr	20	56	tr
sugar refrigerated dough unbaked	1 oz	124	23	tr	42	120	tr
sugar wafers w/ creme filling	1 (0.12 oz)	18	1	tr	2	5	tr

FOOD	PORTION	CALS	CALCI	IRON	POTAS	SOD	ZINC
sugar wafers w/ creme filling sugar free sodium free	1 (0.14 oz)	20	2	tr	2	0	tr
toll house original	1 (0.8 oz)	105	15	1	57	57	tr
vanilla sandwich	1 (0.35 oz)	48	3	tr	9	35	tr
vanilla wafers	1 (0.21 oz)	28	2	tr	6	18	tr
zeppole	1 (0.8 oz)	78	3	tr	9	14	tr
Golden Grahams Treats							
Chocolate Chunk	1 bar (0.8 oz)	90	0	2	25	110	2
Honey Graham	1 bar (0.8 oz)	90	0	2	25	120	2
King Size Chocolate Chunk	1 bar (1.6 oz)	190	0	5	50	220	4
King Size Honey Graham	1 bar (1.6 oz)	180	0	5	45	240	4
Otis Spunkmeyer							
Butter Sugar	1 (2 oz)	250	0	1	–	210	tr
Butter Sugar	1 med (1.3 oz)	160	0	1	0	140	0
Chocolate Chip	1 med (1.3 oz)	170	0	1	0	120	0
Chocolate Chip	1 (2 oz)	250	20	1	–	210	tr
Chocolate Chip	1 bite size (0.75 oz)	100	0	1	–	70	0
Chocolate Chip Pecan	1 med (1.3 oz)	170	0	1	0	110	tr
Chocolate Chip Walnut	1 med (1.3 oz)	180	0	1	0	105	tr
Chocolate Chip Walnut	1 (2 oz)	270	20	1	–	160	1
Chocolate Chip Walnut	1 bite size (0.75 oz)	100	0	1	–	60	tr
Double Chocolate Chip	1 med (1.3 oz)	180	0	1	–	130	tr
Double Chocolate Chip	1 bite size (0.75 oz)	100	0	1	–	75	tr
Oatmeal Raisin	1 med (1.3 oz)	160	0	1	–	130	tr
Oatmeal Raisin	1 bite size (0.75 oz)	90	0	tr	–	75	tr

FOOD	PORTION	CALS	CALCI	IRON	POTAS	SOD	ZINC
Otis Express Double Chocolate Chip	1 (2 oz)	270	20	2	–	200	1
Otis Express Oatmeal Raisin	1 (2 oz)	240	20	2	–	200	1
Otis Express Peanut Butter	1 (2 oz)	270	20	2	–	250	1
Peanut Butter	1 med (1.3 oz)	180	0	1	–	160	tr
White Chocolate Macadamia Nut	1 (2 oz)	280	20	1	–	170	tr
White Chocolate Macadamia Nut	1 med (1.3 oz)	180	0	1	0	110	0

CORIANDER

FOOD	PORTION	CALS	CALCI	IRON	POTAS	SOD	ZINC
seed	1 tsp	5	13	tr	23	1	tr

CORN

FOOD	PORTION	CALS	CALCI	IRON	POTAS	SOD	ZINC
cream style canned	½ cup	93	4	tr	172	365	1
fresh white cooked	½ cup	89	2	1	204	14	tr
fresh white raw	½ cup	66	2	tr	208	12	tr
fresh yellow cooked	1 ear (2.7 oz)	83	2	tr	192	13	tr
fresh yellow cooked	½ cup	89	2	1	204	14	tr
fresh yellow raw	½ cup	66	2	tr	208	12	tr
fresh yellow raw	1 ear (3 oz)	77	2	tr	243	14	tr
fritters	1 (1 oz)	62	21	tr	47	126	tr
frozen cooked	½ cup	67	2	tr	114	4	tr
frozen on-the-cob cooked	1 ear (2.2 oz)	59	2	tr	158	3	tr
on-the-cob w/ butter cooked	1 ear	155	5	tr	360	30	tr
scalloped	½ cup	258	64	1	162	246	1
w/ red & green peppers canned	½ cup	86	5	1	174	396	tr

CORNMEAL

FOOD	PORTION	CALS	CALCI	IRON	POTAS	SOD	ZINC
corn grits cooked	1 cup	146	1	2	54	0	tr
corn grits uncooked	1 cup	579	3	6	213	1	tr
hush puppies	1 (0.75 oz)	74	61	1	32	147	tr
white	1 cup (4.8 oz)	505	7	6	224	4	1

FOOD	PORTION	CALS	CALCI	IRON	POTAS	SOD	ZINC
whole grain	1 cup (4.3 oz)	442	7	4	350	43	2
yellow	1 cup (4.8 oz)	505	7	6	224	4	1
yellow self-rising	1 cup (4.3 oz)	407	440	7	311	1521	2
Aunt Jemima							
Yellow	3 tbsp	102	1	1	51	1	0
Quaker							
Yellow	3 tbsp	102	1	1	51	1	0

CORNSTARCH

FOOD	PORTION	CALS	CALCI	IRON	POTAS	SOD	ZINC
cornstarch	1 cup (4.5 oz)	488	3	1	4	12	tr

COTTAGE CHEESE

FOOD	PORTION	CALS	CALCI	IRON	POTAS	SOD	ZINC
creamed	4 oz	117	68	tr	95	457	tr
creamed	1 cup (7.4 oz)	217	126	tr	177	850	1
creamed w/ fruit	4 oz	140	54	tr	76	457	tr
dry curd	1 cup (5.1 oz)	123	46	tr	47	19	1
dry curd	4 oz	96	36	tr	37	14	1
lowfat 1%	1 cup (7.9 oz)	164	138	tr	193	918	86
lowfat 1%	4 oz	82	69	tr	97	459	tr
lowfat 2%	1 cup (7.9 oz)	203	155	tr	217	918	1
lowfat 2%	4 oz	101	77	tr	109	459	tr

COTTONSEED

FOOD	PORTION	CALS	CALCI	IRON	POTAS	SOD	ZINC
kernels roasted	1 tbsp	51	10	1	135	3	1

COUSCOUS

FOOD	PORTION	CALS	CALCI	IRON	POTAS	SOD	ZINC
cooked	1 cup (5.5 oz)	176	13	1	91	8	tr
dry	1 cup (6.1 oz)	650	42	2	287	17	1

COWPEAS

FOOD	PORTION	CALS	CALCI	IRON	POTAS	SOD	ZINC
catjang dried cooked	1 cup (2.9 oz)	200	44	5	641	32	3
common canned	1 cup	184	48	2	413	718	2
frozen cooked	½ cup	112	20	2	319	5	1

CRAB

FOOD	PORTION	CALS	CALCI	IRON	POTAS	SOD	ZINC
alaska king cooked	1 leg (4.7 oz)	129	80	1	350	1436	10
alaska king cooked	3 oz	82	50	1	222	911	6
alaska king raw	3 oz	71	39	1	173	711	5
alaska king raw	1 leg (6 oz)	144	80	1	351	1438	10
baked	1 (3.8 oz)	160	415	1	598	550	7
blue cooked	3 oz	87	88	1	275	237	4
blue cooked	1 cup	138	140	1	437	376	6

FOOD	PORTION	CALS	CALCI	IRON	POTAS	SOD	ZINC
blue raw	1 crab (7 oz)	18	19	tr	69	62	1
blue raw	3 oz	74	76	1	280	249	3
cake	1 (2 oz)	160	202	1	162	492	2
canned blue	3 oz	84	86	1	318	283	3
dungeness raw	3 oz	73	39	tr	301	251	4
dungeness raw	1 crab (5.7 oz)	140	75	1	577	481	7
soft-shell fried	1 (4.4 oz)	334	55	2	163	1118	1

CRACKER CRUMBS

FOOD	PORTION	CALS	CALCI	IRON	POTAS	SOD	ZINC
chocolate wafer cookie crumbs	½ cup (5.9 oz)	728	56	7	364	980	2
cracker meal	1 cup (4 oz)	440	27	5	132	32	1
graham cracker crumbs	½ cup (4.4 oz)	540	36	5	162	756	1

CRACKERS

FOOD	PORTION	CALS	CALCI	IRON	POTAS	SOD	ZINC
cheese	1 (1 in sq) (1 g)	5	2	tr	1	10	tr
cheese	14 (½ oz)	71	21	1	21	141	tr
cheese low sodium	1 (1 in sq) (1 g)	5	2	tr	1	5	tr
cheese low sodium	14 (½ oz)	71	21	1	15	68	tr
cheese w/ peanut butter filling	1 (0.24 oz)	34	6	tr	17	69	tr
crispbread rye	1 (0.35 oz)	37	3	tr	32	26	tr
melba toast plain	1 (5 g)	19	5	tr	10	41	tr
melba toast pumpernickel	1 (5 g)	19	4	tr	10	45	tr
melba toast rye	1 (5 g)	19	4	tr	10	45	tr
melba toast wheat	1 (5 g)	19	2	tr	7	42	tr
milk	1 (0.42 oz)	55	21	tr	14	71	tr
oyster cracker	1 (1 g)	4	1	tr	1	13	tr
peanut butter sandwich	1 (7 g)	34	7	tr	16	66	tr
rusk toast	1 (0.35 oz)	41	3	tr	25	25	tr
rye w/ cheese filling	1 (0.24 oz)	34	16	tr	24	73	tr
rye wafers plain	1 (0.9 oz)	84	10	1	124	199	1
rye wafers seasoned	1 (0.8 oz)	84	10	1	100	195	1

FOOD	PORTION	CALS	CALCI	IRON	POTAS	SOD	ZINC
saltines	1 (3 g)	13	4	tr	4	38	tr
saltines fat free low sodium	6 (1 oz)	118	7	2	34	191	tr
saltines fat free low sodium	3 (0.5 oz)	59	3	1	17	95	tr
saltines low salt	1 (3 g)	13	4	tr	22	19	tr
snack cracker	1 (3 g)	15	4	tr	4	25	tr
snack cracker low salt	1 (3 g)	15	4	tr	11	11	tr
snack cracker w/ cheese filling	1 (7 g)	33	18	tr	30	98	tr
soup cracker	1 (1 g)	4	1	tr	1	13	tr
wheat w/ cheese filling	1 (0.24 oz)	35	14	tr	21	64	tr
wheat w/ peanut butter filling	1 (0.24 oz)	35	12	tr	21	57	tr
wheat thins	1 (2 g)	9	1	tr	4	16	tr
wheat thins	7 (0.5 oz)	67	7	1	26	113	tr
wheat thins low salt	7 (0.5 oz)	67	7	1	28	40	tr
whole wheat	1 (4 g)	18	2	tr	12	26	tr
whole wheat low salt	1 (4 g)	18	2	tr	12	10	tr
Eden							
Nori Nori Rice	15 (1 oz)	110	40	tr	25	160	0

CRANBERRIES

FOOD	PORTION	CALS	CALCI	IRON	POTAS	SOD	ZINC
cranberry sauce sweetened	½ cup	209	5	tr	35	40	tr
fresh chopped	1 cup	54	8	tr	78	1	tr

CRANBERRY BEANS

FOOD	PORTION	CALS	CALCI	IRON	POTAS	SOD	ZINC
canned	1 cup	216	67	4	675	863	2
dried cooked	1 cup	240	44	4	685	1	2

CRANBERRY JUICE

FOOD	PORTION	CALS	CALCI	IRON	POTAS	SOD	ZINC
cocktail	1 cup	147	8	tr	61	10	tr
cranberry juice cocktail low calorie	6 oz	33	16	tr	39	6	tr

FOOD	PORTION	CALS	CALCI	IRON	POTAS	SOD	ZINC
cranberry juice cocktail frzn as prep	6 oz	102	9	tr	27	6	tr
CRAYFISH							
cooked	3 oz	97	26	3	298	58	1
raw	3 oz	76	20	2	233	45	1
raw	8	24	6	1	74	14	tr
CREAM							
clotted cream	2 tbsp (1 oz)	164	10	tr	15	18	tr
half & half	1 tbsp (0.5 oz)	20	16	tr	19	6	tr
half & half	1 cup (8.5 oz)	315	254	tr	314	98	1
heavy whipping	1 tbsp (0.5 oz)	52	10	tr	11	6	tr
heavy whipping whipped	1 cup (4.1 oz)	411	77	tr	179	89	1
light coffee	1 cup (8.4 oz)	496	14	tr	292	95	1
light coffee	1 tbsp (0.5 oz)	29	14	tr	18	6	tr
light whipping	1 tbsp (0.5 oz)	44	10	tr	15	5	tr
light whipping cream whipped	1 cup (4.2 oz)	345	83	tr	231	82	1
CREAM CHEESE							
cream cheese	1 oz	99	23	tr	34	84	tr
cream cheese	1 pkg (3 oz)	297	68	1	101	251	tr
Breakstone's							
Temp-Tee Whipped	2 tbsp (0.8 oz)	80	0	0	25	70	0
Philadelphia							
Free	1 oz	30	80	0	60	140	1
Regular	1 oz	100	0	0	25	90	0
Soft	2 tbsp (1 oz)	100	20	0	40	100	0
Soft Apple Cinnamon	2 tbsp (1.1 oz)	100	20	0	40	100	0
Soft Cheesecake	2 tbsp (1 oz)	110	20	0	35	95	0
Soft Chives & Onions	2 tbsp (1.1 oz)	110	40	0	60	135	0
Soft Garden Vegetable	2 tbsp (1.1 oz)	110	20	0	35	170	0

FOOD	PORTION	CALS	CALCI	IRON	POTAS	SOD	ZINC
Soft Honey Nut	2 tbsp (1.1 oz)	110	20	0	35	150	0
Soft Pineapple	2 tbsp (1.1 oz)	100	40	0	60	100	0
Soft Salmon	3 tbsp (1.1 oz)	100	20	0	45	200	0
Soft Strawberry	2 tbsp (1.1 oz)	100	40	0	55	100	0
Soft Free	2 tbsp (1.2 oz)	30	150	0	75	200	1
Soft Free Garden Vegetable	2 tbsp (1.2 oz)	30	150	0	80	220	1
Soft Free Strawberries	2 tbsp (1.2 oz)	45	100	0	70	180	1
Soft Light	2 tbsp (1.1 oz)	70	40	0	55	150	0
Soft Light Jalapeno	2 tbsp (1.1 oz)	60	40	0	55	210	0
Soft Light Raspberry	2 tbsp (1.1 oz)	70	40	0	50	125	0
Soft Light Roasted Garlic	2 tbsp (1.1 oz)	70	40	0	550	180	0
Whipped	2 tbsp (0.7 oz)	70	0	0	25	85	0
Whipped Chives	2 tbsp (0.7 oz)	70	20	0	30	130	0
Whipped Smoked Salmon	2 tbsp (0.7 oz)	70	20	0	35	140	0
With Chives	1 oz	90	0	0	25	135	0

CREAM OF TARTAR

FOOD	PORTION	CALS	CALCI	IRON	POTAS	SOD	ZINC
cream of tartar	1 tsp	8	0	tr	495	2	tr

CROAKER

FOOD	PORTION	CALS	CALCI	IRON	POTAS	SOD	ZINC
atlantic breaded & fried	3 oz	188	27	1	289	296	tr
atlantic raw	3 oz	89	13	tr	293	47	tr

CROISSANT

FOOD	PORTION	CALS	CALCI	IRON	POTAS	SOD	ZINC
apple	1 (2 oz)	145	17	1	51	156	1
cheese	1 (2 oz)	236	30	1	76	316	1
plain	1 (2 oz)	232	21	1	67	424	tr
plain	1 mini (1 oz)	115	10	1	34	211	tr
w/ egg & cheese	1 (4.5 oz)	368	244	2	174	551	2
w/ egg cheese & bacon	1 (4.5 oz)	413	151	2	201	889	2
w/ egg cheese & ham	1 (5.3 oz)	474	144	2	272	1081	2
w/ egg cheese & sausage	1 (5.6 oz)	523	144	3	283	1115	2

FOOD	PORTION	CALS	CALCI	IRON	POTAS	SOD	ZINC
CROUTONS							
plain	1 cup (1 oz)	122	23	1	37	209	tr
seasoned	1 cup (1.4 oz)	186	38	1	72	495	tr
CUCUMBER							
fresh raw	1 (11 oz)	38	43	1	434	6	1
fresh raw sliced	½ cup (1.8 oz)	7	7	tr	76	1	tr
kimchee	½ cup (1.8 oz)	36	10	tr	79	173	tr
tzatziki	½ cup (3.4 oz)	72	59	tr	146	197	tr
CUMIN							
seed	1 tsp	8	20	1	38	4	tr
CURRANTS							
black fresh	½ cup	36	31	1	180	1	tr
zante dried	½ cup	204	62	2	642	6	tr
CUSK							
fillet baked	3 oz	106	12	1	477	38	tr
CUSTARD							
baked ready-to-eat	½ cup (5 oz)	148	158	tr	216	109	1
flan mix as prep w/ 2% milk	½ cup (4.7 oz)	135	153	tr	194	68	tr
flan mix as prep w/ whole milk	½ cup (4.7 oz)	150	150	tr	191	65	tr
mix as prep w/ 2 % milk	½ cup (4.7 oz)	148	197	tr	287	200	1
zabaione	½ cup (57.2 g)	135	23	1	16	9	1
CUTTLEFISH							
steamed	3 oz	134	153	9	542	632	3
DANISH PASTRY							
almond	1 (4¼ in) (2.3 oz)	280	61	1	62	236	1
apple	1 (4¼ in) (2.5 oz)	264	33	1	59	251	tr
cheese	1 (3.2 oz)	353	70	2	116	319	1
cinnamon	1 (3.1 oz)	349	37	2	96	326	tr

FOOD	PORTION	CALS	CALCI	IRON	POTAS	SOD	ZINC
cinnamon	1 (4¼ in) (2.3 oz)	262	46	1	81	241	tr
cinnamon nut	1 (4¼ in) (2.3 oz)	280	61	1	62	236	1
fruit	1 (3.3 oz)	335	22	1	110	333	tr
lemon	1 (4¼ in) (2.5 oz)	264	33	1	59	251	tr
raisin	1 (4¼ in) (2.5 oz)	264	33	1	59	251	tr
raisin nut	1 (4¼ in) (2.3 oz)	280	61	1	62	236	1
raspberry	1 (4¼ in) (2.5 oz)	264	33	1	59	251	tr
strawberry	1 (4¼ in) (2.5 oz)	264	33	1	59	251	tr

DATES

FOOD	PORTION	CALS	CALCI	IRON	POTAS	SOD	ZINC
dried chopped	1 cup	489	58	2	1161	5	1
dried whole	10	228	27	1	541	2	tr
jujube dried	1 oz	75	18	1	149	2	tr
California Redi-Date							
Deglet Noor Dried	5–6 (1.4 oz)	120	20	tr	240	0	0

DELI MEATS/COLD CUTS

FOOD	PORTION	CALS	CALCI	IRON	POTAS	SOD	ZINC
barbecue loaf pork & beef	1 oz	49	13	tr	93	378	1
beerwurst beef	1 slice	75	2	tr	42	214	1
beerwurst pork	1 slice	55	2	tr	58	285	tr
berliner pork & beef	1 oz	65	3	tr	80	368	1
bologna beef	1 oz	88	3	tr	44	278	1
bologna beef & pork	1 oz	89	3	tr	51	289	1
bologna pork	1 oz	70	3	tr	80	336	1
braunschweiger pork	1 oz	102	2	3	57	324	1
corned beef loaf	1 oz	43	3	1	29	270	1
dutch brand loaf pork & beef	1 oz	68	24	tr	107	354	tr
headcheese pork	1 oz	60	5	tr	9	356	tr

FOOD	PORTION	CALS	CALCI	IRON	POTAS	SOD	ZINC
honey loaf pork & beef	1 oz	36	5	tr	97	374	1
honey roll sausage beef	1 oz	42	2	1	67	304	1
lebanon bologna beef	1 oz	60	4	1	85	379	1
liver cheese pork	1 oz	86	2	3	64	347	1
luncheon meat beef	1 oz	87	3	1	59	377	1
luncheon meat pork & beef	1 oz	100	5	tr	57	367	tr
luncheon meat pork canned	1 oz	95	2	tr	61	365	tr
luncheon sausage pork & beef	1 oz	74	3	tr	70	335	1
luxury loaf pork	1 oz	40	10	tr	107	347	1
mortadella beef & pork	1 oz	88	5	tr	46	353	1
mother's loaf pork	1 oz	80	12	tr	64	320	tr
new england sausage pork & beef	1 oz	46	2	tr	91	346	1
olive loaf pork	1 oz	67	31	tr	84	421	tr
peppered loaf pork & beef	1 oz	42	15	tr	112	432	1
pepperoni pork & beef	1 slice (0.2 oz)	27	1	tr	19	112	tr
pepperoni pork & beef	1 (9 oz)	1248	25	4	871	5120	6
pickle & pimiento loaf pork	1 oz	74	27	tr	96	394	tr
picnic loaf pork & beef	1 oz	66	13	tr	76	330	1
salami cooked beef & pork	1 oz	71	4	1	56	302	1
salami hard pork	1 slice (⅓ oz)	41	1	tr	—	226	tr
salami hard pork	1 pkg (4 oz)	460	15	1	—	2554	5

FOOD	PORTION	CALS	CALCI	IRON	POTAS	SOD	ZINC
salami hard pork & beef	1 pkg (4 oz)	472	8	2	427	2101	4
salami hard pork & beef	1 slice (0.3 oz)	42	1	tr	38	186	tr
sandwich spread pork & beef	1 tbsp	35	2	tr	16	152	tr
sandwich spread pork & beef	1 oz	67	3	tr	31	287	tr
summer sausage thuringer cervelat	1 oz	98	2	1	65	412	1

DILL

FOOD	PORTION	CALS	CALCI	IRON	POTAS	SOD	ZINC
seed	1 tsp	6	32	tr	25	tr	tr
weed dry	1 tsp	3	18	tr	33	2	tr

DIP
Cheez Whiz

FOOD	PORTION	CALS	CALCI	IRON	POTAS	SOD	ZINC
Medium Cheese & Salsa	2 tbsp (1.2 oz)	100	80	0	95	490	tr
Mild Cheese & Salsa	2 tbsp (1.2 oz)	100	80	0	95	490	tr

DOUGHNUTS

FOOD	PORTION	CALS	CALCI	IRON	POTAS	SOD	ZINC
cake type unsugared	1 (1.6 oz)	198	21	1	60	257	tr
chocolate glazed	1 (1.5 oz)	175	89	1	—	143	tr
chocolate sugared	1 (1.5 oz)	175	89	1	—	143	tr
chocolate coated	1 (1.5 oz)	204	15	1	—	185	tr
creme filled	1 (3 oz)	307	22	2	68	262	1
frosted	1 (1.5 oz)	204	15	1	—	185	tr
honey bun	1 (2.1 oz)	242	26	1	65	205	tr
jelly	1 (3 oz)	289	21	2	67	249	1
old fashioned	1 (1.6 oz)	198	21	1	60	257	tr
sugared	1 (1.6 oz)	192	27	tr	46	181	tr
wheat glazed	1 (1.6 oz)	162	22	1	66	160	tr
wheat sugared	1 (1.6 oz)	162	22	1	66	160	tr
yeast glazed	1 (2.1 oz)	242	26	1	65	205	tr

DRINK MIXERS

FOOD	PORTION	CALS	CALCI	IRON	POTAS	SOD	ZINC
whiskey sour mix	2 oz	55	1	tr	18	66	tr

FOOD	PORTION	CALS	CALCI	IRON	POTAS	SOD	ZINC
DRUM							
freshwater fillet baked	5.4 oz	236	118	2	543	148	1
freshwater baked	3 oz	130	65	1	300	82	1
DUCK							
w/ skin roasted	1 cup (4.9 oz)	472	15	4	286	83	3
w/o skin roasted	1 cup (4.9 oz)	281	17	4	353	91	4
wild w/ skin raw	½ duck (9.5 oz)	571	12	11	672	152	2
wild w/o skin breast raw	½ breast (2.9 oz)	102	3	4	222	47	1
EEL							
fresh cooked	1 fillet (5.6 oz)	375	41	1	555	104	3
fresh cooked	3 oz	200	22	1	297	55	2
raw	3 oz	156	17	tr	232	43	1
EGG							
duck	1 (2.5 oz)	130	45	3	156	102	1
duck 100 year old	1 (1 oz)	49	18	1	43	154	tr
duck salted	1 (1 oz)	54	34	1	52	769	tr
fresh	1	75	25	1	60	63	1
frozen	1	75	25	1	60	63	1
frozen	1 cup	363	120	4	293	307	3
hard cooked	1	77	25	1	63	62	1
hard cooked chopped	1 cup	210	68	2	172	169	1
poached	1	74	25	1	60	140	1
white only	1	17	2	tr	48	55	0
white only	1 cup	121	15	tr	346	399	tr
EGG DISHES							
deviled	2 halves	145	31	1	70	180	1
salad	½ cup	307	189	2	140	565	2
scrambled plain	2 (3.3 oz)	199	54	2	138	211	2
scrambled w/ whole milk & margarine	1 serv	365	157	3	304	616	2
sunny side up	1	91	25	1	61	162	1

FOOD	PORTION	CALS	CALCI	IRON	POTAS	SOD	ZINC
EGG ROLLS							
egg roll wrapper fresh	1	83	13	1	23	162	tr
EGG SUBSTITUTES							
frozen	¼ cup	96	44	1	128	120	1
frozen	1 cup	384	175	5	512	479	2
liquid	1 cup (8.8 oz)	211	133	5	828	444	3
liquid	1½ oz	40	25	1	155	83	1
Second Nature							
No Cholesterol	2 fl oz	60	40	1	—	90	1
No Fat	2 fl oz	40	40	1	—	100	1
No Fat With Garden Vegetables	2.5 fl oz	40	40	1	—	100	1
EGGNOG							
eggnog	1 cup	342	330	1	420	138	1
eggnog	1 qt	1368	1321	2	1678	553	5
eggnog flavor mix as prep w/ milk	9 oz	260	291	tr	369	163	1
EGGPLANT							
cubed cooked	1 cup	28	6	tr	246	3	tr
iman bayildi eggplant w/ onion & tomato	1 serv (15.6 oz)	345	43	2	773	552	1
indian eggplant runi	1 serv	180	30	1	527	228	tr
papoutsakis little shoes	1 serv (15.5 oz)	245	144	2	669	751	2
raw cut up	½ cup (1.4 oz)	11	3	tr	89	1	tr
whole peeled raw	1 (1 lb)	117	34	1	992	14	1
ELK							
roasted	3 oz	124	4	3	279	52	3
EMU							
cooked	3 oz	130	6	6	270	97	4
ENDIVE							
fresh	3.5 oz	9	54	1	346	53	tr
raw chopped	½ cup	4	13	tr	79	6	tr

ENERGY BARS

FOOD	PORTION	CALS	CALCI	IRON	POTAS	SOD	ZINC
Back To Nature							
10th Tee Chocolate Fudge	1 bar	200	40	tr	—	40	tr
1st Tee Chocolate Peanut	1 bar	290	150	2	—	105	tr
1st Tee Oatmeal Raisin	1 bar	280	200	2	—	150	tr
Balance							
Oasis Strawberry Cheesecake	1 bar (1.69 oz)	180	350	6	240	250	5
BeneFit							
Nutrition Bar	1 bar (2 oz)	240	200	6	125	190	5
Better Bar							
Chocolate Coated Caramel Pecan	1 bar (1.8 oz)	180	200	4	30	35	3
Chocolate Coated Peanut	1 bar (1.8 oz)	180	200	4	30	35	3
Yogurt Coated Raspberry	1 bar (1.8 oz)	180	200	4	30	35	3
Breakthru							
Organic Chocolate Fudge	1 bar (2.1 oz)	230	300	5	210	120	4
Organic Cinnamon Crunch	1 bar (2.1 oz)	220	300	5	210	160	4
Organic Honey Graham	1 bar (2.1 oz)	220	300	5	210	160	4
Organic Mocha Fudge	1 bar (2.1 oz)	230	300	5	210	120	4
Centrum							
Energy Chocolate Nougat	1 (1.98 oz)	220	300	5	135	185	6
Energy Chocolate Peanut Butter	1 (1.98 oz)	220	300	5	135	185	6
Clif Bar							
Apricot	1 bar (2.4 oz)	220	300	5	280	90	3
Carrot Cake	1 bar (2.4 oz)	240	250	5	250	150	3
Chocolate Brownie	1 bar (2.4 oz)	240	250	5	260	150	4
Chocolate Almond Fudge	1 bar (2.4 oz)	230	300	5	230	140	4

FOOD	PORTION	CALS	CALCI	IRON	POTAS	SOD	ZINC
Chocolate Chip	1 bar (2.4 oz)	240	250	5	200	170	4
Chocolate Chip Peanut Crunch	1 bar (2.4 oz)	240	250	5	300	290	3
Cookies 'N Cream	1 bar (2.4 oz)	230	300	5	210	180	3
Cranberry Apple Cherry	1 bar (2.4 oz)	220	250	5	240	135	3
Crunchy Peanut Butter	1 bar (2.4 oz)	240	250	5	300	290	5
GingerSnap	1 bar (2.4 oz)	230	300	6	400	140	4
DrSoy							
Double Chocolate	1 bar (1.76 oz)	180	350	18	80	170	15
GeniSoy							
Soy Protein Artic Frost Crispy Chocolate Mint	1 bar (2.2 oz)	230	250	5	290	150	4
Soy Protein Dutch Crunch Sour Apple Crisp	1 bar (2.2 oz)	230	250	5	160	160	4
Soy Protein Fair Trade Arabica Cafe Mocha Fudge	1 bar (2.2 oz)	220	250	5	200	150	4
Soy Protein New York Style Blueberry Cheesecake	1 bar (2.2 oz)	220	250	5	130	160	4
Soy Protein Obsession Fudge Cookies & Cream	1 bar (2.2 oz)	230	250	5	170	250	4
Soy Protein Pure Golden Honey Creamy Peanut Yogurt	1 bar (2.2 oz)	230	250	5	200	160	4
Soy Protein Southern Style Chunky Peanut Butter Fudge	1 bar (2.2 oz)	240	250	5	270	130	4

FOOD	PORTION	CALS	CALCI	IRON	POTAS	SOD	ZINC
Soy Protein UltimateChocolate Fudge Brownie	1 bar (2.2 oz)	230	250	5	250	210	4
Xtreme Carrot Cake Quake	1 bar (1.6 oz)	190	150	5	150	90	4
Xtreme Peanut Butter Fix	1 bar (1.6 oz)	200	200	5	190	190	4
Xtreme Raspberry Rush	1 bar (1.6 oz)	190	100	5	190	90	4
Xtreme Rocky Roadtrip	1 bar (1.6 oz)	190	150	5	180	130	4
Jenny Craig							
Meal Bar Chocolate Peanut	1 bar (2 oz)	220	300	4	170	240	3
Meal Bar Lemon Meringue	1 bar (2 oz)	210	300	4	60	130	3
Meal Bar Milk Chocolate	1 bar (2 oz)	210	300	4	200	180	3
Meal Bar Oatmeal Raisin	1 bar (1.97 oz)	210	300	4	80	75	3
Meal Bar Yogurt Peanut	1 bar (2 oz)	220	300	4	170	270	3
Lean Body For Her							
Chocolate Honey Peanut	1 bar (1.76 oz)	190	250	7	150	135	3
Luna							
Chai Tea	1 bar (1.7 oz)	180	350	6	115	125	5
Chocolate Pecan Pie	1 bar (1.7 oz)	180	350	6	105	125	5
LemonZest	1 bar (1.7 oz)	180	350	6	90	50	5
Nutz Over Chocolate	1 bar (1.7 oz)	180	350	6	105	100	5
S'Mores	1 bar (1.7 oz)	180	350	6	125	125	5
Sesame Raisin Crunch	1 bar (1.7 oz)	170	350	6	130	125	5
Toasted Nuts 'n Cranberry	1 bar (1.7 oz)	170	350	6	100	130	5
Tropical Crisp	1 bar (1.7 oz)	180	350	6	120	135	5

FOOD	PORTION	CALS	CALCI	IRON	POTAS	SOD	ZINC
Met-Rx							
Big 100 Gram Bar Peanut Butter	1 bar (3.5 oz)	340	700	9	—	135	6
Source/One Chocolate Cheesecake	1 bar (2.1 oz)	160	600	7	400	50	5
Nutribar							
Chocolate Covered Belgian Chocolate	1 bar (2.3 oz)	252	350	6	375	255	5
Chocolate Covered Caramel	1 bar (2.3 oz)	261	350	6	375	280	5
Chocolate Covered Chocolate Fudge	1 bar (2.3 oz)	267	350	6	380	300	5
Chocolate Covered Hazelnut	1 bar (2.3 oz)	261	350	6	400	295	5
Chocolate Covered Mocha Almond	1 bar (2.3 oz)	261	350	6	375	280	5
Chocolate Covered Peanut	1 bar (2.3 oz)	262	350	6	375	255	5
Yogurt Covered Peach Apricot	1 bar (2.3 oz)	261	350	6	375	260	5
Yogurt Covered Raspberry	1 bar (2.3 oz)	261	350	6	375	260	5
Yogurt Covered Wildberry	1 bar (2.3 oz)	261	350	6	375	260	5
PermaLean							
Protein Crunch Chocoholic Chocolate	1 bar (1.8 oz)	170	200	tr	100	65	15
Protein Crunch Chocolate Raspberry	1 bar (1.8 oz)	180	200	tr	90	35	15
Protein Crunch Stark Raving Peanutz	1 bar (1.8 oz)	180	200	tr	80	75	15
PowerBar							
Apple Cinnamon	1 bar (2.3 oz)	230	300	6	110	90	5
Banana	1 bar (2.3 oz)	230	300	6	200	90	5
Chocolate	1 bar (2.3 oz)	230	300	6	145	90	5
Essentials Chocolate	1 bar (1.9 oz)	180	500	5	—	105	4

FOOD	PORTION	CALS	CALCI	IRON	POTAS	SOD	ZINC
Harvest Blueberry	1 bar (2.3 oz)	240	150	3	–	80	2
Malt-Nut	1 bar (2.3 oz)	230	300	6	110	90	5
Mocha	1 bar (2.3 oz)	230	300	6	145	90	5
Oatmeal Raisin	1 bar (2.3 oz)	230	300	6	180	120	5
Peanut Butter	1 bar (2.3 oz)	230	300	6	150	110	5
Pria Chocolate Honey Graham	1 bar (1 oz)	110	300	4	–	80	2
Pria Chocolate Peanut Crunch	1 bar (1 oz)	110	300	4	–	80	2
Pria Double Chocolate Cookie	1 bar (1 oz)	110	300	4	–	90	2
Pria French Vanilla Crisp	1 bar (1 oz)	110	300	4	–	80	2
Vanilla Crisp	1 bar (2.3 oz)	230	300	6	110	90	5
Wild Berry	1 bar (2.3 oz)	230	300	6	110	90	5
Slim-Fast							
Crispy Peanut Caramel	1 bar	120	150	3	–	80	1
Dutch Chocolate	1 bar	140	40	5	150	80	4
Meal On-The-Go Apple Cobbler	1 bar	220	300	3	125	150	2
Meal On-The-Go Chocolate Cookie Dough	1 bar	220	350	3	90	180	2
Meal On-The-Go Honey Peanut	1 bar	220	300	3	170	160	2
Meal On-The-Go Milk Chocolate Peanut	1 bar	220	300	3	160	120	2
Meal On-The-Go Oatmeal Raisin	1 bar	220	300	3	170	100	2
Meal On-The-Go Rich Chocolate Brownie	1 bar	220	300	3	180	150	2
Meal On-The-Go Toasted Oat & Spice	1 bar	220	300	3	70	140	2
Peanut Butter	1 bar	150	40	5	150	80	4
Peanut Butter Crunch	1 bar	130	150	3	750	80	1

FOOD	PORTION	CALS	CALCI	IRON	POTAS	SOD	ZINC
Sweet Success							
Chewy Chocolate Brownie	1 bar (1.2 oz)	120	150	3	–	35	1
ZonePerfect							
Honey Peanut	1 bar (1.8 oz)	200	400	3	130	150	8
ENERGY DRINKS							
BeneFit							
Chocolate	1 serv	120	300	6	460	200	5
Vanilla	1 serv	120	300	6	400	220	5
Boost							
Chocolate	1 can (8 oz)	240	300	4	400	130	5
Vanilla	8 oz	240	300	4	400	130	5
GeniSoy							
Soy Protein Shake Chocolate	1 scoop (1.2 oz)	120	250	5	230	170	4
Soy Protein Shake Vanilla	1 scoop (1.2 oz)	130	250	5	70	180	4
Soy Protein Shake Strawberry Banana	1 scoop	130	250	5	70	170	4
Healthy Pleasures							
Chocolate Irish Cream	1 bottle (10.5 oz)	260	500	5	480	320	5
Pounds Off							
Dark Chocolate Ectasy	1 can (11 oz)	200	400	3	590	220	4
French Vanilla	1 can (11 oz)	220	400	3	440	460	4
Resource							
Fruit Beverage	1 pkg (8 oz)	180	135	2	15	55	4
Slim-Fast							
Chocolate as prep w/ fat free milk	1 serv	190	450	6	660	240	5
Chocolate Malt as prep w/ fat free milk	1 serv	190	450	6	650	250	5
JumpStart Chocolate as prep w/ fat free milk	1 serv	240	400	6	620	280	5

FOOD	PORTION	CALS	CALCI	IRON	POTAS	SOD	ZINC
JumpStart Vanilla as prep w/ fat free milk	1 serv	240	400	6	730	300	5
Strawberry as prep w/ fat free milk	1 serv	190	450	6	610	260	5
Vanilla as prep w/ fat free milk	1 serv	190	450	6	610	260	5
Sustacal							
Vanilla	8 oz	240	240	4	490	220	3
Sweet Success							
Creamy Milk Chocolate	1 can	200	350	5	–	230	4
Creamy Milk Chocolate as prep w/ skim milk	1 serv	180	350	5	–	240	4
ENGLISH MUFFIN							
apple cinnamon	1	138	84	1	119	255	1
plain	1	134	99	1	75	265	tr
plain toasted	1	133	99	1	74	262	tr
raisin cinnamon	1	138	84	1	119	255	1
sourdough	1	134	99	1	75	265	tr
w/ butter	1 (2.2 oz)	189	103	2	69	386	tr
w/ cheese & sausage	1 (4 oz)	393	168	2	215	1036	2
w/ egg cheese & canadian bacon	1 (4.8 oz)	289	151	2	199	729	2
w/ egg cheese & sausage	1 (5.8 oz)	487	196	3	294	1135	2
whole wheat	1	134	175	2	139	420	1
EPAZOTE							
fresh	1 tbsp (1 g)	tr	2	tr	5	tr	tr
fresh sprig	1 (2 g)	1	6	tr	13	1	tr
FALAFEL							
falafel	1 (1.2 oz)	57	9	1	99	50	tr
FAT							
beef cooked	1 oz	193	4	tr	34	12	tr
duck	1 tbsp (13 g)	115	0	0	0	0	0
lamb new zealand	1 oz	182	6	tr	15	6	tr

FOOD	PORTION	CALS	CALCI	IRON	POTAS	SOD	ZINC
pork backfat	1 oz	230	1	tr	–	3	tr
pork cooked	1 oz	178	15	tr	–	10	tr
salt pork	1 oz	212	2	tr	19	404	tr
FEIJOA							
fresh	1 (1.75 oz)	25	8	tr	78	2	tr
puree	1 cup	119	41	tr	378	7	tr
FENNEL							
leaves	1 oz	7	31	1	–	25	tr
seed	1 tsp	7	24	tr	34	2	tr
FENUGREEK							
seed	1 tsp	12	6	1	28	2	tr
FIDDLEHEAD FERNS							
fresh	3.5 oz	34	32	1	370	1	1
FIGS							
canned in heavy syrup	3	75	23	tr	85	1	tr
canned in light syrup	3	58	23	tr	86	1	tr
canned water pack	3	42	22	tr	83	1	tr
dried california	½ cup (3.5 oz)	200	150	3	710	11	1
dried cooked	½ cup	140	79	1	391	6	tr
dried whole	10	477	269	4	1332	20	1
fresh	1 med	50	18	tr	116	1	tr
FIREWEED							
leaves chopped	1 cup (0.8 oz)	24	99	1	114	8	1
FISH							
breaded fillet	1 (2 oz)	155	11	tr	149	332	tr
sticks	1 stick (1 oz)	76	6	tr	73	163	tr
taramasalata	2 tbsp	124	6	tr	16	182	tr
FLOUNDER							
battered & fried	3.2 oz	211	17	2	292	484	tr
breaded & fried	3.2 oz	211	17	2	292	484	tr
cooked	3 oz	99	16	tr	292	89	1
cooked	1 fillet (4.5 oz)	148	23	tr	436	133	1

FOOD	PORTION	CALS	CALCI	IRON	POTAS	SOD	ZINC
FLOUR							
buckwheat whole groat	1 cup (4.2 oz)	402	49	5	692	13	4
corn masa	1 cup (4 oz)	416	161	8	340	6	2
cottonseed lowfat	1 oz	94	135	4	500	10	3
peanut defatted	1 cup	196	84	1	774	108	3
peanut defatted	1 oz	92	39	1	361	50	1
peanut lowfat	1 cup	257	78	3	815	0	4
rice brown	1 cup (5.5 oz)	574	17	3	457	13	4
rice white	1 cup (5.5 oz)	578	16	1	120	1	1
rye dark	1 cup (4.5 oz)	415	72	8	934	2	7
rye light	1 cup (3.6 oz)	374	21	2	238	2	2
rye medium	1 cup (3.6 oz)	361	24	2	347	3	2
sesame lowfat	1 oz	95	42	4	113	11	3
triticale whole grain	1 cup (4.6 oz)	439	46	3	606	3	3
white all-purpose	1 cup (4.4 oz)	455	19	6	134	3	1
white bread	1 cup (4.8 oz)	495	21	6	137	3	1
white cake unsifted	1 cup (4.8 oz)	496	19	10	144	3	1
white self-rising	1 cup (4.4 oz)	443	423	6	155	1588	1
white unbleached	1 cup (4.4 oz)	455	19	6	134	3	1
whole wheat	1 cup (4.2 oz)	407	41	5	486	6	4
FRENCH BEANS							
dried cooked	1 cup	228	111	2	655	11	1
FRENCH TOAST							
french toast frozen	1 slice (2 oz)	126	63	1	79	292	tr
plain	1 slice	151	64	1	86	311	tr
sticks	5 (4.9 oz)	513	78	3	127	499	1
w/ butter	2 slices (4.7 oz)	356	73	2	177	513	tr
FRUIT DRINKS							
fruit punch	6 fl oz	87	14	tr	47	41	tr
pineapple & orange drink	8 fl oz	125	13	1	116	9	tr
Fresh Samantha							
Banana Strawberry	1 cup (8 oz)	130	20	1	130	24	0
Carrot Orange	1 cup (8 oz)	100	40	1	150	24	0
Desperately Seeking C	1 cup (8 oz)	110	0	2	120	0	2

FOOD	PORTION	CALS	CALCI	IRON	POTAS	SOD	ZINC
Protein Blast	1 cup (8 oz)	160	40	3	150	24	tr
Super Juice	1 cup (8 oz)	140	20	1	160	0	tr
The Big Bang	1 cup (8 oz)	100	0	1	70	0	0
Odwalla							
Mo Beta	16 fl oz	280	60	5	—	290	5
Pek							
Mango Guava Ecstasy	1 bottle (20 fl oz)	110	250	0	—	20	8
Passionate Peach Grapefruit	8 fl oz	110	250	0	—	20	8

FRUIT MIXED

FOOD	PORTION	CALS	CALCI	IRON	POTAS	SOD	ZINC
dried mixed	11 oz pkg	712	110	8	2332	52	1
dried mixed fruit sweetened	1 cup	245	18	1	327	8	tr
fruit cocktail in heavy syrup	½ cup	93	8	tr	112	7	tr
fruit cocktail juice pack	½ cup	56	10	tr	118	4	tr
fruit cocktail water pack	½ cup	40	6	tr	115	5	tr
fruit salad in heavy syrup	½ cup	94	8	tr	103	7	tr
fruit salad in light syrup	½ cup	73	8	tr	104	7	tr
fruit salad juice pack	½ cup	62	14	tr	144	7	tr
fruit salad water pack	½ cup	37	8	tr	95	4	tr
mixed fruit in heavy syrup	½ cup	92	1	tr	108	5	tr
tropical fruit salad in heavy syrup	½ cup	110	17	1	168	3	tr

FRUIT SNACKS

FOOD	PORTION	CALS	CALCI	IRON	POTAS	SOD	ZINC
fruit leather	1 bar (0.8 oz)	81	7	tr	32	18	tr
fruit leather pieces	1 oz	97	5	tr	48	114	tr
fruit leather pieces	1 pkg (0.9 oz)	92	5	tr	44	109	tr
fruit leather rolls	1 sm (0.5 oz)	49	4	tr	41	8	tr
fruit leather rolls	1 lg (0.7 oz)	73	7	tr	62	13	tr

FOOD	PORTION	CALS	CALCI	IRON	POTAS	SOD	ZINC
GARLIC							
clove	1	4	5	tr	12	1	tr
fresh chopped	1 tsp	4	5	tr	11	0	tr
powder	1 tsp	9	2	tr	31	1	tr
GEFILTE FISH							
sweet	1 piece (1.5 oz)	35	10	1	38	220	tr
GELATIN							
low calorie	½ cup	8	tr	tr	45	9	tr
powder unsweetened	1 pkg (7 g)	23	4	tr	1	14	tr
GIBLETS							
capon simmered	1 cup (5 oz)	238	19	10	222	80	7
chicken floured & fried	1 cup (5 oz)	402	26	15	478	164	9
chicken simmered	1 cup (5 oz)	228	18	9	229	85	7
turkey simmered	1 cup (5 oz)	243	18	10	291	85	5
GINGER							
ground	1 tsp (1.8 g)	6	2	tr	24	1	tr
Eden							
Pickled w/ Shiso Leaves	1 tbsp	15	20	tr	0	340	0
GINKGO NUTS							
canned	1 oz	32	1	tr	51	87	tr
dried	1 oz	99	6	tr	283	4	tr
raw	1 oz	52	1	tr	145	1	tr
GIZZARDS							
chicken simmered	1 cup (5 oz)	222	14	6	259	97	6
turkey simmered	1 cup (5 oz)	236	22	8	306	79	6
GOAT							
roasted	3 oz	122	15	3	344	73	4
GOOSEBERRIES							
canned in light syrup	½ cup	93	20	tr	97	3	tr
fresh	1 cup	67	38	tr	297	1	tr

FOOD	PORTION	CALS	CALCI	IRON	POTAS	SOD	ZINC
GRAPE JUICE							
bottled	1 cup	155	22	1	334	7	tr
frzn sweetened as prep	1 cup	128	9	tr	53	5	tr
GRAPE LEAVES							
canned	1 (4 g)	3	12	tr	1	114	tr
fresh raw	1 (3 g)	3	11	tr	8	tr	tr
GRAPEFRUIT							
fresh pink	½	37	13	tr	158	0	tr
fresh red	½	37	13	tr	158	0	tr
fresh white	½	39	17	tr	175	0	tr
juice pack	½ cup	46	19	tr	209	9	tr
pink sections	1 cup	69	25	tr	296	1	tr
red sections	1 cup	69	25	tr	296	1	tr
unsweetened	1 cup	93	18	1	378	3	tr
water pack	½ cup	44	18	1	161	2	tr
white sections	1 cup	76	28	tr	340	0	tr
GRAPEFRUIT JUICE							
fresh	1 cup	96	22	tr	400	2	tr
frzn as prep	1 cup	102	19	tr	337	2	tr
sweetened	1 cup	116	20	1	405	4	tr
Fresh Samantha							
Juice	1 cup (8 oz)	90	0	tr	110	0	0
GRAPES							
fresh	10	36	5	tr	93	1	tr
thompson seedless in heavy syrup	½ cup	94	13	1	132	7	tr
thompson seedless water pack	½ cup	48	13	1	131	7	tr
GRAVY							
beef	1 cup	124	14	2	189	1305	2
beef	1 can (10 oz)	155	17	2	236	1630	3
brown as prep w/ water	1 cup	75	66	tr	57	1076	tr
chicken	1 cup	189	48	1	260	1375	2
mushroom	1 cup	120	17	2	253	1259	2

FOOD	PORTION	CALS	CALCI	IRON	POTAS	SOD	ZINC
GREAT NORTHERN BEANS							
cooked dried	1 cup	210	121	4	692	4	2
great northern canned	1 cup	300	139	4	919	11	2
Eden							
Organic	½ cup (4.6 oz)	110	73	2	270	65	2
GREEN BEANS							
fresh cooked	½ cup	22	29	1	185	2	tr
frozen cooked	½ cup	18	31	1	76	9	tr
frozen italian cooked	½ cup	18	31	1	76	9	tr
green beans canned	½ cup	13	18	1	74	170	tr
italian canned	½ cup	13	18	1	74	170	tr
italian low sodium canned	½ cup	13	18	1	74	1	tr
low sodium canned	½ cup	13	18	1	74	1	tr
raw	½ cup	17	21	1	115	3	tr
GROUPER							
cooked	1 fillet (7.1 oz)	238	42	2	959	107	1
cooked	3 oz	100	18	1	403	45	tr
raw	3 oz	78	23	1	410	45	tr
GUAVA							
fresh	1	45	18	tr	256	2	tr
guava sauce	½ cup	43	8	tr	268	4	tr
HADDOCK							
fresh cooked	3 oz	95	36	1	339	74	tr
fresh cooked	1 fillet (5.3 oz)	168	64	2	598	131	1
fresh raw	3 oz	74	28	1	264	58	tr
smoked	3 oz	99	41	1	353	649	tr
smoked	1 oz	33	14	tr	116	214	tr
HALIBUT							
atlantic & pacific cooked	½ fillet (5.6 oz)	223	95	2	916	110	1

FOOD	PORTION	CALS	CALCI	IRON	POTAS	SOD	ZINC
atlantic & pacific cooked	3 oz	119	51	1	490	59	tr
atlantic & pacific raw	3 oz	93	40	1	382	46	tr

HAM

FOOD	PORTION	CALS	CALCI	IRON	POTAS	SOD	ZINC
canned extra lean roasted	3 oz	116	5	1	–	965	2
center slice country style lean roasted	4 oz	220	11	1	–	3045	3
chopped canned	1 oz	68	2	tr	81	387	1
ham & cheese loaf	1 oz	73	33	1	166	762	1
ham & cheese spread	1 tbsp	37	33	tr	24	179	tr
ham salad spread	1 tbsp	32	1	tr	22	137	tr
minced	1 oz	75	3	tr	88	353	1
patty cooked	1 patty (2 oz)	203	5	1	–	632	1
prosciutto	1 oz	55	3	tr	145	765	1
sliced extra lean 5% fat	1 oz	37	2	tr	99	405	1
sliced regular 11% fat	1 oz	52	2	tr	94	373	1
steak boneless extra lean	1 (2 oz)	69	2	1	–	720	1

HAM DISHES

FOOD	PORTION	CALS	CALCI	IRON	POTAS	SOD	ZINC
croquettes	1 (3.1 oz)	217	50	2	180	475	2
salad	½ cup	287	33	2	232	671	2

HAM SUBSTITUTES

Yves

FOOD	PORTION	CALS	CALCI	IRON	POTAS	SOD	ZINC
Veggie Ham Deli Slices	1 serv (2.2 oz)	80	40	1	140	480	3

HAMBURGER

FOOD	PORTION	CALS	CALCI	IRON	POTAS	SOD	ZINC
double patty w/ bun	1 reg	544	87	5	363	554	6
double patty w/ cheese & bun	1 reg	457	232	3	308	635	5

FOOD	PORTION	CALS	CALCI	IRON	POTAS	SOD	ZINC
double patty w/ cheese & double bun	1 reg	461	224	4	285	892	4
double patty w/ cheese ketchup mayonnaise onion pickle tomato & bun	1 reg	416	171	3	335	1051	3
double patty w/ ketchup mayonnaise onion pickle tomato & bun	1 reg	649	169	5	389	920	4
double patty w/ ketchup cheese mayonnaise mustard pickle tomato & bun	1 lg	706	240	6	596	1149	7
double patty w/ ketchup mustard mayonnaise onion pickle tomato & bun	1 lg	540	102	6	569	791	6
double patty w/ ketchup mustard onion pickle & bun	1 reg	576	92	6	527	742	6
single patty w/ bacon ketchup cheese mustard onion pickle & bun	1 lg	609	162	5	331	1044	7
single patty w/ bun	1 lg	400	74	4	268	474	4
single patty w/ bun	1 reg	275	63	2	145	387	2
single patty w/ cheese & bun	1 lg	608	91	5	644	1589	6
single patty w/ cheese & bun	1 reg	320	140	2	165	500	2

FOOD	PORTION	CALS	CALCI	IRON	POTAS	SOD	ZINC
single patty w/ ketchup cheese ham mayonnaise pickle tomato & bun	1 lg	745	301	5	539	1713	7
single patty w/ ketchup mustard mayonnaise onion pickle tomato & bun	1 reg	279	63	3	227	504	2
triple patty w/ cheese & bun	1 lg	769	282	8	821	1211	11
triple patty w/ ketchup mustard pickle & bun	1 lg	693	65	8	785	713	11

HAMBURGER SUBSTITUTES
Green Giant
Southwestern Style	1 patty (3.2 oz)	140	80	3	–	370	7

Yves
Veggie Burger	1 (3 oz)	119	60	4	350	480	5

HAZELNUTS
dried	1 oz	191	55	1	131	1	1
dried	1 oz	179	53	1	125	1	1
dry roasted	1 oz	188	55	1	131	1	1
oil roasted	1 oz	187	56	1	132	1	1

HEART
beef simmered	3 oz	148	5	6	198	54	3
chicken simmered	1 cup (5 oz)	268	27	13	192	69	11
lamb braised	3 oz	158	12	5	160	54	3
pork braised	1 cup	215	10	8	–	51	4
pork braised	1	191	9	8	–	45	4
turkey simmered	1 cup (5 oz)	257	19	10	265	79	8
veal braised	3 oz	158	7	4	169	50	2

HEARTS OF PALM
canned	1 cup (5.1 oz)	41	84	5	259	622	2
canned	1 (1.2 oz)	9	19	1	58	141	tr

FOOD	PORTION	CALS	CALCI	IRON	POTAS	SOD	ZINC
HERBS/SPICES							
chinese five spice	1 tsp	7	4	1	23	1	tr
curry powder	1 tsp	6	10	1	31	1	tr
garam masala	1 tsp	8	15	1	29	2	tr
poultry seasoning	1 tsp	5	15	1	10	tr	tr
pumpkin pie spice	1 tsp	6	12	tr	11	1	tr
Eden							
Furikake Seasoning	½ tsp	5	14	tr	10	25	tr
HERRING							
atlantic kippered	1 fillet (1.4 oz)	87	33	1	179	367	1
atlantic cooked	3 oz	172	63	1	356	98	1
atlantic cooked	1 fillet (5 oz)	290	105	2	599	165	2
atlantic pickled	½ oz	39	12	tr	10	131	tr
atlantic raw	3 oz	134	49	1	278	76	1
HICKORY NUTS							
dried	1 oz	187	17	1	124	0	1
HOMINY							
white canned	1 cup (5.6 oz)	482	16	1	14	336	2
HONEY							
honey	1 cup (11.9 oz)	1031	20	2	176	12	1
honey	1 tbsp (0.7 oz)	64	1	tr	11	1	tr
HORSE							
roasted	3 oz	149	7	4	322	47	3
HORSERADISH							
japanese wasabi	¼ tsp	1	2	tr	5	0	tr
wasabi root raw	1 (5.9 oz)	184	216	2	960	29	3
wasabi root raw sliced	1 cup (4.6 oz)	142	166	1	738	22	2
HOT DOG							
beef	1 (2 oz)	180	11	1	95	585	1
beef	1 (1.5)	142	6	1	75	462	1
beef & pork	1 (2 oz)	183	6	1	95	639	1
beef & pork	1 (1.5 oz)	144	6	1	75	504	1
corndog	1	460	101	6	262	972	1

FOOD	PORTION	CALS	CALCI	IRON	POTAS	SOD	ZINC
pork cheesefurter smokie	1 (1.5 oz)	141	25	tr	89	465	1
w/ bun chili	1	297	19	3	166	480	tr
w/ bun plain	1	242	24	2	143	671	2

HOT DOG SUBSTITUTES
Yves

FOOD	PORTION	CALS	CALCI	IRON	POTAS	SOD	ZINC
Good Dog	1 (1.8 oz)	70	40	4	170	460	2
Tofu Dogs	1 (1.3 oz)	45	0	2	90	240	1
Veggie Dogs	1 (1.6 oz)	60	20	3	130	400	2
Veggie Dogs Chili	1 (1.6 oz)	50	20	1	105	360	2
Veggie Dogs Jumbo	1 (2.7 oz)	100	20	5	170	480	4
Veggie Dogs Jumbo Hot N' Spicy	1 (2.7 oz)	106	40	1	190	480	4

HUMMUS

FOOD	PORTION	CALS	CALCI	IRON	POTAS	SOD	ZINC
hummus	1 cup	420	124	4	427	599	3
hummus	⅓ cup	140	41	1	142	200	1

HYACINTH BEANS

FOOD	PORTION	CALS	CALCI	IRON	POTAS	SOD	ZINC
dried cooked	1 cup	228	77	9	653	13	6

ICE CREAM AND FROZEN DESSERTS

FOOD	PORTION	CALS	CALCI	IRON	POTAS	SOD	ZINC
chocolate	½ cup (4 fl oz)	143	72	1	164	50	tr
cone vanilla light soft serve	1 (4.6 oz)	164	153	tr	169	92	tr
dixie cup chocolate	1 (3.5 fl oz)	125	63	1	145	44	tr
dixie cup strawberry	1 (3.5 fl oz)	112	70	tr	109	35	tr
dixie cup vanilla	1 (3.5 fl oz)	116	74	tr	115	46	tr
gelato chocolate hazelnut	½ cup (5.3 oz)	370	179	2	352	49	1
gelato vanilla	½ cup (3 oz)	211	67	tr	77	78	tr
strawberry	½ cup (4 fl oz)	127	79	tr	124	40	tr
sundae caramel	1 (5.4 oz)	303	189	tr	318	195	tr
sundae hot fudge	1 (5.4 oz)	284	207	tr	395	182	tr
sundae strawberry	1 (5.4 oz)	269	161	tr	270	92	tr
vanilla	½ cup (4 fl oz)	132	85	tr	131	53	tr
vanilla soft serve	½ cup	111	138	tr	194	62	tr

ICE CREAM CONES AND CUPS

FOOD	PORTION	CALS	CALCI	IRON	POTAS	SOD	ZINC
sugar cone	1	40	4	tr	14	32	tr
wafer cone	1	17	1	tr	4	6	tr

ICE CREAM TOPPINGS

FOOD	PORTION	CALS	CALCI	IRON	POTAS	SOD	ZINC
marshmallow cream	1 oz	88	1	tr	1	13	tr
marshmallow cream	1 jar (7 oz)	615	6	tr	9	90	tr
pineapple	2 tbsp (1.5 oz)	106	9	tr	133	26	tr
pineapple	1 cup (11.5 oz)	861	75	2	1078	214	2
strawberry	1 cup (11.5 oz)	863	81	3	248	73	2
strawberry	2 tbsp (1.5 oz)	107	10	tr	31	9	tr

ICED TEA

FOOD	PORTION	CALS	CALCI	IRON	POTAS	SOD	ZINC
instant artifically sweetened lemon flavored as prep w/ water	8 oz	5	5	tr	41	24	tr
instant unsweetened lemon flavor as prep w/ water	8 oz	4	5	tr	49	14	tr

ICES AND ICE POPS

FOOD	PORTION	CALS	CALCI	IRON	POTAS	SOD	ZINC
fruit & juice bar	1 (3 fl oz)	75	5	tr	48	3	tr

JAM/JELLY/PRESERVES

FOOD	PORTION	CALS	CALCI	IRON	POTAS	SOD	ZINC
apple butter	1 cup (9.9 oz)	519	13	tr	258	1	tr
apple butter	1 tbsp (0.6 oz)	33	1	tr	16	0	tr
apple jelly	1 pkg (0.5 oz)	38	1	tr	9	5	tr
apple jelly	1 tbsp (0.7 oz)	52	2	tr	12	7	tr
orange marmalade	1 tbsp (0.7 oz)	49	8	tr	7	11	tr
orange marmalade	1 pkg (0.5 oz)	34	5	tr	5	8	tr
strawberry jam	1 tbsp (0.7 oz)	48	4	tr	15	8	tr
strawberry jam	1 pkg (0.5 oz)	34	3	tr	11	6	tr
strawberry preserve	1 pkg (0.5 oz)	34	3	tr	11	6	tr
strawberry preserve	1 tbsp (0.7 oz)	48	4	tr	15	8	tr

FOOD	PORTION	CALS	CALCI	IRON	POTAS	SOD	ZINC
Eden							
Organic Apple Butter	1 tbsp	20	0	0	0	0	0
Whistling Wings							
Blueberry Jam	1 oz	50	5	tr	14	2	tr
Raspberry Jam	1 oz	60	7	tr	29	1	tr
JUTE							
cooked	1 cup	32	184	3	479	10	1
KALE							
chopped cooked	½ cup	21	47	1	148	15	tr
frozen chopped cooked	½ cup	20	90	1	209	10	tr
raw chopped	½ cup	21	46	1	152	15	tr
scotch chopped cooked	½ cup	18	86	1	178	29	tr
KETCHUP							
ketchup	1 tbsp	16	3	tr	72	178	tr
ketchup	1 pkg (0.2 oz)	6	1	tr	29	71	tr
low sodium	1 tbsp	16	3	tr	72	3	tr
KIDNEY							
beef simmered	3 oz	122	15	6	152	114	4
lamb braised	3 oz	117	15	11	151	128	3
pork cooked	3 oz	128	11	5	–	68	4
pork cooked	1 cup	211	18	7	–	112	6
veal braised	3 oz	139	25	3	135	93	4
KIDNEY BEANS							
california red dried cooked	1 cup	219	116	5	741	7	2
canned	1 cup	208	69	3	658	889	1
canned red	1 cup	216	62	3	658	873	1
dried cooked	1 cup	225	0	5	713	4	2
dried red cooked	1 cup	225	50	5	713	4	2
dried royal red cooked	1 cup	218	78	5	669	8	2
Eden							
Organic Cannellini	½ cup (4.6 oz)	100	39	2	250	40	2

FOOD	PORTION	CALS	CALCI	IRON	POTAS	SOD	ZINC
KNISH							
potato	1 lg (7 oz)	332	54	2	358	470	1
potato	1 med (3.5 oz)	166	27	1	179	235	tr
KUMQUATS							
fresh	1	12	8	tr	37	1	tr
LAMB							
cubed lean only braised	3 oz	190	13	2	221	60	6
cubed lean only broiled	3 oz	158	11	2	285	65	5
ground broiled	3 oz	240	19	2	288	69	4
leg lean & fat Choice roasted	3 oz	219	9	2	266	56	4
loin chop w/ bone lean & fat Choice broiled	1 chop (2.3 oz)	201	13	1	209	49	2
loin chop w/ bone lean only Choice broiled	1 chop (1.6 oz)	100	9	tr	175	39	2
new zealand lean & fat cooked	3 oz	259	14	2	138	39	3
new zealand lean only cooked	3 oz	175	11	2	160	43	4
rib chop lean & fat Choice broiled	3 oz	307	16	2	230	64	3
rib chop lean only Choice broiled	3 oz	200	14	2	266	73	4
shank lean & fat Choice braised	3 oz	206	17	2	218	61	7
shank lean & fat Choice roasted	3 oz	191	8	2	277	55	4
shoulder chop w/ bone lean & fat Choice braised	1 chop (2.5 oz)	244	18	2	216	51	4
shoulder chop w/ bone lean only Choice braised	1 chop (1.9 oz)	152	14	1	185	41	4

FOOD	PORTION	CALS	CALCI	IRON	POTAS	SOD	ZINC
sirloin lean & fat Choice roasted	3 oz	248	10	2	256	58	4
LAMB DISHES							
curry	¾ cup	345	24	3	317	258	4
stew	¾ cup	124	54	1	364	140	2
LEMON							
fresh	1 med	22	66	1	157	3	tr
wedge	1	5	16	tr	39	1	tr
LEMON GRASS							
fresh	1 tbsp (5 g)	5	3	tr	35	tr	tr
fresh	1 cup (2.4 oz)	66	44	5	484	4	1
LEMON JUICE							
bottled	1 tbsp	3	2	tr	15	3	tr
fresh	1 tbsp	4	1	0	19	0	tr
frozen	1 tbsp	3	1	tr	14	0	tr
LEMONADE							
as prep w/ water	1 cup	100	8	tr	38	8	tr
powder as prep w/ water	9 fl oz	113	29	tr	1	19	tr
powder w/ artifically sweetened	1 pitcher (67 oz)	40	408	1	6	58	1
LENTILS							
dried cooked	1 cup	231	37	7	731	4	3
yemiser selatta eithopian lentil salad	1 serv (3 oz)	115	19	2	234	536	1
LETTUCE							
arugula	½ cup (0.4 oz)	3	16	tr	37	3	tr
cornsalad field salad	1 cup (1.9 oz)	7	19	1	232	2	tr
iceberg	1 leaf	3	4	tr	32	2	tr
iceberg	1 head (19 oz)	70	102	3	852	48	1
LIMA BEANS							
canned	½ cup	93	35	2	334	309	1
canned large	1 cup	191	50	4	531	809	2

FOOD	PORTION	CALS	CALCI	IRON	POTAS	SOD	ZINC
dried cooked	½ cup	104	27	2	485	14	1
dried large cooked	1 cup	217	32	5	955	4	2
frozen cooked	½ cup	94	19	2	370	26	
frozen fordhook cooked	½ cup	85	19	1	347	45	tr

Eden

FOOD	PORTION	CALS	CALCI	IRON	POTAS	SOD	ZINC
Organic Baby	½ cup (4.6 oz)	100	20	2	290	35	2

LIME

FOOD	PORTION	CALS	CALCI	IRON	POTAS	SOD	ZINC
fresh	1	20	22	tr	68	1	tr

LIME JUICE

FOOD	PORTION	CALS	CALCI	IRON	POTAS	SOD	ZINC
bottled	1 tbsp	3	2	tr	12	2	tr
fresh	1 tbsp	4	2	0	17	0	tr

LINGCOD

FOOD	PORTION	CALS	CALCI	IRON	POTAS	SOD	ZINC
baked	3 oz	93	15	tr	476	64	tr
fillet baked	5.3 oz	164	27	1	846	114	1

LIQUOR/LIQUEUR

FOOD	PORTION	CALS	CALCI	IRON	POTAS	SOD	ZINC
bloody mary	5 oz	116	10	1	216	332	tr
coffee liqueur	1½ oz	174	1	tr	15	4	tr
coffee w/ cream liqueur	1½ oz	154	7	tr	15	43	tr
cosmopolitan	1 (4 oz)	213	2	tr	16	3	tr
daiquiri	2 oz	111	3	tr	13	1	tr
gin	1½ oz	110	0	0	0	1	0
long island ice tea	1 serv (7.5 oz)	159	7	tr	19	12	tr
manhattan	2 oz	128	1	tr	15	2	tr
martini	2½ oz	156	1	tr	13	2	tr
pina colada	4½ oz	262	11	tr	100	9	tr
rum	1½ oz	97	0	tr	1	0	tr
screwdriver	7 oz	174	16	tr	325	2	tr
sloe gin fizz	2½ oz	132	2	0	35	1	0
tequila sunrise	5½ oz	189	10	tr	178	7	tr
vodka	1½ oz	97	0	tr	0	0	0
whiskey	1½ oz	105	0	tr	1	0	tr
whiskey sour	3 oz	123	5	tr	48	10	tr

LIVER

FOOD	PORTION	CALS	CALCI	IRON	POTAS	SOD	ZINC
beef braised	3 oz	137	6	6	200	59	5
beef pan-fried	3 oz	184	9	5	309	90	5

FOOD	PORTION	CALS	CALCI	IRON	POTAS	SOD	ZINC
chicken stewed	1 cup (5 oz)	219	20	12	196	71	6
lamb braised	3 oz	187	7	7	188	48	7
lamb fried	3 oz	202	8	9	299	105	5
pork braised	3 oz	140	9	15	—	42	6
sheep raw	3.5 oz	131	4	12	282	95	4
turkey simmered	1 cup (5 oz)	237	15	11	272	89	4
veal braised	3 oz	140	6	2	174	45	8
veal fried	3 oz	208	10	4	372	112	7
LOBSTER							
northern cooked	1 cup	142	88	1	510	551	4
northern cooked	3 oz	83	52	tr	299	323	2
spiny steamed	3 oz	122	53	1	—	193	6
spiny steamed	1 (5.7 oz)	233	102	2	—	370	12
LOGANBERRIES							
frozen	1 cup	80	38	1	213	1	1
LONGANS							
fresh	1	2	0	0	9	0	0
LOQUATS							
fresh	1	5	2	tr	26	0	0
LOTUS							
Eden							
Root	1 serv (0.3 oz)	35	11	tr	160	25	tr
LUPINES							
dried cooked	1 cup	197	85	2	407	7	2
LYCHEES							
fresh	1	6	0	tr	16	0	tr
MACADAMIA NUTS							
dry roasted w/ salt	10–12 nuts (1 oz)	200	20	1	100	80	tr
oil roasted	1 oz	204	13	1	94	3	tr
MACE							
ground	1 tsp	8	4	tr	8	1	tr
MACKEREL							
atlantic cooked	3 oz	223	13	1	341	71	1
atlantic raw	3 oz	174	10	1	267	76	1

FOOD	PORTION	CALS	CALCI	IRON	POTAS	SOD	ZINC
jack baked	3 oz	171	25	1	442	94	1
jack canned	1 can (12.7 oz)	563	870	7	700	1368	4
jack canned	1 cup	296	458	4	369	720	2
jack fillet baked	6.2 oz	354	52	3	916	194	2
king baked	3 oz	114	34	2	474	172	1
king fillet baked	5.4 oz	207	61	4	859	312	1
pacific baked	3 oz	171	25	1	442	94	1
pacific fillet baked	6.2 oz	354	52	3	916	194	2
spanish cooked	3 oz	134	11	1	471	56	1
spanish cooked	1 fillet (5.1 oz)	230	19	1	808	96	1
spanish raw	3 oz	118	10	tr	379	50	tr
MALTED MILK							
chocolate as prep w/ milk	1 cup	229	304	1	499	172	1
chocolate flavor powder	3 heaping tsp (¾ oz)	79	13	tr	130	53	tr
natural flavor as prep w/ milk	1 cup	237	354	tr	529	223	1
natural flavor powder	3 heaping tsp (¾ oz)	87	63	tr	159	103	tr
MANGO							
fresh	1	135	21	tr	322	4	tr
MANGO JUICE							
Fresh Samantha							
Mango Mama	1 cup (8 oz)	120	0	1	110	0	0
MARJORAM							
dried	1 tsp	2	12	1	9	tr	tr
MARSHMALLOW							
marshmallow	1 reg (0.3 oz)	23	0	tr	0	3	0
marshmallow	1 cup (1.6 oz)	146	1	tr	2	22	tr
MATZO							
egg	1 (1 oz)	111	11	1	43	6	tr
egg & onion	1 (1 oz)	111	10	1	24	81	tr
plain	1 (1 oz)	112	4	1	32	0	tr
whole wheat	1 (1 oz)	99	7	1	89	1	1

FOOD	PORTION	CALS	CALCI	IRON	POTAS	SOD	ZINC
MAYONNAISE							
mayonnaise	1 tbsp	99	2	tr	5	78	tr
mayonnaise	1 cup	1577	40	1	75	1250	tr
MEAT SUBSTITUTES							
Yves							
Veggie Ground Italian	⅓ cup (2 oz)	60	40	3	240	270	3
Veggie Ground Round Italian	⅓ cup (1.9 oz)	60	40	3	240	270	3
Veggie Ground Round Original	2 oz	60	40	3	240	270	3
Veggie Pizza Pepperoni Slices	1 serv (1.7 oz)	70	40	4	140	480	3
Veggie Salami Deli Slices	1 serv (2.2 oz)	90	40	5	150	390	3
MELON							
melon balls frzn	1 cup	55	17	1	484	53	tr
MILK							
1%	1 qt	409	1200	tr	1524	493	4
1%	1 cup	102	300	tr	381	123	1
2%	1 qt	485	1187	tr	1507	487	4
2%	1 cup	121	297	tr	377	122	1
buffalo	7 oz	224	390	tr	200	80	2
buttermilk	1 qt	396	1141	tr	1483	1028	4
buttermilk	1 cup	99	285	tr	371	257	1
buttermilk dried	1 tbsp	25	77	tr	103	34	tr
condensed sweetened	1 cup	982	868	1	1136	389	3
condensed sweetened	1 oz	123	108	tr	142	49	tr
evaporated	½ cup	169	329	tr	382	122	1
evaporated skim	½ cup	99	369	tr	423	147	1
goat	1 cup	168	326	tr	499	122	1
goat	1 qt	672	1303	tr	1995	486	3
human	1 cup	171	79	tr	126	42	tr
indian buffalo	1 cup	236	412	tr	434	127	1
nonfat	1 qt	342	1209	1	1623	505	4
nonfat	1 cup	86	302	tr	406	125	1

FOOD	PORTION	CALS	CALCI	IRON	POTAS	SOD	ZINC
nonfat dried	1 pkg (3.2 oz)	244	837	tr	1552	499	4
whole	1 cup	150	291	tr	370	120	1
Lactaid							
1%	8 fl oz	102	300	tr	381	123	1
Nonfat	8 fl oz	86	302	tr	406	126	1
NutraBalance							
LactaCare	1 pkg (8 oz)	500	572	6	780	240	6

MILK DRINKS

FOOD	PORTION	CALS	CALCI	IRON	POTAS	SOD	ZINC
chocolate milk	1 cup	208	280	1	417	149	1
chocolate milk	1 qt	833	1121	2	1669	596	4
chocolate milk 1%	1 cup	158	287	1	426	152	1
chocolate milk 1%	1 qt	630	1147	2	1702	607	4
chocolate milk 2%	1 cup	179	284	1	422	150	1
strawberry flavor mix as prep w/ whole milk	9 oz	234	292	tr	370	128	1

MILK SUBSTITUTES

FOOD	PORTION	CALS	CALCI	IRON	POTAS	SOD	ZINC
imitation milk	1 cup	150	79	1	279	191	3
imitation milk	1 qt	600	317	4	1116	764	12
EdenBlend							
Organic	8 oz	120	13	1	270	85	1
Edensoy							
Organic Light	8 oz	93	80	1	215	84	1
Organic Light Vanilla	8 oz	120	75	1	196	87	tr
NutraBalance							
NuTaste	1 pkg (8 oz)	80	300	1	46	210	1
Rice Dream							
Organic Original	1 box (8 oz)	120	20	0	54	90	tr
Organic Original Enriched	1 box (8 oz)	120	300	0	60	90	tr
Silk							
Chocolate	1 cup	140	300	1	100	75	1
Vanilla	1 bottle (11 oz)	140	400	1	110	130	1
Soy Dream							
Carob	8 oz	210	40	2	290	150	1
Chocolate Enriched	8 oz	210	300	2	370	150	1
Original	8 oz	140	40	3	270	140	1

FOOD	PORTION	CALS	CALCI	IRON	POTAS	SOD	ZINC
Original Enriched	8 oz	140	300	3	270	140	1
Vanilla	8 oz	170	40	3	290	140	1
Vanilla Enriched	8 oz	140	300	3	270	160	1
White Wave							
Mocha	1 cup	140	200	3	—	50	1
MILKSHAKE							
chocolate	10 oz	360	319	1	567	273	1
strawberry	10 oz	319	320	tr	516	234	1
thick shake chocolate	10.6 oz	356	396	1	672	333	1
thick shake vanilla	11 oz	350	457	tr	572	299	1
vanilla	10 oz	314	344	tr	492	232	1
MILLET							
cooked	1 cup (6.1 oz)	207	5	1	108	3	2
MISO							
miso	½ cup	284	92	4	226	5036	5
Eden							
Organic Genmai	1 tbsp	25	0	tr	80	810	0
MOLASSES							
blackstrap	1 tbsp (0.7 oz)	47	172	4	498	11	tr
blackstrap	1 cup (11.5 oz)	771	2821	57	8174	180	3
molasses	1 tbsp (0.7 oz)	53	41	1	293	7	tr
molasses	1 cup (11.5 oz)	873	671	16	4802	120	1
MONKFISH							
baked	3 oz	82	7	tr	—	20	tr
MOOSE							
roasted	3 oz	114	5	4	284	58	3
MOTH BEANS							
dried cooked	1 cup	207	6	6	538	17	1
MOUSSE							
chocolate	½ cup (7.1 oz)	447	202	1	296	87	1
MUFFIN							
blueberry	1 (2 oz)	158	33	1	70	255	tr

FOOD	PORTION	CALS	CALCI	IRON	POTAS	SOD	ZINC
blueberry mix	1 (1¾ oz)	149	13	1	39	219	tr
corn mix	1 (1.75 oz)	160	37	1	65	397	tr
oat bran wheat free	1 (2 oz)	154	36	2	289	224	1
wheat bran mix	1 (1¾ oz)	138	16	1	73	233	1
MULLET							
striped cooked	3 oz	127	26	1	389	61	1
striped raw	3 oz	99	34	1	304	55	tr
MUNG BEANS							
dried cooked	1 cup	213	55	3	536	4	2
MUNGO BEANS							
dried cooked	1 cup	190	95	3	416	13	2
MUSHROOMS							
chanterelle	3.5 oz	11	8	7	507	3	1
cloud ear dried	1 (5 g)	13	7	tr	34	2	tr
cloud ears dried	1 cup (1 oz)	80	45	2	211	10	tr
fresh raw	1 (½ oz)	5	1	tr	67	1	tr
fresh raw sliced	½ cup	9	2	tr	130	1	tr
fresh sliced cooked	½ cup	21	4	1	277	2	1
fresh whole cooked	1 (0.4 oz)	3	1	tr	43	0	tr
oyster raw	1 lg (5.2 oz)	55	9	3	764	46	1
oyster raw	1 sm (0.5 oz)	6	1	tr	77	5	tr
portabella	1 serv (2 oz)	14	2	tr	137	2	tr
straw canned	1 cup (6.4 oz)	58	18	3	699	699	1
straw dried	1 piece (6 g)	2	1	tr	21	21	tr
tree ear dried	½ cup (0.4 oz)	36	14	1	85	8	1
wood ear dried mok yee	½ cup (0.4 oz)	25	30	12	91	6	tr
Eden							
Shitake Dried	6 (0.4 oz)	35	8	1	200	0	tr
MUSSELS							
blue raw	1 cup	129	39	6	479	429	2
blue raw	3 oz	73	22	3	272	243	1
fresh blue cooked	3 oz	147	28	6	228	313	2
MUSTARD							
dry mustard	1 tsp	15	17	tr	23	tr	tr

FOOD	PORTION	CALS	CALCI	IRON	POTAS	SOD	ZINC
Eden							
Organic Stone Ground	1 tsp	0	0	0	0	65	0
MUSTARD GREENS							
frozen chopped cooked	½ cup	14	75	1	104	19	tr
NATTO							
natto	½ cup	187	191	8	642	6	3
NAVY BEANS							
dried cooked	1 cup	259	128	5	669	2	2
navy canned	1 cup	296	123	5	755	1173	2
NECTARINE							
fresh	1	67	6	tr	288	0	tr
NEUFCHATEL							
neufchatel	1 oz	74	21	tr	32	113	tr
neufchatel	1 pkg (3 oz)	221	64	tr	97	339	tr
Philadelphia							
Neufchatel	1 oz	70	20	0	30	120	0
NOODLE DISHES							
noodle pudding	½ cup	132	51	1	81	222	1
NOODLES							
chow mein	1 cup (1.6 oz)	237	9	2	52	189	1
egg cooked	1 cup (5.6 oz)	213	19	3	45	11	1
japanese soba cooked	1 cup (4 oz)	113	5	1	40	68	tr
japanese somen cooked	1 cup (6.2 oz)	231	14	1	51	283	tr
rice cooked	1 cup (6.2 oz)	192	7	tr	7	33	tr
spinach/egg cooked	1 cup (5.6 oz)	211	30	2	59	19	1
Eden							
Kudzu	2 oz	200	0	1	0	0	0
NOPALES							
cooked	1 cup (5.2 oz)	23	245	1	290	30	tr
raw sliced	1 cup (3 oz)	14	140	1	275	19	tr

FOOD	PORTION	CALS	CALCI	IRON	POTAS	SOD	ZINC
NUTMEG							
ground	1 tsp	12	4	tr	8	tr	tr
NUTRITION SUPPLEMENTS							
Ensure							
Supplement All Flavors	1 can (8 fl oz)	250	300	5	370	200	4
Essential							
Protein Powder	1 serv (0.6 oz)	70	98	3	750	5	1
GeniSoy							
Soy Natural Protein Powder	1 scoop (1 oz)	100	250	5	90	290	4
Met-Rx							
Original	1 pkg (2.5 oz)	250	1000	8	900	370	6
Protein Shake	1 can	200	940	5	370	110	3
NutraBalance							
EggPro	1 tbsp (7.5 g)	30	0	0	84	96	tr
Nutribar							
Shake Chocolate Supreme as prep w/ 2% milk	1 serv (10 oz) (4.6 oz)	262	370	5	790	290	6
Shake Vanilla as prep w/ 2% milk	1 (10 oz)	259	380	4	600	285	6
Pounds Off							
All Flavors	1 bar (2.1 oz)	210	350	18	—	25	15
Resource							
Fructose Sweetened	1 pkg (8 oz)	250	220	2	270	230	3
Liquid Food	1 pkg (8 oz)	250	125	2	380	210	4
Plus Liquid Food	1 pkg (8 oz)	355	167	3	490	300	6
NUTS MIXED							
dry roasted w/ peanuts	1 oz	169	20	1	169	3	1
dry roasted w/ peanuts salted	1 oz	169	20	1	169	223	1
oil roasted w/ peanuts	1 oz	175	31	1	165	3	1

FOOD	PORTION	CALS	CALCI	IRON	POTAS	SOD	ZINC
oil roasted w/ peanuts salted	1 oz	175	31	1	165	217	1
oil roasted w/o peanuts	1 oz	175	30	1	154	3	1
oil roasted w/o peanuts salted	1 oz	175	30	1	154	233	1

OIL

FOOD	PORTION	CALS	CALCI	IRON	POTAS	SOD	ZINC
olive	1 tbsp	119	tr	tr	—	0	tr
olive	1 cup	1909	tr	1	—	tr	tr
peanut	1 cup	1909	tr	tr	tr	tr	tr
peanut	1 tbsp	119	tr	0	0	tr	0
soybean	1 tbsp	120	tr	0	—	0	0
soybean	1 cup	1927	tr	tr	—	tr	0
Eden							
Olive Spanish Extra Virgin	1 tbsp	120	0	0	0	0	0

OKRA

FOOD	PORTION	CALS	CALCI	IRON	POTAS	SOD	ZINC
raw	8 pods	36	77	1	287	8	
raw sliced	½ cup	19	41	tr	151	4	tr
sliced cooked	½ cup	25	50	tr	257	4	tr
sliced cooked	8 pods	27	54	tr	273	5	tr
sliced cooked	½ cup	34	88	1	215	3	1
sliced cooked	1 pkg (10 oz)	94	245	2	597	8	2

OLIVES

FOOD	PORTION	CALS	CALCI	IRON	POTAS	SOD	ZINC
ripe	1 sm	4	3	tr	0	28	tr
ripe	1 lg	5	4	tr	0	38	tr

ONION

FOOD	PORTION	CALS	CALCI	IRON	POTAS	SOD	ZINC
chopped canned	½ cup	21	51	tr	124	416	tr
chopped cooked	½ cup	47	23	tr	174	3	tr
chopped frozen cooked	½ cup	30	17	tr	114	12	tr
chopped frozen cooked	1 tbsp	4	2	tr	16	2	tr
flakes dried	1 tbsp	16	13	tr	81	1	tr
powder	1 tsp	7	8	tr	20	1	tr
raw chopped	1 tbsp	4	2	tr	16	0	tr
raw chopped	½ cup	30	16	tr	125	2	tr

FOOD	PORTION	CALS	CALCI	IRON	POTAS	SOD	ZINC
rings breaded & fried	8 to 9	275	73	tr	129	430	tr
scallions raw chopped	1 tbsp	2	4	tr	17	1	tr
scallions raw sliced	½ cup	16	30	1	138	8	tr
shallots dried	1 tbsp	3	2	tr	15	1	tr
whole canned	1 (2.2 oz)	12	29	tr	70	234	tr
whole frozen cooked	3½ oz	28	27	tr	101	8	tr

ORANGE

FOOD	PORTION	CALS	CALCI	IRON	POTAS	SOD	ZINC
california navel	1	65	56	tr	250	1	tr
california valencia	1	59	48	tr	217	0	tr
florida	1	69	65	tr	254	1	tr
sections	1 cup	85	52	tr	326	0	tr

ORANGE JUICE

FOOD	PORTION	CALS	CALCI	IRON	POTAS	SOD	ZINC
canned	1 cup	104	21	1	436	6	tr
chilled	1 cup	110	24	tr	473	2	tr
fresh	1 cup	111	27	1	496	2	tr
frozen as prep	1 cup	112	22	tr	474	2	tr
orange drink	6 oz	94	12	1	33	31	tr
Fresh Samantha							
Juice	1 cup (8 oz)	100	0	1	120	0	0
NutraShake							
Fortified	1 pkg (4 oz)	50	200	1	216	0	1

OREGANO

FOOD	PORTION	CALS	CALCI	IRON	POTAS	SOD	ZINC
ground	1 tsp	5	24	1	25	tr	tr

OYSTERS

FOOD	PORTION	CALS	CALCI	IRON	POTAS	SOD	ZINC
breaded & fried	6 (4.9 oz)	368	27	4	182	677	16
canned eastern	1 cup	170	111	17	568	277	226
canned eastern	3 oz	58	38	6	195	95	77
eastern cooked	3 oz	117	76	11	389	190	155
eastern cooked	6 med	58	38	6	192	94	76
eastern raw	6 med	58	38	6	192	94	76
eastern raw	1 cup	170	111	17	568	277	226
pacific raw	1 med	41	4	3	84	53	8
pacific raw	3 oz	69	7	4	143	90	14
steamed	3 oz	138	14	8	257	180	28

FOOD	PORTION	CALS	CALCI	IRON	POTAS	SOD	ZINC
steamed	1 med	41	4	2	76	53	8
stew	1 cup	278	331	6	427	928	73

PANCAKE/WAFFLE SYRUP

FOOD	PORTION	CALS	CALCI	IRON	POTAS	SOD	ZINC
maple	1 tbsp (0.8 oz)	52	13	tr	41	2	1
maple	1 cup (11.1 oz)	824	211	4	643	27	13
pancake syrup	1 cup (11 oz)	903	4	tr	7	290	tr
pancake syrup	1 tbsp (0.7 oz)	57	0	tr	0	17	tr
pancake syrup light	1 oz	46	0	0	1	57	tr
pancake syrup w/ butter	1 tbsp (0.7 oz)	59	0	tr	1	20	tr
pancake syrup w/ butter	1 cup (11 oz)	933	6	tr	9	307	tr

PANCAKES

FOOD	PORTION	CALS	CALCI	IRON	POTAS	SOD	ZINC
blueberry	1 (4 in diam)	84	78	1	52	157	tr
buttermilk frozen	1 4 in diam	83	22	1	26	183	tr
buttermilk mix	1 4 in diam	74	48	1	67	239	tr
plain	1 (4 in diam)	86	83	1	50	157	tr
plain frozen	1 4 in diam	83	22	1	26	183	tr
plain mix	1–4 in diam	74	48	1	67	239	tr
potato	1 (4 in diam)	78	10	tr	88	238	tr
sugar free low sodium mix	1 (3 in diam)	44	13	tr	85	58	tr
w/ butter & syrup	2 (8.1 oz)	520	128	3	251	1104	1

PAPAYA

FOOD	PORTION	CALS	CALCI	IRON	POTAS	SOD	ZINC
fresh	1	117	72	tr	780	8	tr
fresh cubed	1 cup	54	33	tr	359	4	tr

PAPAYA JUICE

FOOD	PORTION	CALS	CALCI	IRON	POTAS	SOD	ZINC
nectar	1 cup	142	24	1	78	14	tr

PAPRIKA

FOOD	PORTION	CALS	CALCI	IRON	POTAS	SOD	ZINC
paprika	1 tsp	6	4	1	49	1	tr

PARSLEY

FOOD	PORTION	CALS	CALCI	IRON	POTAS	SOD	ZINC
dry	1 tsp	1	4	tr	11	1	tr
dry	1 tbsp	1	1	tr	25	2	tr
fresh chopped	½ cup	11	41	2	166	17	tr

FOOD	PORTION	CALS	CALCI	IRON	POTAS	SOD	ZINC
PARSNIPS							
fresh cooked	1 (5.6 oz)	130	59	1	588	17	tr
fresh sliced cooked	½ cup	63	29	tr	287	8	tr
raw sliced	½ cup	50	24	tr	251	7	tr
PASTA							
corn cooked	1 cup (4.9 oz)	176	1	tr	43	0	1
elbows cooked	1 cup (4.9 oz)	197	10	2	43	1	1
fresh cooked	2 oz	75	3	1	14	3	tr
fresh spinach cooked	2 oz	74	10	1	21	3	tr
shells small cooked	1 cup (4 oz)	162	8	2	36	1	1
spaghetti cooked	1 cup (4.9 oz)	197	10	2	43	1	1
spinach spaghetti cooked	1 cup (4.9 oz)	182	42	1	81	20	2
spirals cooked	1 cup (4.7 oz)	189	9	2	42	1	1
vegetable cooked	1 cup (4.7 oz)	172	15	1	42	8	1
whole wheat cooked	1 cup (4.9 oz)	174	21	1	62	4	1
whole wheat spaghetti cooked	1 cup (4.9 oz)	174	21	1	62	4	1
Eden							
Organic Extra Fine	2 oz	210	20	1	180	0	1
Organic Gemelli	2 oz	210	20	3	280	0	2
Organic Pesto Gemelli	2 oz	210	20	1	220	0	1
Organic Ribbons Saffron	2 oz	210	20	1	180	0	1
Organic Spaghetti Semolina	2 oz	200	20	1	135	0	1
Organic Spaghetti 50% Whole Grain	2 oz	210	20	2	220	0	1
Organic Spirals Kamut Vegetable	2 oz	210	20	4	210	45	2
Organic Spirals Sesame Rice	2 oz	200	80	2	280	0	2
Organic Spirals Mixed Grain	2 oz	210	20	3	210	15	2
Organic Spirals Spinach	2 oz	210	20	2	320	30	1

FOOD	PORTION	CALS	CALCI	IRON	POTAS	SOD	ZINC
Organic Vegetable Alphabets	2 oz	200	20	1	135	15	1
Spirals Rye	2 oz	200	26	2	300	10	2
PASTA DINNERS							
lasagna	1 piece (2.5 in x 2.5 in)	374	359	3	354	668	3
manicotti	¾ cup (6.4 oz)	273	76	3	303	414	2
rigatoni w/ sausage sauce	¾ cup	260	44	3	286	106	2
spaghetti w/ meatballs & cheese	1 cup	407	164	5	913	696	3
PEACH							
fresh	1	37	5	tr	171	0	tr
fresh sliced	1 cup	73	9	tr	334	1	tr
frozen slices sweetened	1 cup	235	6	1	325	16	tr
halves dried	1 cup	383	45	7	1594	12	1
halves dried	10	311	37	5	1295	9	1
halves in heavy syrup	1 half	60	8	tr	74	5	tr
halves in light syrup	1 half	44	3	tr	79	4	tr
halves juice pack	1 half	34	15	tr	98	3	tr
halves water pack	1 half	18	2	tr	76	3	tr
spiced in heavy syrup	1 fruit	66	5	tr	75	3	tr
spiced in heavy syrup	1 cup	180	15	1	206	9	tr
PEACH JUICE							
nectar	1 cup	134	13	tr	101	17	tr
PEANUT BUTTER							
chunky	1 cup	1520	105	5	1928	1255	7
chunky	2 tbsp	188	13	1	239	156	1
chunky w/o salt	2 tbsp	188	13	1	239	5	1
chunky w/o salt	1 cup	1520	105	5	1928	44	7
smooth	2 tbsp	188	11	1	231	153	1

FOOD	PORTION	CALS	CALCI	IRON	POTAS	SOD	ZINC
smooth	1 cup	1517	88	4	1861	1234	6
smooth w/o salt	2 tbsp	188	11	1	231	5	1
smooth w/o salt	1 cup	1517	88	4	1861	44	6
Skippy							
Reduced Fat Creamy	2 tbsp	190	0	1	—	200	1
PEANUTS							
cooked	½ cup	102	18	tr	58	240	1
dry roasted	1 cup	855	79	3	960	1187	5
dry roasted w/ salt	30 nuts (1 oz)	170	20	1	190	230	1
PEAR							
fresh	1	98	19	tr	208	1	tr
fresh sliced w/ skin	1 cup	97	19	tr	207	1	tr
halves dried	1 cup	472	60	4	959	10	1
halves dried	10	459	59	4	932	10	1
halves in heavy syrup	1 cup	188	12	1	165	13	tr
halves in heavy syrup	1 half	68	4	tr	51	4	tr
halves in light syrup	1 half	45	4	tr	52	4	tr
halves juice pack	1 cup	123	21	1	238	10	tr
PEAR JUICE							
nectar	1 cup	149	11	1	33	9	tr
PEAS							
dried split cooked	1 cup	231	26	3	710	4	2
green canned	½ cup	59	17	1	147	186	1
green canned low sodium	½ cup	59	17	1	147	2	1
green fresh cooked	½ cup	67	22	1	217	2	1
green frozen cooked	½ cup	63	19	1	134	70	1
green raw	½ cup	58	18	1	176	3	1
snap peas fresh cooked	½ cup	34	33	2	192	3	tr

FOOD	PORTION	CALS	CALCI	IRON	POTAS	SOD	ZINC
snap peas frozen cooked	1 pkg (10 oz)	132	150	6	549	12	1
snap peas frozen cooked	½ cup	42	48	2	173	4	tr
PECANS							
dry roasted	1 oz	187	10	1	105	0	2
dry roasted salted	1 oz	187	10	1	105	260	2
halves dry roasted w/ salt	20 (1 oz)	200	20	1	120	110	2
halves dried	1 cup	721	39	2	423	1	6
oil roasted	1 oz	195	10	1	102	0	2
oil roasted salted	1 oz	195	10	1	102	252	2
PECTIN							
powder	¼ pkg (0.4 oz)	39	1	tr	1	24	tr
powder	1 pkg (1.75 oz)	163	4	1	4	100	tr
PEPPER							
black	1 tsp	5	9	1	26	1	tr
cayenne	1 tsp	6	3	tr	36	1	tr
red	1 tsp	6	3	tr	36	1	tr
white	1 tsp	7	6	tr	2	tr	tr
PEPPERS							
ancho dried	1 (0.6 oz)	48	10	2	410	7	tr
banana	1 cup (4.4 oz)	33	17	1	317	16	tr
banana	1 (4 in) (1.2 oz)	9	5	tr	84	4	tr
chili green canned	1 cup (5.5 oz)	29	50	2	157	552	tr
chili green hot	1	18	8	1	153	3	tr
chili green hot chopped	½ cup	30	13	1	255	5	tr
chili red fresh chopped	½ cup	30	13	1	255	5	tr
chili red hot	1 (1.6 oz)	18	8	1	153	3	tr
green	1 (2.6 oz)	20	7	tr	131	1	tr
green chopped	½ cup	13	5	tr	89	1	tr

FOOD	PORTION	CALS	CALCI	IRON	POTAS	SOD	ZINC
green chopped cooked	½ cup	19	6	tr	113	1	tr
green chopped frozen	1 oz	6	3	tr	26	1	tr
green cooked	1 (2.6 oz)	20	7	tr	121	1	tr
green dried	1 tbsp	1	1	tr	13	1	tr
green halves canned	½ cup	13	28	1	102	958	tr
habanero chile	1 tsp	9	5	1	99	2	tr
hungarian	1 (0.9 oz)	8	3	tr	55	tr	tr
jalapeno	1 (0.5 oz)	4	1	tr	30	tr	tr
jalapeno chopped canned	½ cup	17	18	2	92	995	tr
jalapeno sliced	1 cup (3.2 oz)	27	9	1	197	1	tr
pasilla dried	1 (7 g)	24	7	1	156	6	tr
red	1 (2.6 oz)	20	7	tr	131	1	tr
red chopped	½ cup	13	5	tr	69	1	tr
red chopped cooked	½ cup	19	6	tr	113	1	tr
red chopped frozen	1 oz	6	3	tr	26	1	tr
red cooked	1 (2.6 oz)	20	7	tr	121	1	tr
red dried	1 tbsp	1	1	tr	13	1	tr
red halves canned	½ cup	13	28	1	102	958	tr
serrano	1 (6 g)	2	1	tr	19	1	tr
serrano chopped	1 cup (3.7 oz)	34	12	1	320	11	tr

PERCH

FOOD	PORTION	CALS	CALCI	IRON	POTAS	SOD	ZINC
cooked	3 oz	99	87	1	293	67	1
cooked	1 fillet (1.6 oz)	54	47	1	158	36	1
ocean perch atlantic cooked	3 oz	103	117	1	298	82	1
ocean perch atlantic cooked	1 fillet (1.8 oz)	60	69	1	175	48	tr
ocean perch atlantic raw	3 oz	80	91	1	232	64	tr
raw	3 oz	77	68	1	228	52	1

PERSIMMONS

FOOD	PORTION	CALS	CALCI	IRON	POTAS	SOD	ZINC
dried japanese	1	93	8	tr	273	1	tr
fresh japanese	1	118	13	tr	270	3	tr

FOOD	PORTION	CALS	CALCI	IRON	POTAS	SOD	ZINC
PHEASANT							
breast w/o skin raw	½ breast (6.4 oz)	243	6	1	440	60	1
leg w/o skin raw	1 (3.6 oz)	143	31	2	316	48	2
w/ skin raw	½ pheasant (14 oz)	723	50	5	971	161	4
w/o skin raw	½ pheasant (12.4 oz)	470	45	4	921	131	3
PHYLLO DOUGH							
phyllo dough	1 oz	85	3	1	21	137	tr
sheet	1	57	2	1	14	92	tr
Ekizian							
Sheets	½ lb	865	47	9	233	573	2
PICKLES							
dill	1 (2.3 oz)	12	6	tr	75	833	tr
dill low sodium	1 (2.3 oz)	12	6	tr	75	12	tr
dill low sodium sliced	1 slice	1	1	tr	7	1	tr
dill sliced	1 slice	1	1	tr	7	77	tr
kosher dill	1 (2.3 oz)	12	6	tr	75	833	tr
polish dill	1 (2.3 oz)	12	6	tr	75	833	tr
quick sour	1 (1.2 oz)	4	0	tr	8	423	tr
quick sour low sodium	1 (1.2 oz)	4	0	tr	8	6	tr
quick sour sliced	1 slice	1	0	tr	2	85	0
sweet	1 (1.2 oz)	41	1	tr	11	328	tr
sweet low sodium	1 (1.2 oz)	41	1	tr	11	6	tr
sweet sliced	1 slice	7	0	tr	2	56	0
PIE							
apple	⅛ of 9 in pie (4.4 oz)	297	13	1	826	333	tr
apple snack pie	1 (3 oz)	266	127	tr	51	325	tr
banana cream	⅛ of 9 in pie (5.2 oz)	398	110	2	245	355	1
blueberry	⅛ of 9 in pie (5.2 oz)	360	10	2	74	272	tr
butterscotch	⅛ of 9 in pie (4.5 oz)	355	128	2	221	335	1

FOOD	PORTION	CALS	CALCI	IRON	POTAS	SOD	ZINC
cherry	⅙ of 9 in pie (6.3 oz)	486	18	3	138	343	tr
cherry	⅛ of 9 in pie (4.4 oz)	325	15	1	102	308	tr
cherry snack pie	1 (3 oz)	266	127	tr	51	325	tr
chocolate creme	⅙ of 8 in pie (4 oz)	344	41	1	144	153	tr
coconut creme	⅙ of 9 in pie (4.7 oz)	396	113	1	183	356	1
coconut custard	⅙ of 8 in pie (3.6 oz)	271	84	1	182	348	1
custard	⅙ of 9 in pie (4.5 oz)	262	107	1	159	256	1
lemon meringue	⅙ of 9 in pie (4.5 oz)	362	15	1	83	307	tr
lemon meringue	⅛ of 8 in pie (4.5 oz)	303	63	1	100	165	1
lemon snack pie	1 (3 oz)	266	127	tr	51	325	tr
mince	⅙ of 9 in pie (5.8 oz)	477	37	2	335	419	tr
peach	⅙ of 8 in pie (4.1 oz)	261	9	1	146	316	tr
pecan	⅙ of 8 in pie (4 oz)	452	19	1	84	480	1
pumpkin	⅙ of 8 in pie (3.8 oz)	229	66	1	168	308	1
vanilla cream	⅙ of 9 in pie (4.4 oz)	350	113	1	158	327	1

PIE CRUST

FOOD	PORTION	CALS	CALCI	IRON	POTAS	SOD	ZINC
chocolate cookie crumb	⅛ of 9 in pie (1 oz)	139	8	1	48	185	tr
chocolate cookie crumb	9 in crust (7.7 oz)	1130	68	7	375	1502	2
frozen baked	⅛ of 9 in pie (0.6 oz)	82	3	tr	18	104	tr
frozen baked	9 in shell (4.4 oz)	647	26	3	138	815	tr
graham cracker	9 in crust (8.4 oz)	1181	50	5	210	1365	1

FOOD	PORTION	CALS	CALCI	IRON	POTAS	SOD	ZINC
graham cracker	⅛ of 9 in pie (1 oz)	148	6	1	26	171	tr
mix as prep	⅛ of 9 in pie (0.7 oz)	100	12	tr	12	146	tr
mix as prep	9 in crust (5.6 oz)	801	96	3	99	1167	1
puff pastry baked	1 shell (1.4 oz)	223	4	1	25	101	tr
vanilla wafer cracker crumbs	9 in crust (6.1 oz)	937	74	3	140	909	tr
vanilla wafer cracker crumbs	⅛ of 9 in pie (0.8 oz)	119	9	tr	18	116	tr

PIE FILLING

FOOD	PORTION	CALS	CALCI	IRON	POTAS	SOD	ZINC
apple	1 can (21 oz)	599	27	2	268	259	tr
apple	⅛ can (2.6 oz)	74	3	tr	33	32	tr
cherry	⅛ can (2.6 oz)	85	8	tr	78	7	tr
cherry	1 can (21 oz)	683	65	1	625	54	tr
pumpkin pie mix	1 cup	282	99	3	372	561	1

PIEROGI

FOOD	PORTION	CALS	CALCI	IRON	POTAS	SOD	ZINC
pierogi	¾ cup (4.4 oz)	307	156	2	101	369	2

PIG'S EARS AND FEET

FOOD	PORTION	CALS	CALCI	IRON	POTAS	SOD	ZINC
ear simmered	1	184	20	2	—	185	tr
feet pickled	1 lb	921	145	3	—	4187	6
feet pickled	1 oz	58	9	tr	—	262	tr
feet simmered	3 oz	165	38	tr	—	26	1

PIGEON PEAS

FOOD	PORTION	CALS	CALCI	IRON	POTAS	SOD	ZINC
dried cooked	½ cup	102	36	1	322	5	1
dried cooked	1 cup	204	72	2	644	9	2

PIKE

FOOD	PORTION	CALS	CALCI	IRON	POTAS	SOD	ZINC
northern cooked	½ fillet (5.4 oz)	176	113	1	514	76	1
northern cooked	3 oz	96	62	1	282	42	1
northern raw	3 oz	75	48	tr	220	33	1
walleye baked	3 oz	101	120	1	424	56	1
walleye fillet baked	4.4 oz	147	175	2	618	81	1

FOOD	PORTION	CALS	CALCI	IRON	POTAS	SOD	ZINC
PIMIENTOS							
canned	1 tbsp	3	1	tr	19	2	tr
canned	1 slice	0	0	tr	2	0	0
PINE NUTS							
pignolia dried	1 oz	146	7	3	170	1	1
pignolia dried	1 tbsp	51	3	1	60	0	tr
pinyon dried	1 oz	161	2	1	178	20	1
PINEAPPLE							
chunks in heavy syrup	1 cup	199	35	1	264	3	tr
chunks juice pack	1 cup	150	34	1	304	4	tr
chunks sweetened frozen	½ cup	104	11	tr	122	2	tr
crushed in heavy syrup	1 cup	199	35	1	264	3	tr
fresh diced	1 cup	77	11	1	175	1	tr
fresh slice	1 slice	42	6	tr	95	1	tr
slices in heavy syrup	1 slice	45	8	tr	60	1	tr
slices in light syrup	1 slice	30	8	tr	61	1	tr
slices juice pack	1 slice	35	8	tr	70	1	tr
slices water pack	1 slice	19	9	tr	74	1	tr
tidbits in heavy syrup	1 cup	199	35	1	264	3	tr
tidbits in juice	1 cup	150	34	1	304	4	tr
tidbits in water	1 cup	79	37	1	313	3	tr
PINEAPPLE JUICE							
canned	1 cup	139	42	1	334	2	tr
frozen as prep	1 cup	129	28	1	340	3	tr
PINK BEANS							
dried cooked	1 cup	252	88	4	858	3	2
PINTO BEANS							
canned	1 cup	186	89	4	723	998	2
dried cooked	1 cup	235	82	4	800	3	2
Eden							
Organic Spicy	½ cup (4.6 oz)	125	80	3	380	195	2

FOOD	PORTION	CALS	CALCI	IRON	POTAS	SOD	ZINC
PISTACHIOS							
dried	1 cup	739	173	9	1399	7	2
dry roasted	1 oz	172	20	1	275	2	tr
dry roasted salted	1 cup	776	90	4	1242	1040	2
dry roasted salted	47 nuts (1 oz)	160	40	1	290	120	1
PIZZA							
cheese	12 in pie	1121	929	5	875	2680	7
cheese	⅛ of 12 in pie	140	116	1	110	336	1
cheese meat & vegetables	⅛ of 12 in pie	184	101	2	178	382	1
cheese meat & vegetables	12 in pie	1472	805	12	1423	3054	9
pepperoni	12 in pie	1445	517	7	1220	2133	4
pepperoni	⅛ of 12 in pie	181	65	1	153	267	1
PLANTAINS							
fresh uncooked	1 (6.3 oz)	218	5	1	893	7	tr
sliced cooked	½ cup	89	2	tr	358	4	tr
PLUMS							
fresh	1	36	2	tr	113	0	tr
fresh sliced	1 cup	91	6	tr	284	1	tr
purple in heavy syrup	1 cup	320	24	2	234	50	tr
purple in heavy syrup	3	119	12	1	121	26	tr
purple in light syrup	1 cup	158	24	2	233	50	tr
purple in light syrup	3	83	13	1	123	26	tr
purple juice pack	3	55	9	tr	147	1	tr
purple juice pack	1 cup	146	25	1	389	3	tr
purple water pack	3	39	6	tr	120	1	tr
purple water pack	1 cup	102	17	tr	314	2	tr
POLLACK							
altantic fillet baked	5.3 oz	178	116	1	689	166	1
atlantic baked	3 oz	100	65	1	388	94	1

FOOD	PORTION	CALS	CALCI	IRON	POTAS	SOD	ZINC
POMPANO							
florida cooked	3 oz	179	36	1	541	65	1
florida raw	3 oz	140	19	1	324	55	1
POPCORN							
air-popped	1 cup (0.3 oz)	31	1	tr	24	0	tr
caramel coated	1 cup (1.2 oz)	152	15	1	38	72	tr
caramel coated w/ peanuts	⅔ cup (1 oz)	114	19	1	101	84	tr
cheese	1 cup (0.4 oz)	58	12	tr	29	98	tr
oil popped	1 cup (0.4 oz)	55	1	tr	25	97	tr
POPOVER							
home recipe as prep w/ 2% milk	1 (1.4 oz)	87	38	1	65	82	tr
home recipe as prep w/ whole milk	1 (1.4 oz)	90	37	1	64	82	tr
POPPY SEEDS							
poppy seeds	1 tsp	15	41	0	20	1	tr
PORK							
boston blade roast lean & fat cooked	3 oz	229	24	1	–	57	3
boston blade steak lean & fat cooked	3 oz	220	31	1	–	59	4
center loin roast lean bone in cooked	3 oz	169	21	1	–	56	2
center loin chop lean bone in cooked	3 oz	172	20	1	–	53	2
center rib chop lean & fat bone in cooked	3 oz	213	21	1	–	34	2

FOOD	PORTION	CALS	CALCI	IRON	POTAS	SOD	ZINC
center rib roast lean & fat bone in cooked	3 oz	217	24	1	—	39	2
fresh ham rump lean roasted	3 oz	175	6	1	—	55	3
fresh ham rump lean & fat roasted	3 oz	214	10	1	—	53	2
fresh ham shank lean roasted	3 oz	183	6	1	—	54	3
fresh ham shank lean & fat roasted	3 oz	246	13	1	—	50	3
fresh ham whole lean roasted	3 oz	179	6	1	—	54	3
fresh ham whole lean roasted diced	1 cup	285	9	2	—	86	4
fresh ham whole lean & fat roasted	3 oz	232	12	1	—	51	3
fresh ham whole lean & fat roasted diced	1 cup	369	19	1	—	81	4
ground cooked	3 oz	252	19	1	—	62	3
loin chop lean bone in braised	3 oz	191	20	1	—	53	3
loin chop lean bone in broiled	3 oz	199	20	1	—	68	3
loin roast lean bone in roasted	3 oz	210	25	1	—	25	3
loin whole lean & fat braised	3 oz	203	18	1	—	41	2
loin whole lean & fat broiled	3 oz	206	16	1	—	53	2
loin whole lean & fat roasted	3 oz	211	16	1	—	50	2
lungs braised	3 oz	84	7	14	—	69	2
pancreas cooked	3 oz	186	14	2	—	36	4

FOOD	PORTION	CALS	CALCI	IRON	POTAS	SOD	ZINC
ribs country style lean & fat braised	3 oz	252	25	1	—	50	3
shoulder arm picnic lean & fat roasted	3 oz	269	16	1	—	60	3
shoulder whole lean & fat roasted	3 oz	248	20	1	—	58	3
shoulder whole lean & fat roasted diced	1 cup	394	32	2	—	92	5
shoulder whole lean roasted	3 oz	196	15	1	—	64	4
shoulder whole lean roasted diced	1 cup	311	24	2	—	101	6
sirloin chop lean & fat bone in braised	3 oz	208	15	1	—	43	2
sirloin roast lean & fat bone in cooked	3 oz	222	20	1	—	51	2
spareribs braised	3 oz	338	40	2	—	79	2
spleen braised	3 oz	127	11	19	—	91	3
tail simmered	3 oz	336	11	1	—	21	1
tenderloin lean roasted	3 oz	139	5	1	—	48	2
top loin chop boneless lean & fat cooked	3 oz	198	18	1	—	36	2
top loin roast bonless lean & fat cooked	3 oz	192	4	1	—	37	2

POTATO

FOOD	PORTION	CALS	CALCI	IRON	POTAS	SOD	ZINC
au gratin mix as prep	½ cup	160	146	1	483	528	1
baked skin only	1 skin (2 oz)	115	20	4	332	12	tr

FOOD	PORTION	CALS	CALCI	IRON	POTAS	SOD	ZINC
baked topped w/ cheese sauce	1	475	310	3	1167	381	2
baked topped w/ cheese sauce & bacon	1	451	309	3	1179	973	2
baked topped w/ cheese sauce & broccoli	1	402	334	3	1440	484	2
baked topped w/ cheese sauce & chili	1	481	409	6	1570	701	4
baked topped w/ sour cream & chives	1	394	105	3	1383	182	tr
baked w/ skin	1 (6.5 oz)	220	20	3	844	16	1
baked w/o skin	1 (5 oz)	145	8	1	610	8	tr
boiled	½ cup	68	4	tr	295	3	tr
french fries	10 strips	111	4	1	229	15	tr
french fries thick cut	10 strips	109	5	1	240	23	tr
hashed brown	½ cup	170	12	1	340	27	tr
instant mashed flakes as prep w/ whole milk & butter	½ cup	118	52	tr	245	349	tr
instant mashed flakes not prep	½ cup	78	5	tr	239	24	tr
mashed	½ cup	111	27	tr	303	309	tr
microwaved	1 (7 oz)	212	22	3	903	16	1
microwaved w/o skin	½ cup	78	4	tr	321	5	tr
o'brien	1 cup	157	70	1	516	421	1
potato pancakes	1 (1.3 oz)	101	9	1	291	188	tr
potato puffs	½ cup	138	19	1	236	462	tr
potato salad	½ cup	179	24	1	317	661	tr
raw w/o skin	1 (3.9 oz)	88	8	1	608	7	tr
scalloped mix	½ cup	105	70	1	461	409	tr

POTATO STARCH

FOOD	PORTION	CALS	CALCI	IRON	POTAS	SOD	ZINC
potato starch	1 oz	96	10	tr	4	1	tr

FOOD	PORTION	CALS	CALCI	IRON	POTAS	SOD	ZINC
POUT							
ocean baked	3 oz	86	11	tr	–	66	1
ocean fillet baked	4.8 oz	139	18	tr	–	107	2
PRETZELS							
dutch twist	4 (2.1 oz)	229	21	3	68	1029	1
pretzels	1 oz	108	10	1	42	486	tr
rods	4 (2 oz)	229	21	3	68	1029	1
sticks	120 (2 oz)	229	21	3	68	1029	1
twists	10 (2.1 oz)	229	21	3	68	1029	1
whole wheat	2 sm (1 oz)	103	8	1	122	58	tr
whole wheat	2 med (2 oz)	205	16	2	244	115	tr
PRUNE JUICE							
canned	1 cup	181	30	3	706	11	1
PRUNES							
canned in heavy syrup	5	90	15	tr	194	2	tr
canned in heavy syrup	1 cup	245	40	1	528	6	tr
dried	10	201	43	2	626	3	tr
dried	1 cup	385	82	4	1200	6	1
dried cooked w/ sugar	½ cup	147	25	1	371	2	tr
dried cooked w/o sugar	½ cup	113	24	1	354	2	tr
PUDDING							
banana	1 pkg (5 oz)	180	120	tr	156	278	tr
banana mix as prep w/ 2% milk	½ cup (4.9 oz)	142	154	tr	193	232	1
banana mix as prep w/ whole milk	½ cup (4.9 oz)	157	151	tr	189	231	tr
bread pudding	½ cup (4.4 oz)	212	143	1	282	291	1
bread w/ raisins	½ cup	180	124	2	266	185	1
chocolate	1 pkg (5 oz)	189	128	1	256	183	1
chocolate mix	½ cup (5 oz)	150	161	1	240	148	1
corn	⅔ cup	181	67	1	268	92	1

FOOD	PORTION	CALS	CALCI	IRON	POTAS	SOD	ZINC
instant banana as prep w/ 2% milk	½ cup (5.2 oz)	152	150	tr	192	435	tr
instant banana as prep w/ whole milk	½ cup (5.2 oz)	167	147	tr	189	434	tr
instant chocolate	½ cup (5.2 oz)	149	153	tr	247	418	1
instant lemon	½ cup (5.2 oz)	155	149	tr	190	394	tr
instant vanilla	½ cup (5 oz)	147	146	tr	185	407	tr
lemon mix	½ cup (5.1 oz)	163	11	tr	7	94	tr
rice as prep w/ whole milk	½ cup (5.1 oz)	175	149	1	186	158	1
rice w/ raisins	½ cup	246	125	2	265	270	1
tapioca	1 pkg (5 oz)	169	119	tr	148	168	tr
tapioca mix	½ cup (5 oz)	147	149	tr	190	172	tr
vanilla	1 pkg (4 oz)	146	99	tr	128	153	tr
vanilla mix as prep w/ 2% milk	½ cup (4.9 oz)	141	153	tr	194	224	1
vanilla mix as prep w/ whole milk	½ cup (4.9 oz)	155	150	tr	190	223	tr
yorkshire	1 serv (3 oz)	177	37	tr	45	168	tr

PUDDING POPS

FOOD	PORTION	CALS	CALCI	IRON	POTAS	SOD	ZINC
chocolate	1 (1.6 oz)	72	66	tr	105	77	tr
vanilla	1 (1.6 oz)	75	61	tr	65	50	tr

PUMMELO

FOOD	PORTION	CALS	CALCI	IRON	POTAS	SOD	ZINC
fresh	1	228	23	1	1317	7	tr
sections	1 cup	71	7	tr	411	2	tr

PUMPKIN

FOOD	PORTION	CALS	CALCI	IRON	POTAS	SOD	ZINC
canned	½ cup	41	32	2	251	6	tr
seeds dried	1 oz	154	12	4	229	5	2
seeds roasted	1 oz	148	12	4	229	5	2
seeds roasted	1 cup	1184	97	34	1829	40	17
seeds salted & roasted	1 oz	148	12	4	229	144	2

FOOD	PORTION	CALS	CALCI	IRON	POTAS	SOD	ZINC
seeds salted & roasted	1 cup	1184	97	34	1829	1294	17
seeds whole roasted	1 oz	127	16	1	261	5	3
seeds whole roasted	1 cup	285	35	2	588	12	7
seeds whole roasted salted	1 oz	127	16	1	261	191	3
whole roasted salted	1 cup	285	35	2	588	268	7
QUAIL							
breast w/o skin raw	1 (2 oz)	69	5	1	146	31	2
QUINOA							
quinoa not prep	1 cup (6 oz)	636	102	16	1258	36	6
RABBIT							
domestic w/o bone roasted	3 oz	167	16	2	325	40	2
RADISHES							
moo namul saengche korean salad	1 serv (3.7 oz)	34	19	tr	247	547	tr
red raw	10	7	9	tr	104	11	tr
red sliced	½ cup	10	12	tr	134	14	tr
Eden							
Daikon Dried Shredded	2 tbsp	45	60	1	420	20	tr
Daikon Pickled	2 slices	5	0	0	25	250	0
RAISINS							
golden seedless	1 cup	437	76	3	1082	17	tr
seedless	1 cup	434	71	3	1089	17	tr
RASPBERRIES							
canned in heavy syrup	½ cup	117	14	1	120	4	tr
fresh	1 cup	61	27	1	187	0	1
fresh	1 pint	154	69	2	474	0	1
frozen sweetened	1 cup	256	38	2	285	1	tr
frozen sweetened	1 pkg (10 oz)	291	43	2	324	1	1

FOOD	PORTION	CALS	CALCI	IRON	POTAS	SOD	ZINC
RASPBERRY JUICE							
Fresh Samantha							
Raspberry Dream	1 cup (8 oz)	120	20	1	120	0	0
RELISH							
hamburger	1 tbsp	19	1	tr	11	164	tr
hamburger	½ cup	158	5	1	93	1338	tr
hot dog	½ cup	111	7	2	95	1332	tr
hot dog	1 tbsp	14	1	tr	12	164	tr
sweet	½ cup	159	4	1	30	990	tr
sweet	1 tbsp	19	0	tr	4	122	tr
RENNIN							
tablet	1 (0.9 g)	1	34	tr	3	234	tr
RHUBARB							
fresh	½ cup	13	52	tr	175	2	tr
frozen	½ cup	60	132	tr	73	1	tr
frozen as prep w/ sugar	½ cup	139	174	tr	115	2	tr
RICE							
brown long grain cooked	1 cup (6.8 oz)	216	20	1	84	10	1
brown medium grain cooked	1 cup (6.8 oz)	218	20	1	154	2	1
glutinous cooked	1 cup (6.1 oz)	169	3	tr	17	9	1
pilaf	½ cup	84	21	1	206	362	1
spanish	¾ cup	363	22	2	369	1339	1
white long grain cooked	1 cup (5.5 oz)	205	16	2	55	2	1
white long grain instant cooked	1 cup (5.8 oz)	162	13	1	7	5	tr
white medium grain cooked	1 cup (6.5 oz)	242	6	3	54	0	1
white short grain cooked	1 cup (6.5 oz)	242	2	3	48	0	1
ROCKFISH							
pacific cooked	1 fillet (5.2 oz)	180	18	1	774	114	1

FOOD	PORTION	CALS	CALCI	IRON	POTAS	SOD	ZINC
pacific cooked	3 oz	103	10	tr	442	65	tr
pacific raw	3 oz	80	8	tr	344	51	tr

ROLL

brown & serve	1 (1 oz)	85	34	1	38	148	tr
cheese	1 (2.3 oz)	238	78	1	—	236	tr
cinnamon raisin	1 (2¾ in)	223	43	1	67	229	tr
cinnamon w/ frosting	1	109	10	1	19	250	tr
crescent	1 (1 oz)	98	6	1	45	341	tr
dinner	1 (1 oz)	85	34	1	38	148	tr
hamburger	1 (1½ oz)	123	60	1	60	241	tr
hard	1 (3½ in)	167	54	2	61	310	1
hotdog	1 (1½ oz)	123	60	1	60	241	tr
kaiser	1 (3½ in)	167	54	2	61	310	1
whole wheat	1 (1 oz)	75	30	1	77	135	1

ROSE HIP

fresh	1 oz	26	73	tr	83	42	tr

ROSEMARY

dried	1 tsp	4	15	tr	11	1	tr

RUTABAGA

cooked mashed	½ cup	41	50	1	344	22	tr
raw cubed	½ cup	25	33	tr	236	14	tr

SAGE

ground	1 tsp	2	12	tr	7	tr	tr

SALAD

chef w/o dressing	1½ cups	386	317	3	330	279	5
tossed w/o dressing	¾ cup	16	13	tr	179	27	tr
tossed w/o dressing	1½ cups	32	26	1	356	53	tr
tossed w/o dressing w/ cheese & egg	1½ cups	102	100	tr	371	119	tr
tossed w/o dressing w/ chicken	1½ cups	105	37	1	447	209	tr
tossed w/o dressing w/ pasta & seafood	1½ cups (14.6 oz)	380	73	3	600	1572	2
tossed w/o dressing w/ shrimp	1½ cups	107	60	tr	404	487	1

FOOD	PORTION	CALS	CALCI	IRON	POTAS	SOD	ZINC
waldorf	½ cup	79	12	tr	78	49	tr
SALAD DRESSING							
french	1 tbsp	67	2	tr	12	214	tr
french reduced calorie	1 tbsp	22	2	tr	13	128	tr
italian	1 tbsp	69	1	0	2	116	tr
russian	1 tbsp	76	3	tr	24	133	tr
thousand island	1 tbsp	59	2	tr	18	109	tr
SALMON							
chinook baked	3 oz	196	24	1	429	51	tr
chinook smoked	1 oz	33	3	tr	49	220	tr
chinook smoked	3 oz	99	9	1	149	666	tr
chum baked	3 oz	131	12	1	467	54	1
pink w/ bone canned	1 can (15.9 oz)	631	969	4	1982	2514	4
pink w/ bone canned	3 oz	118	181	1	277	471	1
salmon cake	1 (3 oz)	241	203	1	290	602	1
sockeye cooked	½ fillet (5.4 oz)	334	11	1	582	102	1
sockeye cooked	3 oz	183	6	1	582	102	1
sockeye raw	3 oz	143	5	tr	332	40	tr
sockeye w/ bone canned	3 oz	130	203	1	321	458	1
sockeye w/ bone canned	1 can (12.9 oz)	566	883	4	1392	1987	4
Bumble Bee							
Keta	½ cup (3.5 oz)	160	150	tr	290	490	1
Red	½ cup (3.5 oz)	180	150	tr	290	490	1
SALT/SEASONED SALT							
salt	1 tbsp (18 g)	0	4	tr	1	6976	tr
salt	1 tsp (6 g)	0	1	tr	0	2325	tr
Eden							
Atlantic Sea Salt	¼ tsp	0	tr	0	tr	467	0
Brittany Sea Salt	¼ tsp	0	tr	0	tr	552	0

FOOD	PORTION	CALS	CALCI	IRON	POTAS	SOD	ZINC
SANDWICHES							
chicken fillet plain	1	515	60	5	358	957	2
chicken fillet w/ cheese lettuce mayonnaise & tomato	1	632	258	4	334	1238	3
croque monsieur	1 (12.4 oz)	765	1089	3	437	1018	5
fish fillet w/ tartar sauce	1	431	84	3	339	615	tr
fish fillet w/ tartar sauce & cheese	1	524	185	4	353	939	1
fried egg w/ cheese	1	340	225	3	188	804	2
fried egg w/ cheese & ham	1	348	212	3	209	1005	2
ham w/ cheese	1	353	130	3	290	772	1
roast beef submarine sandwich w/ tomato lettuce & mayonnaise	1	411	41	3	330	845	4
roast beef w/ cheese	1	402	183	5	345	1634	5
roast beef plain	1	346	54	4	316	792	3
steak w/ tomato lettuce salt & mayonnaise	1	459	91	5	525	798	5
submarine w/ salami ham cheese lettuce tomato onion & oil	1	456	189	3	394	1650	3
tuna salad submarine sandwich w/ lettuce & oil	1	584	74	3	335	1294	2
SARDINES							
atlantic in oil w/ bone	2	50	92	1	95	121	tr

FOOD	PORTION	CALS	CALCI	IRON	POTAS	SOD	ZINC
atlantic in oil w/ bone	1 can (3.2 oz)	192	351	3	365	465	1
pacific in tomato sauce w/ bone	1 can (13 oz)	658	887	9	1262	1532	5
pacific in tomato sauce w/ bone	1	68	91	1	130	157	1

SAUCE

FOOD	PORTION	CALS	CALCI	IRON	POTAS	SOD	ZINC
cheese mix as prep w/ milk	1 cup	307	570	tr	554	1566	1
fish sauce vietnamese nuoc mam	1 tbsp	6	8	tr	52	1390	tr
hoisin	1 tbsp	35	5	tr	19	258	tr
oyster	1 tbsp	8	5	tr	9	437	tr
sour cream mix as prep w/ milk	1 cup	509	546	1	733	1007	1
stroganoff mix as prep	1 cup	271	521	1	672	1829	1
sweet & sour mix as prep	1 cup	294	41	2	66	779	tr
teriyaki	1 tbsp	15	4	tr	41	690	tr
white mix as prep w/ milk	1 cup	241	424	tr	443	796	1
Cheez Whiz							
Cheese	2 tbsp (1.2 oz)	90	100	0	105	540	1
Cheese Jalapeno Pepper	2 tbsp (1.2 oz)	90	100	0	90	510	1
Cheese Mild Salsa	2 tbsp (1.2 oz)	100	100	0	85	530	1
Cheese Squeezable	2 tbsp (1.2 oz)	100	60	0	30	470	tr

SAUERKRAUT

FOOD	PORTION	CALS	CALCI	IRON	POTAS	SOD	ZINC
canned	½ cup	22	36	2	201	780	tr
Eden							
Organic	½ cup	25	40	1	160	580	0

FOOD	PORTION	CALS	CALCI	IRON	POTAS	SOD	ZINC
SAUSAGE							
bratwurst pork cooked	1 link (3 oz)	256	38	1	180	473	2
brotwurst pork & beef	1 link (2.5 oz)	226	34	1	197	778	1
italian pork cooked	1 (3 oz)	268	20	1	253	765	2
kielbasa pork	1 oz	88	12	tr	77	305	1
knockwurst pork & beef	1 (2.4 oz)	209	7	1	136	687	1
polish pork	1 (8 oz)	739	26	3	538	1989	4
pork cooked	1 link (½ oz)	48	4	tr	47	168	tr
vienna canned	7 (4 oz)	315	12	1	114	1077	2
vienna canned	1 (½ oz)	45	2	tr	16	152	tr
SAUSAGE SUBSTITUTES							
nonmeat sausage	1 patty (38 g)	97	24	1	88	137	1
nonmeat sausage	1 link (25 g)	64	16	1	58	222	tr
Yves							
Veggie Breakfast Links	1 (1.6 oz)	60	40	1	110	390	2
Veggie Breakfast Patties	1 (2 oz)	70	60	3	290	350	2
SAVORY							
ground	1 tsp	4	30	1	15	tr	tr
SCALLOP							
breaded & fried	2 lg	67	13	tr	103	144	tr
raw	3 oz	75	21	tr	274	137	1
SCUP							
fresh baked	3 oz	115	44	1	313	46	1
SEA CUCUMBER							
dried	1 oz	74	87	3	101	1411	1
fresh	1 oz	20	81	4	12	143	tr
SEAWEED							
agar dried	1 oz	87	78	6	321	29	1
irishmoss fresh	1 oz	14	21	3	18	19	1
kelp fresh	1 oz	12	48	1	25	66	tr
kombu fresh	1 oz	12	48	1	25	66	tr
laver fresh	1 oz	10	20	1	101	14	tr

FOOD	PORTION	CALS	CALCI	IRON	POTAS	SOD	ZINC
nori fresh	1 oz	10	20	1	101	14	tr
nori sheet dried	1 (8 x 8 in)	5	7	1	45	18	tr
tangle fresh	1 oz	12	48	1	25	66	tr
wakame fresh	1 oz	13	43	1	14	249	tr
Maine Coast							
Alaria	⅓ cup (7 g)	18	90	2	522	301	tr
Dulse	⅓ cup (7 g)	18	10	3	547	122	tr
Dulse Flakes	1 oz	75	60	9	2217	493	1
Kelp	⅓ cup (7 g)	17	70	5	784	312	tr
Kelp Crunch	1 bar (1 oz)	129	170	5	344	109	5
Kelp Crunch Peanut-Raisin	1 bar (1 oz)	129	170	5	344	109	5
Laver	⅓ cup (7 g)	22	10	2	188	113	tr

SEMOLINA

FOOD	PORTION	CALS	CALCI	IRON	POTAS	SOD	ZINC
dry	1 cup (5.9 oz)	601	28	7	311	2	2

SESAME

FOOD	PORTION	CALS	CALCI	IRON	POTAS	SOD	ZINC
seeds	1 tsp	16	4	tr	11	1	tr
sesame butter	1 tbsp	95	154	3	93	2	1
tahini from roasted & toasted kernels	1 tbsp	89	64	1	62	17	1
tahini from stone ground kernels	1 tbsp	86	63	tr	62	11	1
tahini from unroasted kernels	1 tbsp	85	20	1	64	0	1
Eden							
Organic Seaweed Gomasio	1 serv (1.5 oz)	10	0	0	0	35	0
Organic Gomasio	½ tsp	10	0	0	0	40	0
Organic Gomasio Garlic	½ tsp	10	0	0	0	35	0

SHAD

FOOD	PORTION	CALS	CALCI	IRON	POTAS	SOD	ZINC
american baked	3 oz	214	51	1	418	56	tr

SHARK

FOOD	PORTION	CALS	CALCI	IRON	POTAS	SOD	ZINC
batter-dipped & fried	3 oz	194	52	1	132	103	tr
raw	3 oz	111	29	1	136	67	tr

FOOD	PORTION	CALS	CALCI	IRON	POTAS	SOD	ZINC
SHEEPSHEAD FISH							
cooked	3 oz	107	32	1	435	62	1
cooked	1 fillet (6.5 oz)	234	70	1	952	136	1
raw	3 oz	92	18	tr	344	61	tr
SHERBET							
orange	½ cup (4 fl oz)	132	52	tr	92	44	tr
orange	½ gal	2158	827	2	1585	706	11
orange	1 bar (2.75 fl oz)	91	36	tr	63	30	tr
SHRIMP							
breaded & fried	3 oz	206	57	1	191	292	1
canned	1 cup	154	75	4	269	216	2
canned	3 oz	102	50	2	179	143	1
cooked	4 large	22	9	1	40	49	tr
cooked	3 oz	84	33	3	154	190	1
jambalaya	¾ cup	188	67	3	422	83	1
raw	4 large	30	15	1	52	42	tr
raw	3 oz	90	44	2	157	126	1
SMELT							
rainbow cooked	3 oz	106	65	1	316	65	2
rainbow raw	3 oz	83	51	1	247	51	1
SNACKS							
cheese puffs	1 oz	157	16	1	47	298	tr
corn puffs cheese	1 bag (8 oz)	1256	131	5	376	2383	1
corn twists cheese	1 oz	157	16	1	47	298	tr
corn twists cheese	1 bag (8 oz)	1256	131	5	376	2383	1
oriental mix	1 oz	155	22	1	147	235	1
pork skins	1 oz	154	8	tr	36	521	tr
trail mix	1 oz	131	22	1	194	65	1
trail mix	1 cup (5.3 oz)	693	117	5	1028	343	5
trail mix tropical	1 oz	115	16	1	201	3	tr
trail mix w/ chocolate chips	1 cup (5.1 oz)	707	159	5	946	177	5
trail mix w/ chocolate chips	1 oz	137	31	1	184	34	1

FOOD	PORTION	CALS	CALCI	IRON	POTAS	SOD	ZINC
Chex Mix							
Bold'n Zesty	1 pkg (1.7 oz)	230	0	7	90	610	0
Cheddar Cheese	1 pkg (1.7 oz)	220	0	7	135	550	0
Hot'n Spicy	1 pkg (1.7 oz)	210	0	7	35	90	0
Traditional	1 pkg (1.7 oz)	210	0	7	85	680	0
Dakota Gourmet							
Amazing Corn Classic	1 pkg (1 oz)	360	6	2	768	813	1
Amazing Corn Cool Ranch	1 pkg (1 oz)	367	31	2	754	1073	1
Amazing Corn Mesquite BBQ	1 pkg (1 oz)	369	11	2	764	725	1
Toasted Corn Heart Smart	1 pkg (1.75 oz)	177	7	1	388	470	1
Trail Mix Heart Smart	1 pkg (1.75 oz)	172	32	1	271	156	1
Pumpkorn							
Caramel	⅓ cup	150	20	5	—	85	2
Chili	⅓ cup	150	20	5	—	100	2
Curry	⅓ cup	150	20	5	—	100	2
Maple Vanilla	⅓ cup	150	20	5	—	100	2
Mesquite	⅓ cup	150	20	5	—	110	2
Original	⅓ cup	150	20	5	—	110	2
SNAIL							
cooked	3 oz	233	96	9	590	350	3
escargot cooked	5	25	5	1	95	25	tr
raw	3 oz	117	48	4	295	175	1
SNAKE							
fresh	3 oz	78	15	3	303	57	3
SNAPPER							
cooked	3 oz	109	34	tr	444	48	tr
cooked	1 fillet (6 oz)	217	69	tr	887	96	1
raw	3 oz	85	27	tr	355	54	tr
SODA							
cola	12 oz	151	9	tr	4	14	0
cream	12 oz	191	19	tr	4	43	tr
diet cola	12 oz	2	12	tr	0	21	tr
diet cola w/ equal	12 oz	2	12	tr	0	21	tr

FOOD	PORTION	CALS	CALCI	IRON	POTAS	SOD	ZINC
diet cola w/ saccharin	12 oz	2	14	tr	7	57	tr
ginger ale	12 oz can	124	12	tr	5	25	tr
grape	12 oz	161	12	tr	3	57	tr
lemon lime	12 oz	149	9	tr	4	41	tr
orange	12 oz	177	19	tr	9	49	tr
pepper type	12 oz	151	12	tr	2	38	tr
root beer	12 oz	152	19	tr	3	49	tr
Yoo-Hoo							
Original	9 fl oz	150	100	tr	250	200	tr

SOLE

FOOD	PORTION	CALS	CALCI	IRON	POTAS	SOD	ZINC
battered & fried	3.2 oz	211	17	2	292	484	tr
breaded & fried	3.2 oz	211	17	2	292	484	tr
cooked	1 fillet (4.5 oz)	148	23	tr	436	133	1
cooked	3 oz	99	16	tr	292	89	1

SOUFFLE

FOOD	PORTION	CALS	CALCI	IRON	POTAS	SOD	ZINC
spinach	1 cup	218	230	1	202	763	1

SOUP

FOOD	PORTION	CALS	CALCI	IRON	POTAS	SOD	ZINC
asparagus cream of as prep w/ milk	1 cup	161	175	1	359	1041	1
asparagus cream of as prep w/ water	1 cup	87	29	1	173	981	1
beef noodle as prep w/water	1 cup	84	15	1	99	952	2
beef stew soup	1 cup (8.8 oz)	221	32	3	527	461	6
black bean turtle	1 cup	241	103	5	801	6	1
black bean turtle soup	1 cup	218	84	5	739	922	1
black bean as prep w/water	1 cup	116	45	2	273	1198	1
brunswick stew soup	1 cup (8.5 oz)	232	39	2	509	438	2
celery cream of as prep w/ milk	1 cup	165	186	1	309	1010	tr

FOOD	PORTION	CALS	CALCI	IRON	POTAS	SOD	ZINC
celery cream of as prep w/ water	1 cup	90	40	1	123	949	tr
celery cream of not prep	1 can (10¾ oz)	219	98	2	299	2308	tr
cheese as prep w/ milk	1 cup	230	288	1	340	1020	1
cheese as prep w/ water	1 cup	155	142	1	154	959	1
cheese not prep	1 can (11 oz)	377	345	2	374	2331	2
chicken broth as prep w/ water	1 cup	39	9	1	210	776	tr
chicken broth mix	1 pkg (0.2 oz)	16	11	tr	19	1116	tr
chicken broth mix as prep w/ water	1 cup	21	15	tr	25	1484	tr
chicken cream of as prep w/ milk	1 cup	191	180	1	273	1046	1
chicken cream of as prep w/ water	1 cup	116	34	1	87	986	1
chicken gumbo as prep w/ water	1 cup	56	24	1	75	955	tr
chicken noodle as prep w/ water	1 cup	75	17	1	55	1107	tr
chicken noodle mix as prep w/ water	1 cup	53	32	1	31	1284	tr
chicken rice as prep w/ water	1 cup	251	17	1	100	814	tr
clam chowder manhattan as prep w/ water	1 cup	77	26	2	188	1029	1
clam chowder new england as prep w/ water	1 cup	95	43	1	146	914	1
clam chowder new england as prep w/ milk	1 cup	163	187	1	300	992	1

FOOD	PORTION	CALS	CALCI	IRON	POTAS	SOD	ZINC
consomme w/ gelatin not prep	1 can (10½ oz)	71	21	1	373	1550	1
consomme w/ gelatin as prep w/ water	1 cup	29	8	1	153	637	tr
corn & cheese chowder	¾ cup	215	220	1	337	386	1
french onion as prep w/ water	1 cup	57	26	1	69	1053	1
french onion mix not prep	1 pkg (1.4 oz)	115	55	1	260	3493	tr
greek lemon	¾ cup	63	22	1	45	386	tr
hot & sour	1 serv (14 oz)	173	50	1	197	475	1
minestrone as prep w/water	1 cup	83	34	1	312	911	1
mushroom cream of as prep w/ milk	1 cup	203	178	1	270	1076	1
mushroom cream of as prep w/ water	1 cup	129	46	1	101	1031	1
onion mix as prep w/ water	1 cup	28	13	tr	63	848	tr
onion soup gratinee	1 serv	492	637	2	528	1325	3
oyster stew as prep w/ milk	1 cup	134	167	1	235	1040	10
oyster stew as prep w/ water	1 cup	59	22	1	49	980	10
pasta e fagioll	1 cup (8.8 oz)	194	62	3	522	790	1
pepperpot as prep w/ water	1 cup	103	23	1	152	970	1
potato cream of as prep w/ milk	1 cup	148	166	1	323	1060	1
potato cream of as prep w/ water	1 cup	73	20	tr	137	1000	1
ratatouille	1 cup (7.5 oz)	266	56	1	485	329	tr
scotch broth as prep w/ water	1 cup	80	15	1	159	1012	2

FOOD	PORTION	CALS	CALCI	IRON	POTAS	SOD	ZINC
split pea w/ ham as prep w/ water	1 cup	189	22	2	399	1008	1
tomato as prep w/ milk	1 cup	160	159	2	450	932	tr
tomato as prep w/ water	1 cup	86	13	2	263	872	tr
tomato mix as prep w/ water	1 cup	102	54	tr	295	943	tr
vegetarian vegetable as prep w/ water	1 cup	72	21	1	209	823	tr
vichyssoise	1 cup	148	166	1	323	1060	1
vietnamese pho beef noodle	1 serv (7.8 oz)	480	44	4	334	43	3
Boston Market							
Chicken Broth Reduced Sodium	1 cup	15	0	1	—	760	1

SOUR CREAM

FOOD	PORTION	CALS	CALCI	IRON	POTAS	SOD	ZINC
sour cream	1 cup (8 oz)	493	268	tr	331	123	1
sour cream	1 tbsp (0.4 oz)	26	14	tr	17	6	tr

SOY

FOOD	PORTION	CALS	CALCI	IRON	POTAS	SOD	ZINC
soy milk	1 cup	79	10	1	338	30	1

SOY SAUCE

FOOD	PORTION	CALS	CALCI	IRON	POTAS	SOD	ZINC
shoyu	1 tbsp	9	3	tr	32	1029	tr
soy sauce	1 tbsp	7	1	tr	27	1024	tr
tamari	1 tbsp	11	4	tr	38	1005	tr
Eden							
Shoyu	1 tbsp	15	0	0	85	1010	0

SOYBEANS

FOOD	PORTION	CALS	CALCI	IRON	POTAS	SOD	ZINC
dried cooked	1 cup	298	175	9	886	1	2
dry roasted	½ cup	387	232	3	1173	2	4
roasted	½ cup	405	119	3	1264	140	3
roasted & toasted	1 oz	129	39	1	417	1	1
roasted & toasted	1 cup	490	149	5	1588	4	4

FOOD	PORTION	CALS	CALCI	IRON	POTAS	SOD	ZINC
roasted & toasted salted	1 oz	129	39	1	417	54	1
roasted & toasted salted	1 cup	490	149	5	1588	176	4
sprouts raw	½ cup	43	23	1	169	5	tr
sprouts steamed	½ cup	38	28	1	167	5	tr
sprouts stir fried	1 cup	125	82	tr	567	14	2
Dakota Gourmet							
Soy Nuts	1 oz	129	72	1	367	217	1
Eden							
Organic Black	½ cup (4.6 oz)	120	80	3	310	30	2

SPAGHETTI SAUCE

FOOD	PORTION	CALS	CALCI	IRON	POTAS	SOD	ZINC
marinara sauce	1 cup	171	44	2	1061	1572	1
spaghetti sauce	1 cup	272	70	2	957	1236	1
Eden							
Organic Lightly Seasoned	½ cup (4.4 oz)	80	80	1	530	320	0

SPANISH FOOD

FOOD	PORTION	CALS	CALCI	IRON	POTAS	SOD	ZINC
burrito w/ apple	1 lg (5.4 oz)	484	32	2	218	443	tr
burrito w/ apple	1 sm (2.6 oz)	231	15	1	104	211	tr
burrito w/ beans	2 (7.6 oz)	448	113	5	653	986	2
burrito w/ beans & cheese	2 (6.5 oz)	377	214	2	496	1166	2
burrito w/ beans & chili peppers	2 (7.2 oz)	413	100	5	580	1043	3
burrito w/ beans & meat	2 (8.1 oz)	508	105	5	656	1335	4
burrito w/ beans cheese & beef	2 (7.1 oz)	331	131	4	410	990	2
burrito w/ beans cheese & chili peppers	2 (11.8 oz)	663	288	8	810	2060	6
burrito w/ beef	2 (7.7 oz)	523	84	6	739	1492	5
burrito w/ beef & chili peppers	2 (7.1 oz)	426	87	4	499	1116	4
burrito w/ beef cheese & chili peppers	2 (10.7 oz)	634	223	8	667	2091	8

FOOD	PORTION	CALS	CALCI	IRON	POTAS	SOD	ZINC
burrito w/ cherry	1 sm (2.6 oz)	231	15	1	104	211	tr
burrito w/ cherry	1 lg (5.4 oz)	484	32	2	218	443	tr
chimichanga w/ beef	1 (6.1 oz)	425	63	5	587	910	5
chimichanga w/ beef & cheese	1 (6.4 oz)	443	238	4	203	956	3
chimichanga w/ beef & red chili peppers	1 (6.7 oz)	424	71	4	613	1169	3
chimichanga w/ beef cheese & red chili peppers	1 (6.3 oz)	364	218	3	330	895	5
enchilada w/ cheese	1 (5.7 oz)	320	324	1	240	784	3
enchilada w/ cheese & beef	1 (6.7 oz)	324	228	3	574	1320	3
enchirito w/ cheese beef & beans	1 (6.8 oz)	344	217	2	560	1251	3
frijoles w/ cheese	1 cup (5.9 oz)	226	188	2	605	882	2
nachos w/ cheese	6 to 8 (4 oz)	345	272	1	172	816	2
nachos w/ cheese & jalapeno peppers	6 to 8 (7.2 oz)	607	620	2	292	1736	3
nachos w/ cheese beans ground beef & peppers	6 to 8 (8.9 oz)	568	384	3	451	1800	4
nachos w/ cinnamon & sugar	6 to 8 (3.8 oz)	592	85	3	75	439	tr
taco	1 sm (6 oz)	370	221	2	473	802	4
taco salad	1½ cups	279	192	2	416	763	3
taco salad w/ chili con carne	1½ cups	288	246	3	393	886	3
taco shell baked	1 med (0.5 oz)	61	21	tr	23	48	tr
taco shell baked w/o salt	1 med (½ oz)	61	21	tr	23	2	tr
tostada w/ beans & cheese	1 (5.1 oz)	223	211	2	403	543	2
tostada w/ beans beef & cheese	1 (7.9 oz)	334	190	2	490	870	3
tostada w/ beef & cheese	1 (5.7 oz)	315	217	3	572	896	4

FOOD	PORTION	CALS	CALCI	IRON	POTAS	SOD	ZINC
tostada w/ guacamole	2 (9.2 oz)	360	424	2	649	789	4
SPINACH							
canned	½ cup	25	135	2	370	29	tr
cooked	½ cup	21	122	3	419	63	1
frozen cooked	½ cup	27	139	1	283	82	1
malabar cooked	1 cup (1.5 oz)	10	55	1	113	24	tr
raw chopped	½ cup	6	28	1	156	22	tr
raw chopped	1 pkg (10 oz)	46	202	6	1139	160	1
SPOT							
baked	3 oz	134	15	tr	541	32	1
SPROUTS							
lentil sprouts	½ cup	40	9	1	122	4	1
mung bean	½ cup	16	7	tr	77	3	tr
mung bean cooked	½ cup	13	7	tr	63	6	tr
pea	½ cup	77	21	1	229	12	1
radish	½ cup	8	10	tr	16	1	tr
SQUASH							
acorn cooked mashed	½ cup	41	32	1	321	3	tr
acorn cubed baked	½ cup	57	45	1	446	4	tr
butternut cooked mashed frozen	½ cup	47	23	1	160	2	tr
butternut baked	½ cup	41	42	1	290	4	tr
crookneck raw sliced	½ cup	12	14	tr	138	1	tr
crookneck sliced cooked	½ cup	18	24	tr	173	1	tr
crookneck sliced frozen cooked	½ cup	24	19	tr	243	6	tr
crookneck sliced canned	½ cup	14	13	1	104	5	tr
hubbard baked	½ cup	51	17	tr	365	8	tr
hubbard cooked mashed	½ cup	35	12	tr	252	6	tr
scallop raw sliced	½ cup	12	12	tr	118	1	tr
scallop sliced cooked	½ cup	14	14	tr	126	1	tr

FOOD	PORTION	CALS	CALCI	IRON	POTAS	SOD	ZINC
seeds dried	1 cup	747	59	21	1114	24	10
seeds dried	1 oz	154	12	4	229	5	2
seeds roasted	1 oz	148	12	4	229	5	2
seeds roasted	1 cup	1184	97	34	1829	40	17
seeds salted & roasted	1 oz	148	12	4	229	5	2
seeds salted & roasted	1 cup	1184	97	34	1829	1294	17
seeds whole roasted	1 oz	127	16	1	261	5	3
seeds whole roasted	1 cup	285	35	2	588	12	7
seeds whole saled roasted	1 oz	127	16	1	261	191	3
seeds whole salted roasted	1 cup	285	35	2	588	368	7
spaghetti cooked	½ cup	23	17	tr	91	14	tr

SQUID

FOOD	PORTION	CALS	CALCI	IRON	POTAS	SOD	ZINC
fried	3 oz	149	33	1	237	260	1
raw	3 oz	78	27	1	209	37	1

STARFRUIT

FOOD	PORTION	CALS	CALCI	IRON	POTAS	SOD	ZINC
fresh	1	42	6	tr	207	2	tr

STRAWBERRIES

FOOD	PORTION	CALS	CALCI	IRON	POTAS	SOD	ZINC
fresh	1 pint	97	45	1	530	4	tr
fresh	1 cup	45	21	1	247	2	tr
frozen unsweetened	1 cup	52	23	1	220	3	tr
frozen sweetened sliced	1 cup	245	29	1	249	8	tr
frozen sweetened sliced	1 pkg (10 oz)	273	31	2	277	9	tr
frozen whole sweetened	1 cup	200	29	1	249	3	tr
frozen whole sweetened	1 pkg (10 oz)	223	32	1	277	3	tr
in heavy syrup	½ cup	117	16	1	109	5	tr

FOOD	PORTION	CALS	CALCI	IRON	POTAS	SOD	ZINC
STUFFING/DRESSING							
bread	½ cup (3½ oz)	195	74	2	152	534	tr
bread as prep w/ water & fat	½ cup	251	46	1	63	627	tr
bread as prep w/ water egg & fat	½ cup	107	31	1	80	319	tr
cornbread	½ cup	179	26	1	62	455	tr
sausage	½ cup	292	17	1	96	258	1
SUCKER							
white baked	3 oz	101	76	1	414	44	1
SUGAR							
brown packed	1 cup (7.7 oz)	828	167	4	762	86	tr
brown unpacked	1 cup (5.1 oz)	546	123	3	502	57	tr
maple	1 piece (1 oz)	100	26	tr	78	3	2
powdered	1 tbsp (0.3 oz)	31	0	0	0	0	0
powdered unsifted	1 cup (4.2 oz)	467	1	tr	3	2	tr
white	1 cup (7 oz)	773	2	tr	4	3	tr
white	1 tsp (4 g)	15	0	0	0	0	0
SUNFISH							
pumpkinseed baked	3 oz	97	87	1	381	87	2
SUNFLOWER							
seeds dried	1 oz	162	33	2	196	1	1
seeds dried	1 cup	821	168	10	992	4	7
seeds dry roasted	1 oz	165	20	1	241	1	2
seeds dry roasted	1 cup	745	90	5	1088	4	7
seeds dry roasted salted	1 cup	745	90	5	1088	975	7
seeds dry roasted salted	1 oz	165	20	1	241	195	2
seeds oil roasted	1 cup	830	76	9	652	4	7
seeds oil roasted salted	1 oz	175	16	2	137	201	1
seeds oil roasted salted	1 cup	830	76	9	6528	804	7
seeds toasted	1 oz	176	16	2	139	1	2
seeds toasted	1 cup	826	76	9	658	4	7

FOOD	PORTION	CALS	CALCI	IRON	POTAS	SOD	ZINC
seeds toasted salted	1 oz	176	16	2	139	204	2
seeds toasted salted	1 cup	826	76	9	658	817	7
sunflower butter	1 tbsp	93	19	1	12	82	1
sunflower butter w/o salt	1 tbsp	93	19	1	12	1	1
Dakota Gourmet							
Honey Roasted Kernels	1 pkg (1 oz)	158	28	2	164	56	1
Lightly Salted Kernels	1 pkg (1 oz)	168	28	2	164	85	1
SunGold							
SunButter	2 tbsp	200	20	1	—	120	2

SUSHI

FOOD	PORTION	CALS	CALCI	IRON	POTAS	SOD	ZINC
california roll	1 piece (0.8 oz)	28	13	tr	37	37	tr
sashimi	1 serv (6 oz)	198	25	1	668	718	tr
tuna roll	1 piece (0.7 oz)	23	2	tr	24	33	tr
vegetable roll	1 piece (1.2 oz)	27	20	tr	60	47	tr
vinegared ginger	⅓ cup (1.6 oz)	48	8	tr	189	6	tr
yellowtail roll	1 piece (0.6 oz)	25	12	tr	14	32	tr

SWEET POTATO

FOOD	PORTION	CALS	CALCI	IRON	POTAS	SOD	ZINC
baked w/ skin	1 (3½ oz)	118	32	1	397	12	tr
candied	3½ oz	144	27	1	198	73	tr
canned in syrup	½ cup	106	16	1	189	38	tr
canned pieces	1 cup	183	44	2	625	107	tr
frozen cooked	½ cup	88	31	tr	332	7	tr
mashed	½ cup	172	35	1	301	21	tr

SWEETBREADS

FOOD	PORTION	CALS	CALCI	IRON	POTAS	SOD	ZINC
beef braised	3 oz	230	14	2	209	51	4
lamb braised	3 oz	199	10	2	247	44	2

SWORDFISH

FOOD	PORTION	CALS	CALCI	IRON	POTAS	SOD	ZINC
cooked	3 oz	132	5	1	314	98	
raw	3 oz	103	4	1	245	76	

FOOD	PORTION	CALS	CALCI	IRON	POTAS	SOD	ZINC
SYRUP							
corn dark	1 cup (11.5 oz)	925	58	1	144	608	tr
corn dark	1 tbsp (0.7 oz)	56	4	tr	9	31	tr
corn light	1 cup (11.5 oz)	925	10	tr	13	395	tr
corn light	1 tbsp (0.7 oz)	56	1	tr	1	24	0
malt	1 cup (13 oz)	1222	234	4	1229	134	1
malt	1 tbsp (0.8 oz)	76	15	tr	77	8	tr
maple	1 cup (11.1 oz)	824	211	4	643	27	13
maple	1 tbsp (0.8 oz)	52	13	tr	41	2	1
sorghum	1 tbsp (0.7 oz)	61	31	1	210	2	tr
sorghum	1 cup (11.6 oz)	957	495	13	3300	28	1
Eden							
Organic Barley Malt	1 tbsp	60	0	0	65	0	0
Whistling Wings							
Blueberry	1 oz	45	5	tr	19	1	tr
Raspberry	1 oz	60	3	tr	25	2	tr
TANGERINE							
in light syrup	½ cup	76	9	tr	99	8	tr
juice pack	½ cup	46	14	tr	165	7	
TANGERINE JUICE							
canned sweetened	1 cup	125	45	1	443	2	tr
fresh	1 cup	106	44	tr	440	2	tr
frozen sweetened as prep	1 cup	110	18	tr	273	2	tr
Fresh Samantha							
Fresh Juice	1 cup (8 oz)	110	40	tr	130	0	0

FOOD	PORTION	CALS	CALCI	IRON	POTAS	SOD	ZINC
TAPIOCA							
pearl dry	½ cup (2.7 oz)	272	15	1	9	1	tr
TARRAGON							
ground	1 tsp	5	18	1	48	1	tr
TEA/HERBAL TEA							
brewed tea	6 oz	2	0	tr	66	5	tr
chamomile brewed	1 cup	2	5	tr	21	2	tr
instant unsweetened as prep w/ water	8 oz	2	5	tr	47	8	tr
Eden							
Organic Genmaicha Tea	1 cup	0	0	0	0	0	0
Organic Kukicha Tea	1 cup	0	0	0	0	0	0
Silk							
Chai	1 cup	140	300	1	—	50	1
TEMPEH							
tempeh	½ cup	165	77	2	305	5	2
THYME							
ground	1 tsp	4	26	2	11	1	tr
TILEFISH							
cooked	½ fillet (5.3 oz)	220	39	tr	768	88	1
cooked	3 oz	125	22	tr	435	50	tr
raw	3 oz	81	22	tr	368	45	tr
TOFU							
firm	¼ block (3 oz)	118	166	8	192	11	1
firm	½ cup	183	258	13	298	17	2
fresh fried	1 piece (0.5 oz)	35	48	1	19	2	tr
koyadofu dried frozen	1 piece (⅓ oz)	82	62	2	3	1	1
regular	¼ block (4 oz)	88	122	6	141	8	1
regular	½ cup	94	130	7	150	9	1

FOOD	PORTION	CALS	CALCI	IRON	POTAS	SOD	ZINC
TOMATO							
fresh cooked	½ cup	32	7	1	335	13	tr
fresh green	1	30	16	1	251	16	tr
fresh red	1 (4.5 oz)	26	6	1	273	11	tr
fresh red chopped	1 cup	35	12	1	372	16	tr
paste	½ cup	110	46	4	1221	86	1
puree	1 cup	102	37	2	1051	532	1
puree w/o salt	1 cup	102	37	2	1051	49	1
red whole canned	½ cup	24	32	1	265	195	tr
sauce	½ cup	37	17	1	452	738	tr
sauce w/ mushrooms	½ cup	42	16	1	464	552	tr
sauce w/ onion	½ cup	52	20	1	504	672	tr
stewed	1 cup	80	27	1	249	460	tr
stewed	½ cup	34	47	1	307	325	tr
stewed w/ green chiles	½ cup	18	24	tr	129	481	tr
wedges in tomato juice	½ cup	34	34	1	329	285	tr
Eden							
Organic Diced	½ cup	30	20	tr	330	5	0
Organic Diced w/ Green Chilies	½ cup	30	20	tr	250	35	0
TOMATO JUICE							
tomato juice	6 oz	32	16	1	400	658	tr
tomato juice	½ cup	21	10	1	268	441	tr
TONGUE							
beef simmered	3 oz	241	6	3	153	51	4
lamb braised	3 oz	234	8	2	134	57	3
pork braised	3 oz	230	16	4	–	93	4
TORTILLA							
corn	1 (6 in diam)	56	44	tr	39	40	tr
corn w/o salt	1–6 in diam (.9 oz)	56	44	tr	39	3	tr
flour w/o salt	1–8 in diam (1.2 oz)	114	44	1	46	167	tr

FOOD	PORTION	CALS	CALCI	IRON	POTAS	SOD	ZINC
TRITICALE							
dry	1 cup (6.7 oz)	645	71	5	637	10	7
triticale not prep	1 oz	94	11	2	127	7.4	1
TROUT							
baked	3 oz	162	47	2	393	57	1
rainbow cooked	3 oz	129	73	2	539	29	1
seatrout baked	3 oz	113	19	tr	372	63	tr
TUNA							
light in oil	1 can (6 oz)	399	23	2	354	606	2
light in oil	3 oz	169	11	1	176	301	1
light in water	3 oz	99	10	1	202	287	1
light in water	1 can (5.8 oz)	192	19	3	391	558	1
skipjack baked	3 oz	112	32	1	444	40	1
white in oil	1 can (6.2 oz)	331	8	1	593	704	1
white in oil	3 oz	158	4	1	283	336	tr
yellowfin baked	3 oz	118	17	1	–	40	1
TUNA DISHES							
tuna salad	1 cup	383	35	2	365	824	1
tuna salad	3 oz	159	15	1	151	342	tr
TURKEY							
back w/ skin roasted	½ back (9 oz)	637	87	6	682	191	10
bologna	1 oz	57	24	tr	56	249	tr
breast	1 slice (0.75 oz)	23	1	tr	58	301	tr
breast w/ skin roasted	4 oz	212	24	2	323	70	2
ground cooked	3 oz	188	21	2	222	68	2
leg w/ skin roasted	2.5 oz	147	23	2	199	55	3
leg w/ skin roasted	1 (1.2 lbs)	1133	176	13	1530	420	23
neck simmered	1 (5.3 oz)	274	56	3	226	84	11
pastrami	2 oz	80	5	1	147	698	1
pastrami	1 pkg (8 oz)	320	20	4	589	2372	5
prebasted breast w/ skin roasted	½ breast (1.9 lbs)	1087	75	6	2141	3434	13
prebasted breast w/ skin roasted	1 breast (3.8 lbs)	2175	149	11	4281	6868	26

FOOD	PORTION	CALS	CALCI	IRON	POTAS	SOD	ZINC
prebasted thigh w/ skin roasted	1 thigh (11 oz)	494	25	5	758	1371	13
roast boneless seasoned light & dark meat roasted	1 pkg (1.7 lbs)	1213	40	13	2332	5320	20
roll light & dark meat	1 oz	42	9	tr	77	166	1
roll light meat	1 oz	42	11	tr	71	139	tr
salami cooked	1 pkg (8 oz)	446	44	4	553	2278	4
salami cooked	2 oz	111	11	1	138	569	1
skin roasted	from ½ turkey (9 oz)	1096	87	4	396	132	5
skin roasted	1 oz	141	11	1	51	17	1
turkey loaf breast meat	2 slices (1.5 oz)	47	3	tr	118	608	tr
turkey loaf breast meat	1 pkg (6 oz)	187	12	1	473	2433	2
w/ skin roasted	½ turkey (4 lbs)	3857	488	33	5207	1269	55
wing w/ skin roasted	1 (6.5 oz)	426	44	3	494	114	4

TURKEY DISHES

FOOD	PORTION	CALS	CALCI	IRON	POTAS	SOD	ZINC
gravy & turkey	1 cup (8.4 oz)	160	33	2	—	1328	2
gravy & turkey	1 pkg (5 oz)	95	20	1	—	786	1

TURKEY SUBSTITUTES

Yves

FOOD	PORTION	CALS	CALCI	IRON	POTAS	SOD	ZINC
Veggie Turkey Deli Slices	1 serv (2.2 oz)	85	40	4	169	480	3

TURMERIC

FOOD	PORTION	CALS	CALCI	IRON	POTAS	SOD	ZINC
ground	1 tsp	8	4	1	56	1	tr

TURNIPS

FOOD	PORTION	CALS	CALCI	IRON	POTAS	SOD	ZINC
canned greens	½ cup	17	138	2	165	325	tr
cooked mashed	½ cup (4.2 oz)	47	58	1	391	25	tr
cubed cooked	½ cup (3 oz)	33	41	tr	277	17	tr
frozen greens cooked	½ cup	24	125	2	184	12	tr

FOOD	PORTION	CALS	CALCI	IRON	POTAS	SOD	ZINC
greens chopped cooked	½ cup	15	99	1	146	21	tr
greens raw chopped	½ cup	7	53	tr	83	11	tr
raw cubed	½ cup (2.4 oz)	25	39	tr	236	14	tr

VEAL

FOOD	PORTION	CALS	CALCI	IRON	POTAS	SOD	ZINC
cutlet lean only braised	3 oz	172	7	1	329	57	3
cutlet lean only fried	3 oz	156	6	1	375	65	3
ground broiled	3 oz	146	14	1	287	70	3
loin chop w/ bone lean & fat braised	1 chop (2.8 oz)	227	22	1	224	64	3
loin chop w/ bone lean only braised	1 chop (2.4 oz)	155	22	1	205	58	3
shoulder w/ bone lean only braised	3 oz	169	31	1	271	83	6
sirloin w/ bone lean & fat roasted	3 oz	171	11	1	299	71	3
sirloin w/ bone lean only roasted	3 oz	143	12	1	310	72	3

VEAL DISHES

FOOD	PORTION	CALS	CALCI	IRON	POTAS	SOD	ZINC
parmigiana	4.2 oz	279	137	3	531	545	3

VEGETABLE JUICE

FOOD	PORTION	CALS	CALCI	IRON	POTAS	SOD	ZINC
vegetable juice cocktail	6 fl oz	34	20	1	351	664	tr
vegetable juice cocktail	½ cup	22	13	1	234	442	tr

VEGETABLES MIXED

FOOD	PORTION	CALS	CALCI	IRON	POTAS	SOD	ZINC
buddha's delight	1 serv (16 oz)	174	109	2	668	1368	2
mixed vegetables frozen cooked	½ cup	54	22	1	154	32	tr

FOOD	PORTION	CALS	CALCI	IRON	POTAS	SOD	ZINC
mixed vegetables canned	½ cup	39	22	1	239	122	tr
peas & carrots canned	½ cup	48	29	1	128	332	1
peas & carrots frozen cooked	½ cup	38	18	1	127	55	tr
peas & carrots low sodium canned	½ cup	48	29	1	128	332	1
peas & onions canned	½ cup	30	10	1	57	265	tr
succotash	½ cup	111	16	1	393	16	1
succotash frozen cooked	½ cup	79	13	1	225	38	tr

VENISON

FOOD	PORTION	CALS	CALCI	IRON	POTAS	SOD	ZINC
roasted	3 oz	134	6	4	285	46	2

VINEGAR

Eden

FOOD	PORTION	CALS	CALCI	IRON	POTAS	SOD	ZINC
Organic Brown Rice	1 tbsp	2	0	0	0	0	0

WAFFLES

FOOD	PORTION	CALS	CALCI	IRON	POTAS	SOD	ZINC
buttermilk frozen	1 4 in sq (1.2 oz)	88	77	1	43	262	tr
plain	1 (7 in diam)	218	191	2	119	383	1
plain frozen	1 4 in sq (1.2 oz)	88	77	1	43	262	tr
plain mix as prep	1 (7 in diam) (2.6 oz)	218	93	1	134	458	tr

WALNUTS

FOOD	PORTION	CALS	CALCI	IRON	POTAS	SOD	ZINC
black dried chopped	1 cup	759	72	4	655	2	4
english dried	1 oz	182	27	1	142	3	1
english dried chopped	1 cup	770	113	3	602	12	3
halves	14 (1 oz)	190	40	1	130	tr	1

WATER

FOOD	PORTION	CALS	CALCI	IRON	POTAS	SOD	ZINC
ice cubes	3	0	1	tr	0	2	tr
tap water	8 oz	0	5	tr	0	7	tr

FOOD	PORTION	CALS	CALCI	IRON	POTAS	SOD	ZINC
Reebok							
Fitness Water Berry	1 bottle (24 oz)	30	50	0	70	0	1
Fitness Water Natural	1 bottle (24 oz)	0	50	0	70	0	1
San Pellegrino							
Mineral Water	1 liter (33.8 oz)	0	204	tr	3	41	tr
WATER CHESTNUTS							
chinese sliced canned	½ cup	35	3	1	82	6	tr
WATERMELON							
cut up	1 cup	50	13	tr	186	3	tr
wedge	⅟₁₆	152	38	1	560	10	tr
WHEAT							
sprouted	1 cup (3.8 oz)	214	30	2	183	17	2
WHEAT GERM							
plain toasted	¼ cup (1 oz)	108	13	3	268	1	5
plain toasted	1 cup	431	50	10	1070	4	19
w/ brown sugar & honey toasted	1 oz	107	9	2	201	1	4
w/ brown sugar & honey toasted	1 cup	426	38	8	803	3	14
Kretschmer							
Honey Crunch	¼ cup	105	13	2	273	2	4
WHEY							
acid dry	1 tbsp (3 g)	10	59	tr	66	28	tr
acid fluid	1 cup (8 fl oz)	59	253	tr	352	118	1
sweet dry	1 tbsp (8 g)	26	59	tr	155	80	tr
sweet fluid	1 cup (8 fl oz)	66	115	tr	396	132	tr
WHIPPED TOPPINGS							
cream pressurized	1 cup (2.1 oz)	154	61	tr	88	78	tr
cream pressurized	1 tbsp (3 g)	8	3	tr	4	4	tr
nondairy frozen	1 tbsp	13	tr	tr	1	1	tr

FOOD	PORTION	CALS	CALCI	IRON	POTAS	SOD	ZINC
nondairy pressurized	1 tbsp (4 g)	11	tr	tr	1	2	tr
nondairy pressurized	1 cup	184	4	tr	13	43	tr
WHITE BEANS							
canned	1 cup	306	191	8	1189	13	3
dried regular cooked	1 cup	249	161	7	1003	11	2
dried small cooked	1 cup	253	131	5	828	4	2
WHITEFISH							
smoked	1 oz	39	5	tr	118	285	tr
smoked	3 oz	92	15	tr	360	866	tr
WHITING							
cooked	3 oz	98	53	tr	369	113	tr
raw	3 oz	77	41	tr	212	61	1
WILD RICE							
cooked	1 cup (5.7 oz)	166	5	1	166	5	2
Haddon House							
Extra Fancy	¼ cup (1.6 oz)	170	0	1	120	0	2
WINE							
port	3.5 oz	156	4	tr	–	4	tr
red	3½ oz	74	8	tr	115	6	tr
rose	3½ oz	73	9	tr	102	5	tr
sweet dessert	2 oz	90	5	tr	54	5	tr
white	3½ oz	70	9	tr	82	5	tr
WINGED BEANS							
dried cooked	1 cup	252	244	7	481	22	2
YAM							
fresh cubed cooked	½ cup	79	9	tr	455	6	tr
YAMBEAN							
cooked	¾ cup	38	11	1	135	4	tr

FOOD	PORTION	CALS	CALCI	IRON	POTAS	SOD	ZINC
YARDLONG BEANS							
dried cooked	1 cup	202	72	5	539	9	2
YAUTIA (TANNIER)							
fresh sliced	1 cup (4.7 oz)	132	12	1	807	28	1
root raw	1 (10.7 oz)	299	27	3	1824	64	2
YEAST							
baker's compressed	1 cake (0.6 oz)	18	3	1	102	5	2
YELLOW BEANS							
canned	½ cup	13	18	1	74	170	tr
canned low sodium	½ cup	13	18	1	74	1	tr
dried cooked	1 cup	254	110	4	576	8	2
fresh cooked	½ cup	22	29	1	185	2	tr
fresh raw	½ cup	17	21	1	115	3	tr
frozen cooked	½ cup	18	31	1	76	9	tr
YOGURT							
coffee lowfat	8 oz	194	389	tr	498	149	2
fruit lowfat	8 oz	225	314	tr	402	121	2
fruit lowfat	4 oz	113	157	tr	201	60	1
plain	8 oz	139	274	tr	351	105	1
plain lowfat	8 oz	144	415	tr	531	159	2
plain no fat	8 oz	127	452	tr	579	174	2
vanilla lowfat	8 oz	194	389	tr	498	149	2
YOGURT FROZEN							
vanilla soft serve	½ cup (4 fl oz)	114	103	tr	152	63	tr
ZUCCHINI							
canned italian style	½ cup	33	19	1	312	427	tr
frozen cooked	½ cup	19	19	1	218	2	tr
raw sliced	½ cup	9	10	tr	161	2	tr
sliced cooked	½ cup	14	12	tr	228	2	tr

INDEX

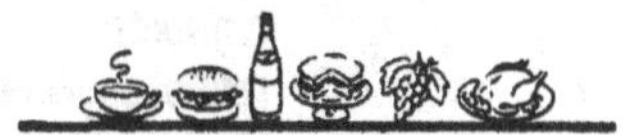

t = table
q = quiz